CYTOHISTOLOGY OF SMALL TISSUE SAMPLES

Published in association with the Papanicolaou Society of Cytopathology

Series Editors: Kim Geisinger MD
Department of Pathology, Wake Forest University School of Medicine, Winston-Salem, NC, USA

Martha B. Pitman MD
Department of Pathology, Massachusetts General Hospital, Boston, MA, USA

Forthcoming Titles

Lung and Mediastinal Cytohistology, Ali and Yang

Head and Neck Cytohistology, Baloch, Faquin, Elsheikh, and Vielh

Musculoskeletal Cytohistology, Bedrossian, Palombini, and Layfield

Breast Cytohistology, Cangiarella, Simsir, and Tabbara

Uterine Cytohistology, Raab, Longacre, Post, Kurtycz, and Geisinger

Body Fluid Cytohistology, Michael, Chhieng, and Bedrossian

CYTOHISTOLOGY OF SMALL TISSUE SAMPLES

CYTOHISTOLOGY: ESSENTIALS AND BASIC CONCEPTS

Prabodh K. Gupta MBBS, MD, FIAC

Zubair W. Baloch MD, PhD

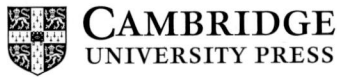
CAMBRIDGE
UNIVERSITY PRESS

CAMBRIDGE UNIVERSITY PRESS
Cambridge, New York, Melbourne, Madrid, Cape Town, Singapore,
São Paulo, Delhi, Dubai, Tokyo, Mexico City

Cambridge University Press
The Edinburgh Building, Cambridge CB2 8RU, UK

Published in the United States of America by Cambridge University Press, New York

www.cambridge.org
Information on this title: www.cambridge.org/9780521883580

First published 2011

Printed in the United Kingdom at the University Press, Cambridge

A catalog record for this publication is available from the British Library

Library of Congress Cataloging-in-Publication Data

Gupta, Prabodh K.
    Cytohistology : essential and basic concepts / Prabodh K. Gupta, Zubair W. Baloch.
        p. ; cm. – (Cytohistology of small tissue samples)
    Includes bibliographical references and index.
    ISBN 978-0-521-88358-0 (Hardback)
    1. Cytodiagnosis.   2. Histology, Pathological.   I. Baloch, Zubair W.   II. Title.   III. Series: Cytohistology of
small tissue samples.
    [DNLM: 1. Cytodiagnosis–methods.   2. Cell Physiological Phenomena.   3. Cytological Techniques–methods.
4. Pathology, Clinical–methods. QY 95]
RB43.G87 2011
616.07′582–dc22

                                                                                                        2010029088

ISBN 978-0-521-88358-0 Hardback

This book is dedicated to our numerous students, trainees, cytotechnologists, and colleagues who have taught us much of what we know.

PKG
ZWB

In celebration of the life and teachings of the late
John Kingsbury Frost MD
(1922–1990)
Dedicated teacher and a friend.
He leaves behind the Basic Concepts that shall enrich the lives of many students of cytopathology.
PKG
ZWB

CONTENTS

CONTRIBUTORS

Carlos W. M. Bedrossian MD, PhD(Hon), FIAC
Rush University Medical Center,
Chicago, IL, USA

Gary W. Gill BA, CT (ASCP)
Corporate Compliance officer, DCL Medical Laboratories,
Indianapolis, IN, USA

ABBREVIATIONS

ASC-H	atypical squamous cells suspect high grade
ASPS	alveolar soft part sarcoma
BAL	bronchoalveolar
BES	balanced electrolyte solution
BSA	bovine serum albumin
BSS	balanced salt solution
CCP	ciliocytophthoria
CD	clusters of differentiation
CGH	comparative genomic hybridization
CIS	carcinoma in situ
CISH	chromogenic in situ hybridization
CMA	chromosomal microanalysis
DF	dermatofibroma
DTTF	diagnostic true tissue fragment
EBC	evidence-based criteria
EGFR	Epidermal Growth Factor Receptor
E-LMS	epithelioid leiomyosarcoma
EMA	epithelial membrane antigen
EMSS	epithelioid monophasic synovial sarcoma
ES	epithelioid sarcoma
EUS	endoscopic ultrasound
FISH	fluorescent in situ hybridization
FNA	fine needle aspirations
GCT	germ cell tumors
GFAP	glial fibrillary acidic proteins
GIST	gastrointestinal stromal tumor
HCG	human chorionic gonadotropin

HPC	hemangiopericytoma
HSP	heat shock proteins
IAP	inhibitor of apoptosis proteins
LBC	liquid-based cytology
LBP	liquid-based preparation
LCA	leucocyte Common Antigens
LOH	loss of heterozygosity
LSC	laser scanning cytometry
MFH	malignant fibrous histiocytoma
MH	mesothelial hyperplasia
MM	malignant mesothelioma
N:C	Nucleocytoplasmic Ratio
NFP	neurofilament proteins
NSGCT	non-seminomatous germ cell tumors
PCP	*Pneumocystis jiroveci* pneumonia
PEComa	perivascular epithelioid cell tumor
PEG	polyethylene glycol
PNET	peripheral neuroectodermal tumor
PP	post-partum
PTO	post-test odds
SBRCT	small blue round cell tumors
SFT	solitary fibrous tumor
SLCL	small cell lung cancer
TBS	The Bethesda System
TdT	terminal deoxynucleotidyl transferase
TMA	tissue microarray
TP	terminal plate

PREFACE

Learn from yesterday, live for today, hope for tomorrow. The important thing is to not stop questioning
Albert Einstein

This monograph is a compilation of the Concepts Basic to General Cytopathology written by the late John K. Frost MD, published in 1959 by Johns Hopkins University Press, Baltimore. It was produced for use by the various students of cytopathology. The last (fourth) edition was printed in 1972. The original book of "concepts" has been translated into Chinese and Persian languages and is considered a "Bible" for understanding the fundamentals of clinical cytopathology.

This book is a conceptual document and not a comprehensive account of cytohistology. It integrates the fundamental concepts of diagnostic cytohistology as developed over decades of observations and insights which have stood the test of time. They are regarded as the most valuable for *accurate interpretation and diagnosis of the cytologic specimens*. In the modern practice of medicine, microscopic interpretation and biologic behavior are often poorly connected. These factual conclusions, however slim, contribute to the crux of diagnosis and patient care, including grading and staging of most tumors. This monograph is intended to improve cytodiagnoses.

The book is organized into seven chapters. A brief history of cytohistology is presented followed by a detailed discussion of "normal" cells derived from the various body sites and preparations; malignant cell transformation, functional differentiation of various tissues, and diagnostic pitfalls are presented in that order. A chapter by Mr. Gary W. Gill on Fixation and Specimen Processing is included. A final chapter by Dr. Carlos Bedrossian is an overview that briefly discusses the ancillary techniques used for the refinement of cytologic interpretation. This chapter on the multidisciplinary approach to cytopathology is enriched by contributions from Dr. Fernando Schmitt,

Dr. Ben Davidson, Dr. Claire Michael, Dr. Bjorn Risberg, and Dr. J. Reis Filho.

Although originally intended to be used with a set of representative glass slides corroborating the features described in the book, in the present monograph the original form has been suitably modified while retaining its integrity. A number of photomicrographs illustrating the salient features seen in the glass slides have been incorporated. The text has also been updated, reflecting some of our opinions and concepts as well as including the morphologic alterations seen by the recent introduction of various cytologic specimen collection and preparation techniques.

The cytologic descriptions in this manual are based upon the features as observed in the routine Papanicolaou polychromatic and Diff-Quik™ stains; however, when other stains have been used, this is mentioned. The line illustrations are conceptual and depict the critical/reproducible diagnostic cytomorphologic features that need to be scrutinized in the specimens. These were drawn and lettered by the late Dr. Frost; penned inscriptions and text have been carefully updated to facilitate interpretation without losing the original flair. Photomicrographs have been included to further enhance the learning experience and improve the teaching value. Most illustrations represent conventional smears and concentration techniques (Millipore®filters, Cytospins®, ThinPrep®, and SurePath™). The majority of these photomicrographs represent our (PG, ZB) collection; magnifications and resolutions observable by high dry microscope objectives and proper optical alignment are reproduced. Some of the key figures are from Dr. Frost's archival files kept at the Johns Hopkins Cytopathology Laboratory, Baltimore. A few illustrations are selected from the collections of Dr. Yener S. Erozan MD, Professor Emeritus, Johns Hopkins University, Baltimore, and former staff members including the late Drs. David H. Hollander MD and William Howdon MD. We thank Mr. Allen Green for his valuable secreterial assistance. Special thanks to Mr. Christopher Miller of the Cambridge University Press for his help and willingness to work with us and keep us on track.

We believe this book will serve as a valuable primer to all students of cytopathology including cytotechnologists and pathologists in training; experienced persons may consult it when the cells do not speak loudly enough or in a muffled voice.

PKG

ZWB

Philadelphia PA

October 2010

1 HISTORICAL PERSPECTIVE

The first documented evidence in English literature of cell examination in disease processes appears during the nineteenth century, when malignant cells from a mammary carcinoma were recognized and reported by Professor Johannes Müller of the University of Berlin (Figure 1.1). (Professor Müller trained a number of medical pioneers including Rudolf Virchow, Friedrich Henle, Robert Koch, Paul Ehrlich, and Theodor Schwann.) Alfred Donné is credited with identifying abnormal cells in vaginal smears, and published the first cytology atlas in 1845 containing photomicrographs of cells. In the same year, Lebert published an atlas with 250 cytology figures. He is believed to have laid the foundation of modern cytology. In 1852, Babo developed a centrifuge that he used to study specimens from the body cavity fluids and urinary tract (Figure 1.2).

In 1850, Gottlieb documented cancer cells in detail in an atlas. He wrote:

In cancer ... the cells present peculiarities. The characteristic cancer cells are spherical, ovoid, irregularly polyhedral, and frequently exhibit caudate prolongations. They possess finely granular contents, with a round or oval nucleolated nucleus as large as or larger than a pus-corpuscle. Sometimes cancer cells are double the ordinary size or more and not infrequently contain several nuclei, or even other cells constituting parent or endogenous cells.

Lionel S. Beale – Professor of Pathology, Physiology and Medicine at King's College London – should truly be

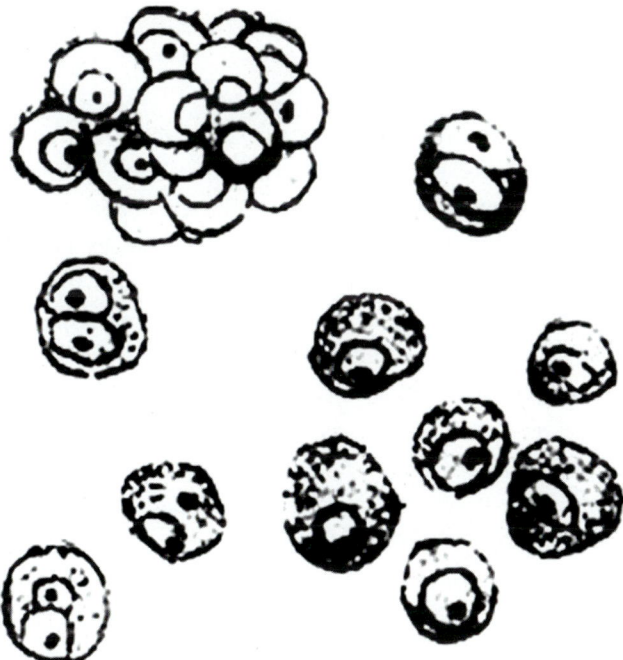

Figure 1.1 Malignant cells mammary carcinoma, Professor Johannes Muller, nineteenth century.

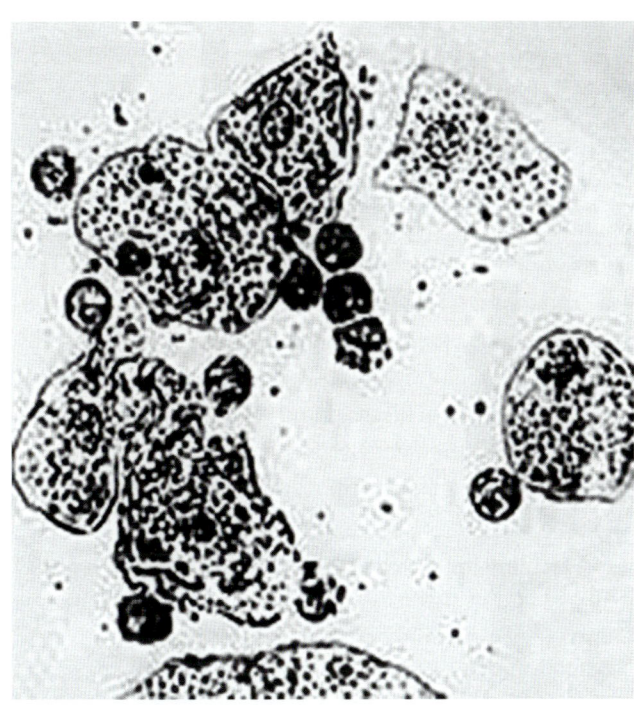

Figure 1.2 Urinary bladder cells, centrifuge specimen, Babo (1852).

Cytohistology: Essential and Basic Concepts, Prabodh Gupta and Zubair Baloch. Published by Cambridge University Press. © Cambridge University Press 2011.

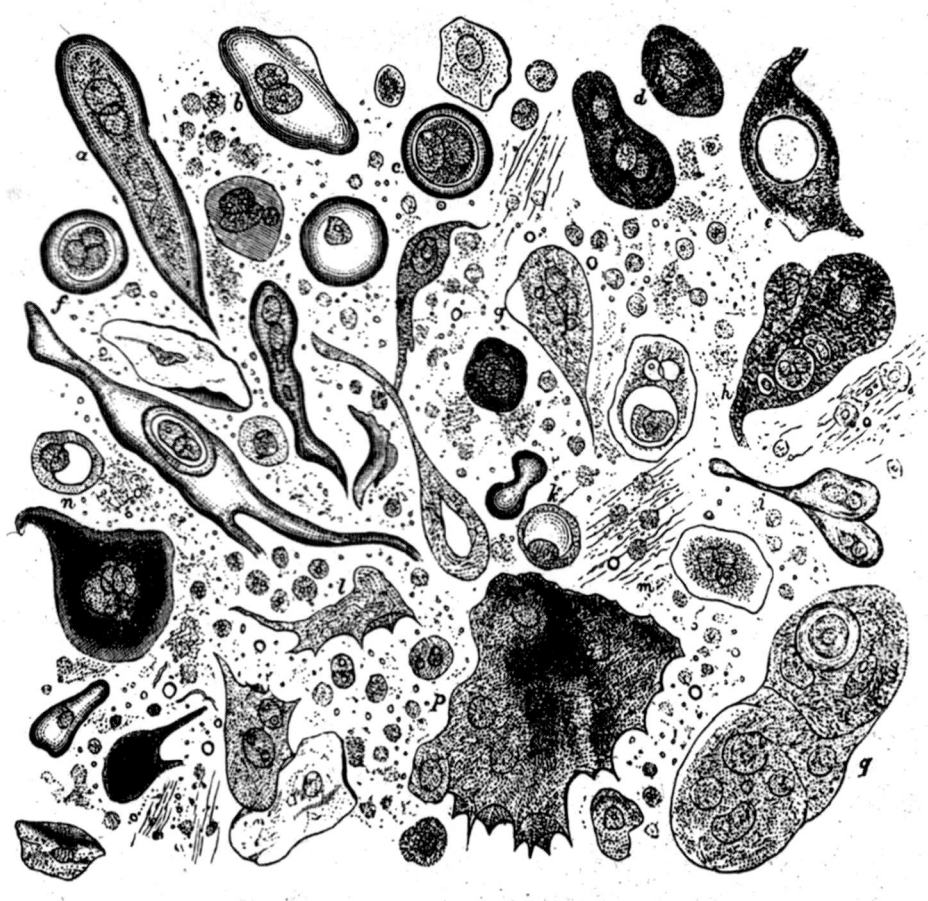

Figure 1.3 Laryngeal carcinoma cells. Wood carving, Lionel Beale (1861).

considered the father of cytology. He examined urinary specimens with water and glycerin and reported papillary fragments with cancer cells. In 1861, Beale published a paper on the examination of sputum from a case of laryngeal carcinoma (Figure 1.3). This wood carving is considered among the finest illustrations of tumor cells, nearly a quarter of a century before the birth of George Papanicolaou. Upon his death in 1906 at the age of 76 years, William Osler commented upon Dr. Beale's contributions and influence in medicine in an obituary published in *The Lancet*.

Paul Ehrlich is credited with introducing stains used in cytology and in tissue examinations. He developed aniline and basic dyes used in hematology. The first atlas of urine sediments was published in Germany in 1896. In 1900, Widal and Ravaut published a cytology review of nonneoplastic effusions using Romanowsky stains.

The present era of cytology was started by George Papanicolaou. In association with Charles Stockard in 1917, he published the first paper describing hormonal changes in the vaginal smears of guinea pigs. While at Cornell Medical Center, New York, Dr. Papanicolaou delivered his seminal paper entitled "New cancer diagnosis" at the Third Race Betterment Conference held at Battle Creek, Michigan. This is considered the beginning of modern cytology in the United States. Dr. Papanicolaou introduced the alcohol-based polychromatic stain for use with wet-fixed cellular specimens. One of his earlier colored illustrations (Figure 1.4) – made by Hashime Murayama, a well recognized artist of that era – depicts the accuracy and attention to detail of the great master. Murayama also illustrated the lecture delivered by George Papanicolaou at Battle Creek.

These observations have stood the test of time. Harvard University Press published the *Color Atlas* in 1954, in a ring-binder, facilitating periodic update in the newly emerging field. Students and trainees of Dr. Papanicolaou further promoted the practice of cytology. Mrs. Ruth

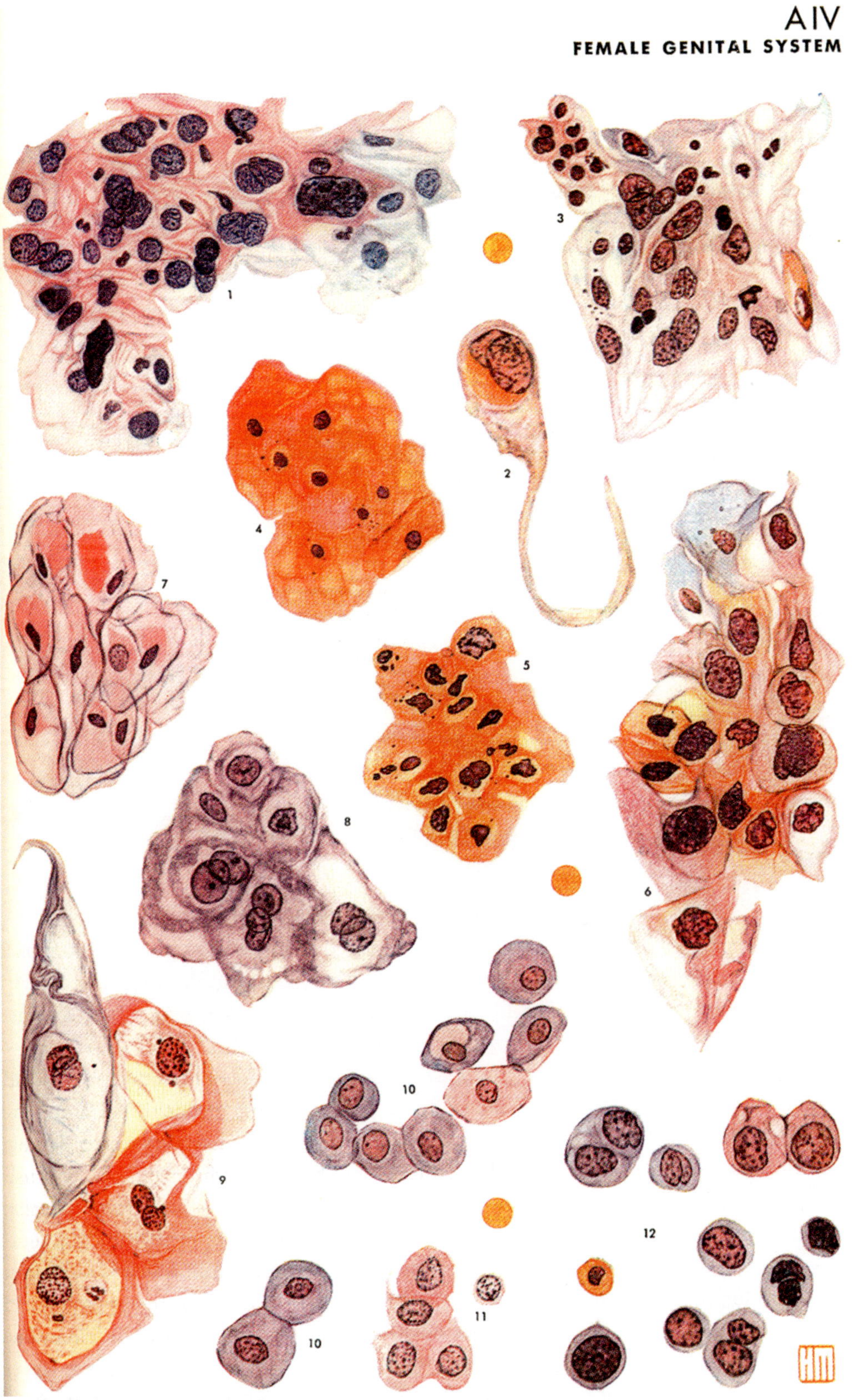

AIV
FEMALE GENITAL SYSTEM

Figure 1.4 Female genital system drawings, George Papanicolaou (1954). (Reproduced with permission: *Atlas of Exfoliative Cytology*, George N Papanicolaou Commonwealth Funds, Harvard University Press, 1954.)

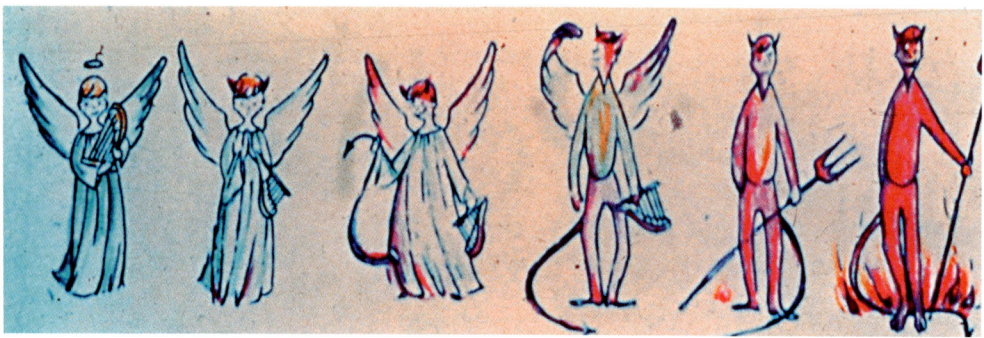

Figure 1.5 Concept of developing cervical cancer – angel and devil, Hugh Grady/Emil Novak, early 1940s. (Reproduced with permission: *Gynecological and Obstetrical Pathology, 1st Edition*, Emil Novak, W.B. Saunders, 1940.)

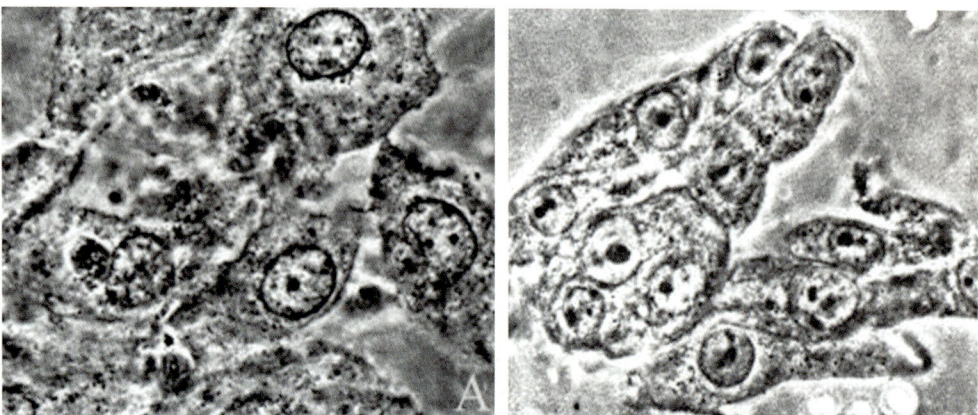

Figure 1.6 Cervical cells carcinoma, Peter Stoll (1969). (Reproduced with permission: *Gynecological Vital Cytology*, Peter Stoll, Spinger-Verlag, 1969.)

Graham was Papanicolaou's cytotechnologist and she became the head of the cytology laboratory at the Massachusetts General Hospital in Boston. She is credited with describing the "third type" or carcinoma in-situ cell after Dr. Papanicolaou observed the fiber and tadpole forms in squamous cell carcinoma. At nearly the same time, the concept of developing cervical cancer (Figure 1.5) was graphically depicted by Dr. Emil Novak.

Parenthetically, there is documentation that Dr. Aurel Babés of Romania independently recognized cancer cells in cervical smears at practically the same time as Papanicolaou. Drs. Bernard Naylor, George Wied, Leopold G. Koss, James W. Reagan, Stanley R. Patten, and John K. Frost – to name a few – continued to follow and further expand the field of cytopathology. Incidentally, in the late 1950s, John Frost is credited with introducing the word "cytopathology."

Drs. George Wied and Stanley Patten conducted the earlier studies on morphometry and automation. The introduction of computers and the neural network further advanced this now rapidly evolving field. Work on flow cytometry applicable to cytopathology was initiated in the laboratories of Drs. Koss and Patten. Exfoliated cells in health and disease were studied using phase-contrast microscopy (Figure 1.6).

Drs. Guelfo Sani and colleagues used fluorescent dyes for the study of exfoliated cells (Figure 1.7). Notice the remarkable concepts of developing cervical cancer as seen microscopically.

Although the cytologic examination of gynecological and non-gynecological cellular specimens gained acceptance and much popularity in the United States, evaluation of fine needle aspirations (FNA) failed to gain ground. In the 1930s, the first large series on needle aspiration evaluation using #18 gauge needles was published by Hayes Martin and associates from Memorial Hospital in New York. It appears that Dr. James Ewing, the pathologist at Memorial, was skeptical of FNA utilization in cytology and perhaps impeded its acceptance in the US. Interestingly, Dr. Ewing diagnosed his own bladder cancer by urine

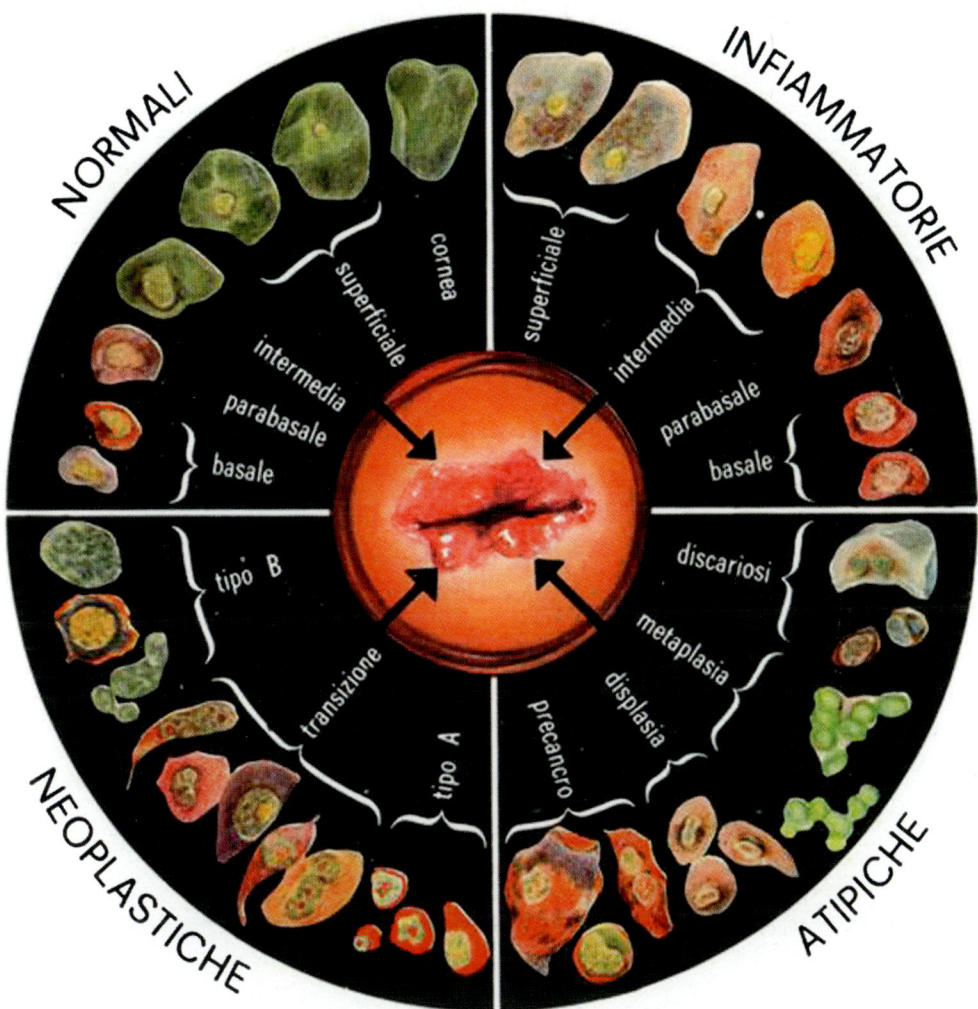

Figure 1.7 Normal and pathologic cervical cells as seen by fluorescence microscopy, Guelfo Sani (1963). (Reproduced with permission: *Fluorescence Microscopy in the Diagnosis of Cancer*, Guelfo Sani, Ugo Citti, Giuliano Caramazza, and Pietro Quinto, Charles C. Thomas Publisher Ltd., 1964.)

cytology. In Europe, hematologists were quite familiar with bone marrow specimens and utilization of Romanowsky stains. They were able to recognize tumor cells in the bone marrow aspirates and expanded their studies to include other organs such as thyroid, breast, and lung. Dr. Paul Lopes-Cardozo published a book on clinical cytology in 1954 and his *Atlas on Clinical Cytology* in 1976. In 1952, Nils Söderström published his experience with thyroid aspirations. Drs. Franzen Sixten, Joseph Zajicek, and Trosten Löwhagen – all from the Karolinska Institute in Stockholm, Sweden – should be attributed with popularizing the present use of FNAs.

Methylene Blue was used as a quick stain for FNA specimens over a number of years, in preference to the Romanowsky procedure which required a number of staining steps. A major improvement occurred in 1971 with the introduction of the Diff-Quik stain, permitting FNA to truly become a bedside diagnostic procedure. The Ultrafast Papanicolaou stain introduced a few years ago combines the properties of Papanicolaou and the convenience of Diff-Quik stains.

FURTHER READING

Babés, A. (1928). "Diagnostic du cancer du col utérin par les frottiss". *Presse Méd* **36**: 451–4.

Beale, L. S. (1861). "Results of the chemical and microscopical examination of solid organs and secretions. Examination of sputum from a case of cancer of the pharynx and the adjacent parts". *Arch Med (Lond)* **2**: 44.

George N. Papanicolaou Commonwealth Funds. (1954). *Atlas of Exfoliative Cytology*. Cambridge, MA, Harvard University Press.

Grace, C., H. Yang, *et al.* (2001). "Application of ultrafast Papanicolaou stain to body fluid cytology". *Acta Cytol* **45**: 180–5.

Graham, R. M. (1950). *The Cytologic Diagnosis of Cancer*. Vincent Memorial Laboratory, Vincent Memorial Hospital. Philadelphia, PA, WB Saunders Company.

Guelf, S., U. Citti, *et al.* (1964). *Fluorescence Microscopy in the Diagnosis of Cancer.* Springfield, IL, Charles C. Thomas.

Lopez-Cardozo, P. (1976). *Atlas of Clinical Cytology.* Leiden, Targa b.v.'s Hertogenbosch.

Martin, H. E., E. B. Ellis. (1930). "Biopsy by needle puncture and aspiration". *Ann Surg* **92**: 169–81.

Obituary. *Lancet* 1906; **1**: 1004.

Papanicolaou G. H. (1928). "New cancer diagnosis". *Proceedings of the 3rd Race Betterment Conference.* Battle Creek, MI, RBF, pp. 528–34.

Söderström, N. (1952). "Puncture of goiters for aspiration biopsy: a preliminary report". *Acta Med Scand* **144**: 237–44.

Stoll, P. (1969). *Gynecological Vital Cytology.* Berlin, Springer-Verlag.

2 NORMAL CELL MORPHOLOGY – EUPLASIA (CELLS IN NORMAL HEALTH AND PHYSIOLOGIC STATE)

THE CELL AS A WHOLE

(a) General features

The cell is an independently functioning, structural unit of an organism. It almost always contains a nucleus and cytoplasm; some cells (mature erythrocytes) do not have a recognizable nucleus. *One or more than one type of cells when organized as part of a purposeful, working arrangement in the body form a tissue.* Clonal derivation of the *euplastic* (healthy, normal, and physiologically responsive) cells and tissues imparts certain predictable morphologic and physiologic characteristics to the cells and tissues. These characteristics are diagnostically important. Familiarity and recognition of the cellular and tissue attributes is essential for proper evaluation and diagnosis of "normal" cells and tissues.

Cellular reactions to the body can be conveniently divided into the *growth* and the *functional* activities. These include: physiologically healthy or resting *(euplastic)*, dying or dead or physiologically regressive *(retroplastic)*, stimulated or reactive *(proplastic)*, and stimulated with uncertain or autonomous growth *(neoplastic)* activities.

Cellular activity level is primarily reflected in nuclear morphology. An evaluation and familiarity with the various nuclear constituents evident in a well-prepared cellular specimen including nuclear envelope (membrane), chromatin, parachromatin distribution and clearing, and nucleoli are the most critical components of clinical cytopathology. Morphological changes in one or more of these nuclear components often mirror the underlying disease process.

While the growth cycle is reflected in the nuclear features, functional differentiation of the cell is observed primarily within the cytoplasm. In most instances, this cytoplasmic mantle surrounding the nucleus determines the type or the anatomic nature of the site and the tissue of the cell origin. The nuclei of an intermediate cell from the cervix and an astrocyte from the central nervous system are morphologically similar, as are the nuclei of parabasal and intermediate cells from the cervix. Similarly, various types of bronchial epithelial cells can only be characterized by the cytoplasmic appearance, nuclei of both the ciliated and non-ciliated cells being morphologically identical (Figures 2.1 and 2.2).

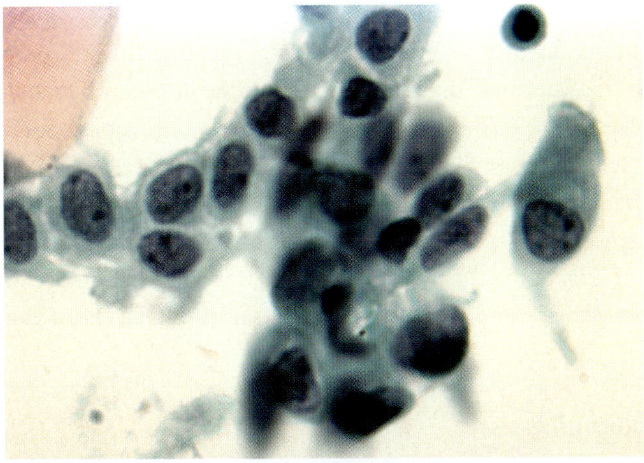

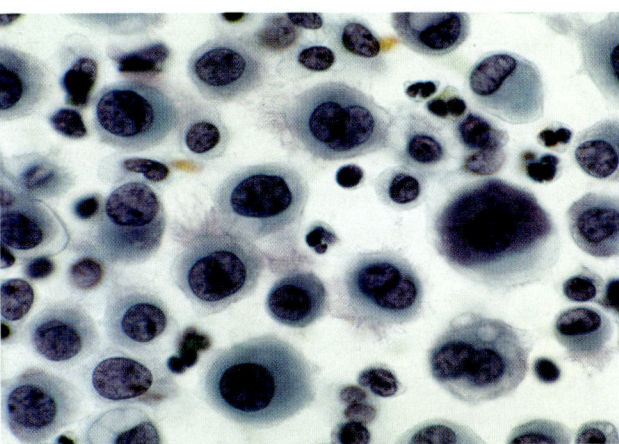

Figure 2.1 Cervical specimen depicting uniform nuclear features among columnar and cuboidal endocervical cells. LBP, Pap stain.

Figure 2.2 Bronchial cells. Ciliated and non-ciliated forms can be distinguished by the cytoplasmic features. Bronchial wash, Pap stain.

Cytohistology: Essential and Basic Concepts, Prabodh Gupta and Zubair Baloch. Published by Cambridge University Press. © Cambridge University Press 2011.

Proper evaluation, interpretation, and recognition of normal (euplastic) cells are fundamental to the diagnostic cytopathology; in this context, the value of quality of cyto-preparations cannot be minimized. "Normal," baseline cells represent resting phase and a reflection of the various physiological transient changes. Depending upon the tissue (nerve cells and lymphocytes vs. adipocytes and myocytes), various cells may reveal morphologic alterations that can be overlapping and mimicking "atypical" or "neoplastic" features. There is both a morphological and functional overlap between the physiological adaptive (i.e. pregnancy, obesity) and "early" reactive changes (oral contraceptives, environmental, physical, and biochemical irritants) observed in cellular specimens. For example, fat cells (adipocytes) can vary considerably in size depending upon the lipids accumulation and physical effects. Smooth muscle cells of the uterus during pregnancy similarly can demonstrate considerable hypertrophy and hyperplasia. It must be appreciated that there is a continuum in the tissue changes, and even a clonal group of cells may reflect different cellular changes simultaneously.

The classic features of "normal" cells are valuable when evaluating biologic behavior among cells derived from the same clone, such as in a tissue fragment or micro-biopsy often seen in cytologic preparations. Quite commonly, cells obtained from a clonal "normal" area such as a cervix, mesothelium, bronchial mucosa or the urothelium, although occurring singly and unattached, preserve and display similar and morphological characteristics. It must be recognized that these cells are in the same growth phase and are preserved identically.

Normal (euplastic, resting) cell. The normal resting or healthy (euplastic) cell exhibits certain cytomorphologic characteristics, including roundness, uniformity, predictability, and symmetry (Figure 2.3A,B).

Recognition of these fundamental cytological features of the euplastic or healthy cell is critical in the evaluation and diagnosis of the cellular samples in health and disease processes. In small tissue fragments, micro-biopsies and histopathology samples, surprisingly these crucial features are evaluated subconsciously, and one is able to separate "normal" from "abnormal" almost instantaneously. Such quick decisions are a common occurrence in interpretations of routine histopathology sections such as cervical and bronchial biopsies and other tissues (Tables 2.1 and 2.2). It must be recognized that this assessment is helpful when the cells are derived from a single clone and occur together, situated on a single basement membrane and interconnected by cytoplasmic processes (Figure 2.4). Certain physical,

(A)

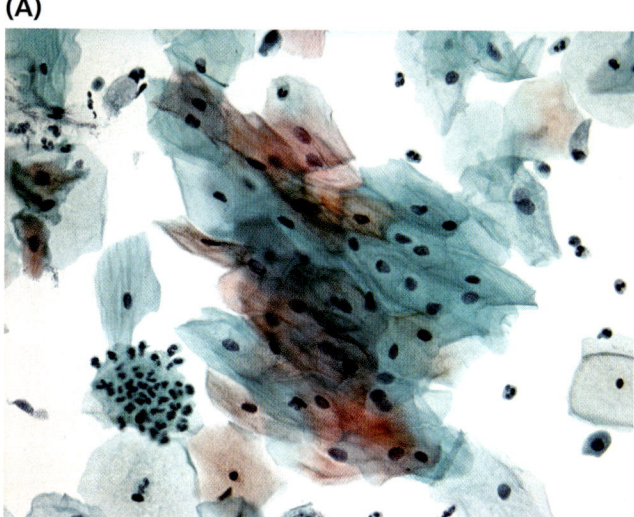

(B)

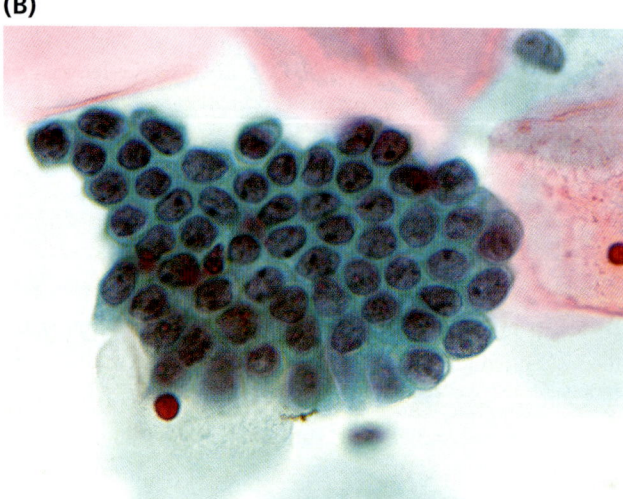

Figure 2.3 (A) and (B) show the morphologic features of euplastic cells. Notice the chromatin, parachromatin, and nuclear membrane features. Vaginocervical smear, Pap stain.

metabolic or physiological processes can alter this attribute of the "normal" tissues. For example, the normal squamous cells of the epidermis, although polyhedral in shape, associated with tone filaments and intercellular bridges can often be seen to mold against each other, becoming flattened and wafer-like as a result of mechanical pressures. Similarly, the fat cells in the subcutaneous region as well as the osteocytes immediately adjacent to the periosteal layer of the bone can be reshaped by physical forces.

Roundedness

Healthy cells naturally tend to acquire a round or rounded shape, especially when devoid of any convergent physical forces. As an example, the mesothelial cells exfoliated in the effusion fluids acquire a rounded appearance (Figure 2.5).

Table 2.1 Diagnostic cytomorphologic features helpful in differentiating between true tissue fragments and non-tissue fragments

Diagnostic true tissue fragment (DTTF)	Similar structures
	Clumps, aggregates, clusters, conglomerates, morula, pseudo-acini, pseudo-papillae. It must be appreciated that these represent three planes of focus and not necessarily three superimposed sheets
	Diagnostic features
No windows	Intercellular spaces – windows
Fence-like outer border	Generally loop-to-loop pattern
Obtuse angle between cells	Acute angle between cells
Tight intercellular junctions	Loose junctions
True acini (three–dimensional structures with top (*en-face* viewing) and inner layer with true luminal border)	No true acini No distinct epithelial sheet No true inner border No true bottom layer
True polypoid or papillary fragment epithelial center sheet – lumen with inner stroma and core	No true sheet No luminal border No stroma

Table 2.2 Salient cytomorphologic features helpful in differentiating between endocervical and endometrial cells

Features	Endocervical cell	Endometrial cell
Cytoplasm	Variable	Scant
Cytoplasmic border	Distinct	Indistinct
Nuclei	Oval or round	Irregular
Multiple	Frequently	Usually single
Chromatin	Granular	Clumped
Size variation	Variable	Little
Preservation	Good	Poor/variable

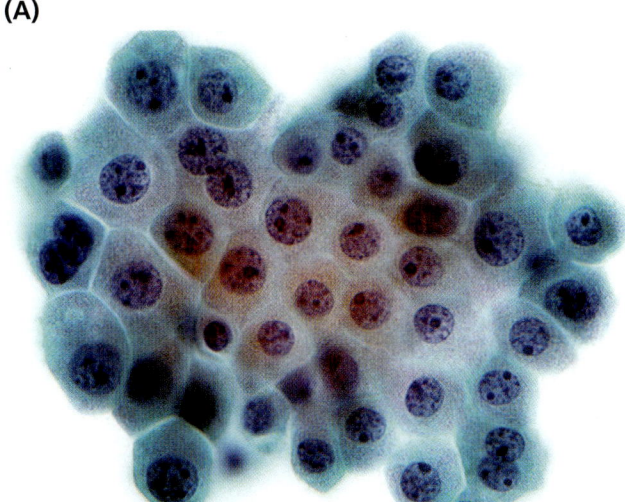

(A)

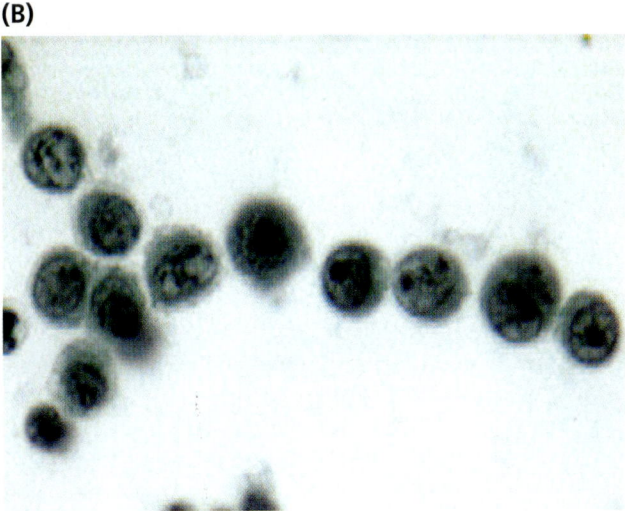

(B)

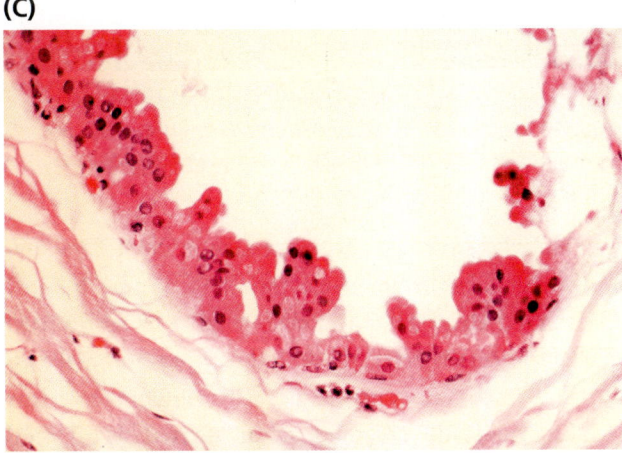

(C)

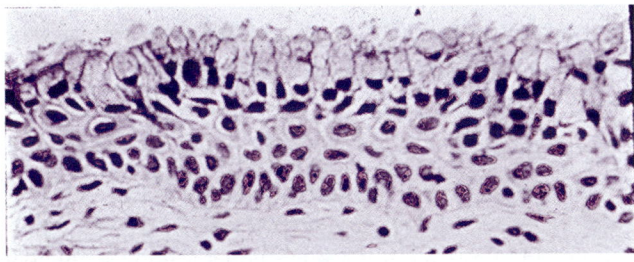

Figure 2.4 Endocervical and reserve cells showing cellular changes resulting from hormonal and physiological effects. These cells are resting on a basement membrane and reveal features of benign cells. Cervical biopsy, H/E stain.

Figure 2.5 (A–C) Roundedness in the cell and nuclear organelles. Metaplastic cells (apocrine cells) in breast cyst, fine needle aspiration. (A) cytospin slide. (B) mesothelial cells abdominal fluid, cytospin, Pap stain. (C) histologic section of a breast cyst lined by apocrine cells, H/E.

(A)

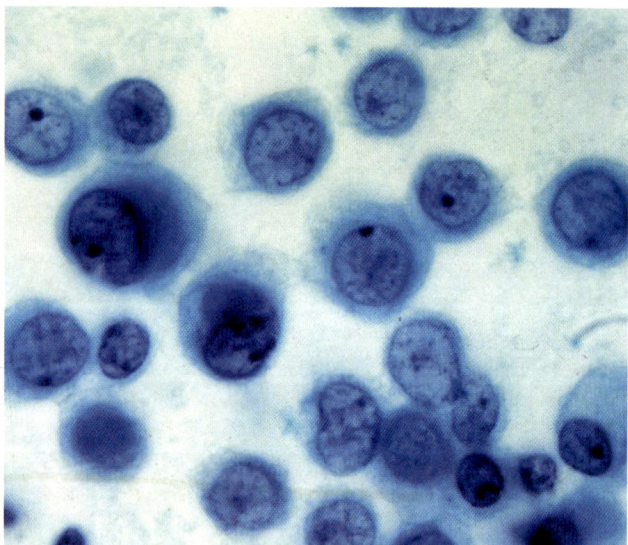

(B)

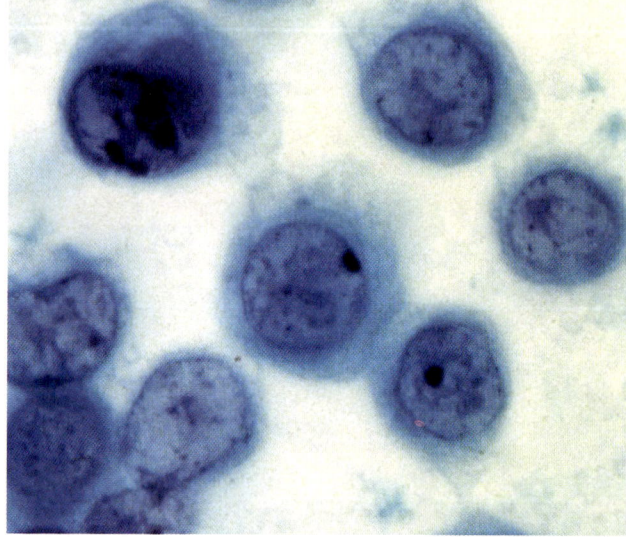

Figure 2.6 Pleural fluid, refrigerated for 3 days. Notice the well-preserved round nuclei of mesothelial cells on low power (A) and preservation of their nuclear details on high power (B). Millipore filter preparation, Pap stain.

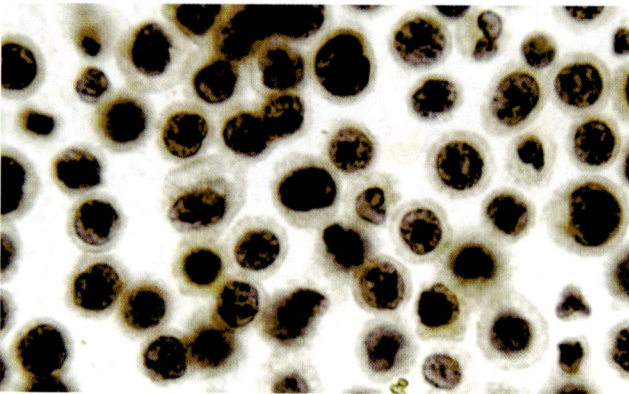

Figure 2.7 Pleural fluid with gastric adenocarcinoma cells after 3 days of refrigeration. Notice the hyperchromasia and lack of distinction between malignant and benign mesothelial cells. Millipore filter, Pap stain.

Similarly, urothelial cells suspended in the fluid within the urinary bladder for some time also acquire blunted edges and a rounded appearance. It must be appreciated that this feature is determined by the cytokeratin make up of the cell to a certain degree, i.e. cells with low molecular weight cytokeratin are more often affected by physical forces. They are often retained to variable degrees in other benign and malignant cells (Figures 2.6 and 2.7).

Uniformity
This refers to the cell size, shape, texture, and nuclear structure. Cells within the same micro-fragment exhibit identical morphometric and textural characteristics. Nuclear chromatin, irrespective of its basic morphological appearance (granular, meshy, or fibrillary) tends to be uniform, i.e. minimal variation in shape and size, as well as its distribution within the nuclear sap. Similarly, the shape of the nuclear membrane (outer rim of the nuclear envelope) is uniformly round or oval (Figure 2.8). However, this can be altered by physiological and physiochemical forces, such as secretion within the cytoplasm or by the neighboring cells and structures (best studied in living cells by phase contrast microscopy). Morphological changes can occur due to specimen fixation and preservative used; commonly utilized 95% ethanol provides the least amount of morphologic alterations, thus making cellular interpretation meaningful.

Predictability
Euplastic cells derived from the same site and assembled as a tissue fragment demonstrate certain morphological features which are extremely reliable in assessing their biologic nature. These include the size, shape, polarity, and location of the nuclei; orientation of the cytoplasmic vacuoles; size and shape of the cells; size of the nuclei; shape of the nuclear envelope; the nucleocytoplasmic (N:C) ratios; the thickness of the nuclear membrane; the size, location, and distribution of chromatin material as well as pattern; the texture of parachromatin shape; and the number of nucleoli (Figure 2.9). Among euplastic cells, all cellular components are predictable (as discussed below). Under certain physiological conditions the cells can show some deviation in their predictable behavior; however, this is minimal (i.e. less than one to four or six times variation in the size of nuclei and number of nucleoli).

(A)

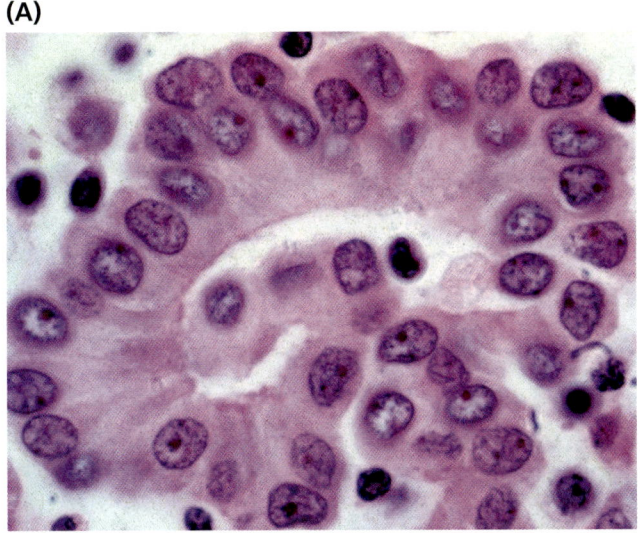

(B)

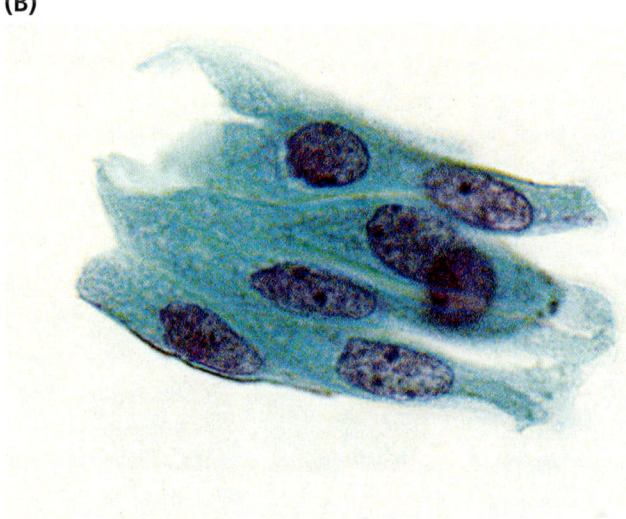

Figure 2.8 (A, B) Mesothelial cells (A), and endocervical cells (B) depict uniformity among the various cells and their constituents. Pleural fluid, cell block H/E; (A) LBP; (B) Pap stain.

(A)

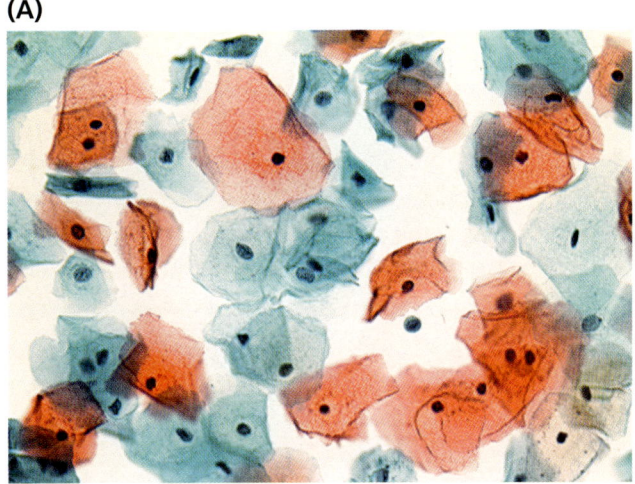

(B)

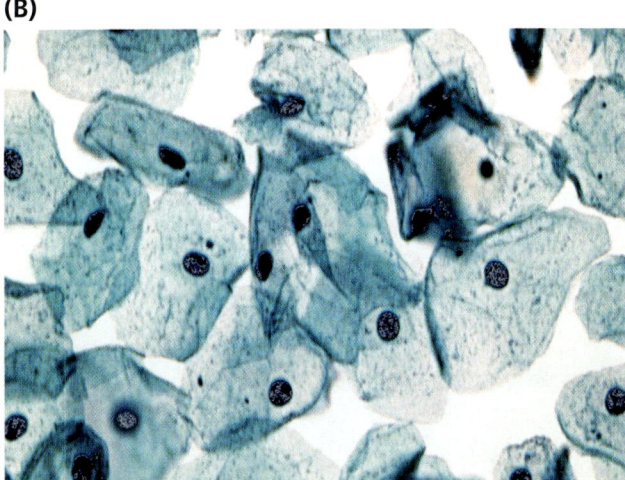

Figure 2.9 (A, B) These two pictures represent cervical samples showing uniformity among superficial and intermediate cells (A) and nuclei of intermediate cells (B). LBP, Pap stain.

(b) Nuclear structures

Size and shape

The nuclei in benign cells tend to be of the size (10–12 micron) of a well-preserved neutrophil. A few euplastic cells, such as megakaryocytes and ganglion cells, may show some extreme deviation in nuclear size. However, the nuclei of euplastic, unstressed cells, whether they are bronchial or endocervical columnar, hepatocytes, or gastric epithelial or mesothelial and mesenchymal, generally conform to the same nuclear size and shape (Figures 2.10–2.12). The presence of neutrophils, red blood cells or an intermediate cell nucleus provide an important surrogate for size comparison.

Hematoxylinophilia or chromasia

This is direct reflection of the DNA content and associated proteins within the nucleus. The nuclear chromasia is imparted by the chromosomal material, the chromatin network and chromatin rim. Among benign cells, the degree of nuclear chromasia or hematoxylinophilia is essentially identical.

Chromatin pattern

The chromatinic material, whether granular, fibrillary, or meshy, tends to be identical among euplastic cells derived from the same source.

Parachromatinic material

Among the euplastic cells, finely assimilated chromosome material is present in the nuclear sap or parachromatin.

(A)

(B)

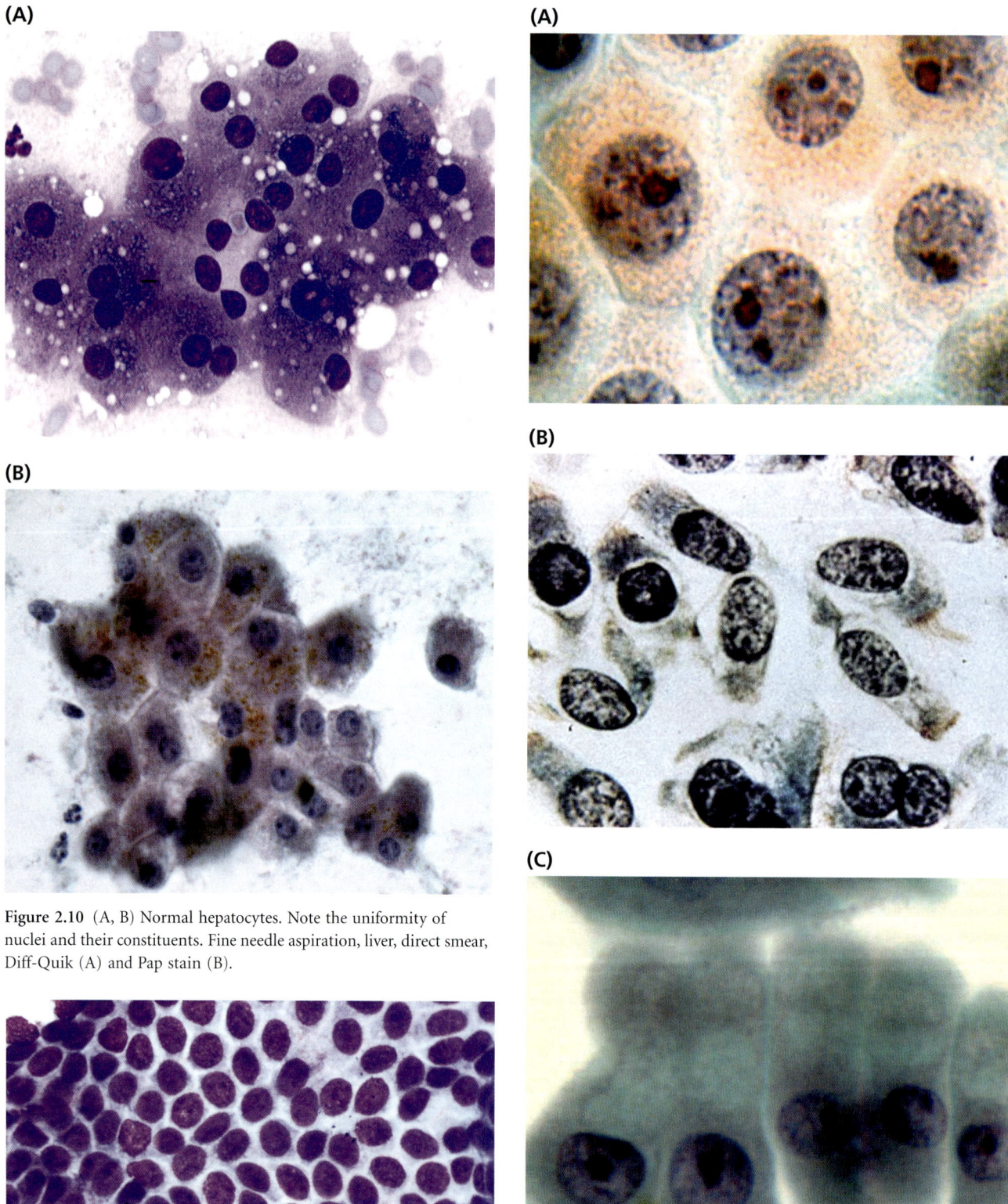

Figure 2.10 (A, B) Normal hepatocytes. Note the uniformity of nuclei and their constituents. Fine needle aspiration, liver, direct smear, Diff-Quik (A) and Pap stain (B).

Figure 2.11 Normal mesothelial cells. Note the nuclear features of benign cells. Peritoneal fluid, direct smear, Diff-Quik stain.

(A)

(B)

(C)

Figure 2.12 (A–C) These cells depict the chromatin pattern among euplastic or normal cells. (A) hepatocytes show granularity; (B) bronchial cells reveal a lacy pattern; whereas the metaplastic cell (C) reveals a homogenous chromatin distribution. (A) fine needle aspiration liver; (B) bronchial brush; (C) breast cyst aspiration. Conventional smears, Pap stain.

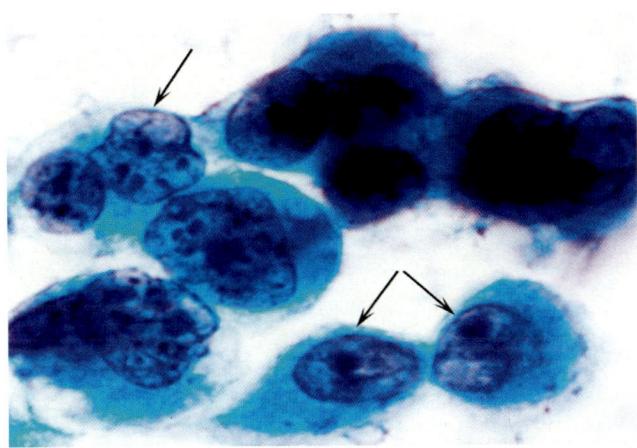

Figure 2.13 Nucleoli obscured by chromatin material (arrows), adenocarcinoma pancreas, fine needle aspiration, conventional smear, Pap stain. In the liquid-based preparations the chromatin pattern generally tends to be paler, making recognition of the nucleoli more obvious. The nucleoli in euplastic cells are all round or rounded; however, on occasion they may appear slightly elongated or oval in shape. Most important is the number of nucleoli in euplastic cells. The variation in the number of nucleoli among euplastic cells derived from the same source and occurring as a microbiopsy or tissue fragment (discussed later) usually follow this general rule: if one cell has two nucleoli, the adjacent cell in the same tissue fragment may have four plus one, i.e. $(2n+1)$, = five nucleoli, but not more. It may not always be possible to precisely determine the morphological nature of the nucleus that may be obscured by the associated chromatin or its location (Figures 2.7, 2.13, 2.14).

Parachromatin haze, its granularity and texture tends to be uniform and identical among euplastic cells.

Chromatinic network

Although uniform and essentially identical in all euplastic cells from the same source/clone, the chromatinic network may show extreme degrees of irregularities, clearing, and condensation (hyperchromasia) among nuclei which are either degenerating (retroplasic) or neoplastic in nature (nuclear rim), or the inner layer of the nuclear envelope, which is recognizable as the nuclear membrane by light microscopy and formed by a condensation of chromatinic material. In euplastic cells, the margin chromatin material throughout this rim is uniform in thickness, showing a predictability from cell to cell, thus helping in the proper recognition of the biological nature of these cells, i.e. euplastic vs. neoplastic (Figure 2.12).

Nucleolus

The presence of a nucleolus within the nucleus essentially indicates metabolic activity and cellular proliferation. The round or rounded nucleoli can be extremely variable in size

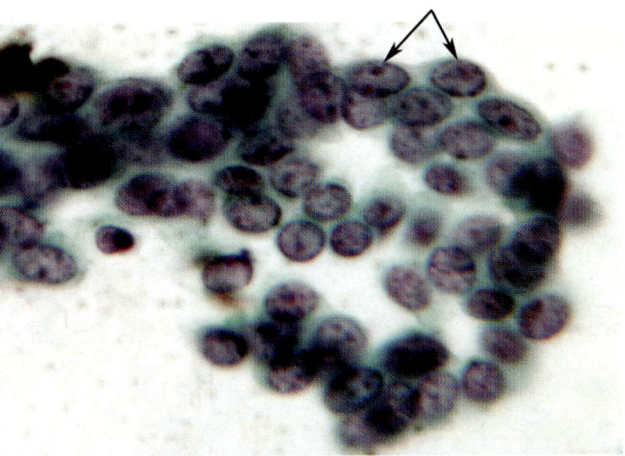

Figure 2.14 Nucleoli partially obscured by chromatin material (arrows). Reserve cells, bronchial brush specimen, direct smear, Pap stain.

and number. The prominence of nucleoli or their size per se is of no help in determining the biological nature of the cells, although extreme size (>6–8 micron) may be associated with neoplastic proliferation. The nuclei in euplastic cells generally are eosinophilic, as seen with the Papanicolaou stain. However, they can show varying degrees of basophilia resulting from the overlying chromatin network (Figures 2.13 and 2.14).

Symmetry

This refers to the distribution of intranuclear contents. If the nucleus is divided into four quadrants by two imaginary lines, the nuclear contents in the two quadrants across from each other are symmetrical, i.e. the chromatinic distributions, nuclear sap, and nuclear clearing tend to be symmetrical and predictable (Figure 2.15).

Cytoplasmic structure

In general, the cytoplasm of euplastic cells tends to be abundant, being at least twice as much as the size of the nucleus in most cells. Exceptions include lymphocytes and some other cells including basal/reserve cells, where the nucleus cytoplasmic ratio can be extremely high. The cytoplasmic basophilia commonly observed in Papanicolaou stains reflects the presence of ribonucleic acid (RNA) and ribosomal proteins, and tends to be more intense among more active and immature cells. However, this feature should not entirely be relied upon as a euplastic criterion (Figures 2.13 and 2.14). Mature squamous cells orient parallel to the basement membrane.

(A)

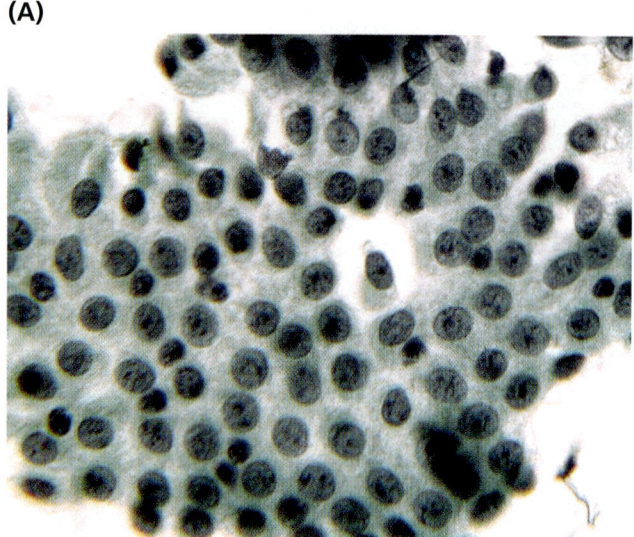

(B)

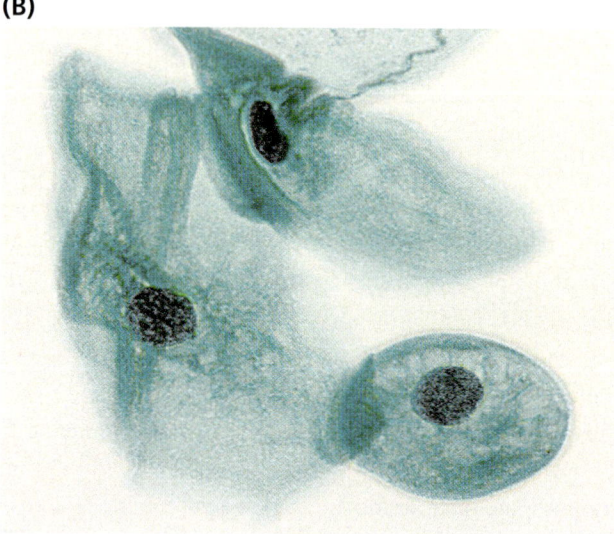

Figure 2.15 (A, B) Nuclear organelle symmetry, while the endocervical cells occurring in a small tissue fragment appear symmetrical (A), similar nuclear features are preserved among intermediate squamous cells (B). Vaginocervical smear, Pap stain.

SQUAMOUS CELLS (STRATIFIED EPITHELIUM)

General features

When differentiating along the epidermal axis, these cells are generally large (15–25 micron), flat with abundant cytoplasm. They have a round or oval nucleus with a variable reticular chromatin pattern. The nucleus is often centrally placed with a symmetrical distribution of cytoplasm. Depending upon the maturation of the cells within the epithelium, the tinctorial characteristics as well as morphological features of the cytoplasm of the squamous cells may change. With the Papanicolaou polychromatic

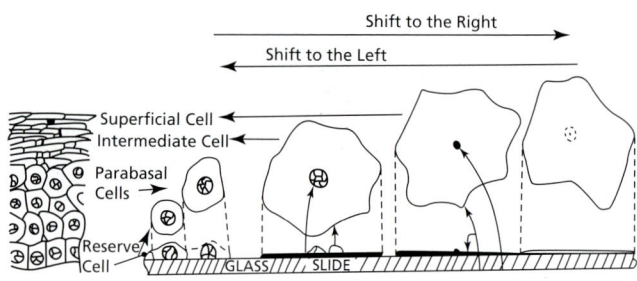

Figure 2.16 This line drawing depicts the general characteristics of squamous epithelial cells. Reserve cells cannot be recognized with certainty in the exfoliated squamous cells such as from the cervix and bronchus. They may be observed in brush and scraped specimens. Maturation shift is generally not observed; use of hormonal contraceptives and lack of vaginal component in the smears renders this alteration unreliable.

stain, many squamous cells tend to be eosinophilic and take on a shade of red or orange. The cytoplasmic coloration should not be used as criteria for diagnosing squamous cells. Similar cytoplasmic orangophilia can appear if the cells are air-dried or if they contain intracytoplasmic mucopolysaccharide material.

Hyperkeratotic

Hyperkeratotic squamous cells are generally observed in squamous epithelium exposed to chronic external environmental stimulation or various irritative processes (Figures 2.16 and 2.17). The most mature and outermost cell in the squamous epithelium generally appears as elongated, flat and parallel to the underlying surface epithelium with tapering cytoplasm; the edges and the tips may appear blurred. These cells also show a gradual centrifugal thinning of the cytoplasm. Occasionally, a central pallor or a bulge may be observed in the cells. The location of the original nucleus may be only partially visible or appear as ill-defined hematoxynophilic granules or a ghost image.

Hyperkeratrotic squamous cells can also develop in epidermal inclusion cysts or sub-areolar abscess in the breast (Fig. 2.17A, B). Occasionally, cavitary chronic infection, undulating catheter, and calculi and prostheses may produce hyperkeratotic squamous cells. It must be appreciated, however, that the presence of hypermature keratinized cells per se is not indicative or diagnostic for a neoplastic lesion, and may be covering or associated with a more serious underlying epithelial change. As such, the presence of hypermature or hyperkeratotic cells should be properly documented and additional studies recommended as appropriate. Figure 2.18A and B show the association of hypermature cells with an accompanying squamous cancer.

(A)

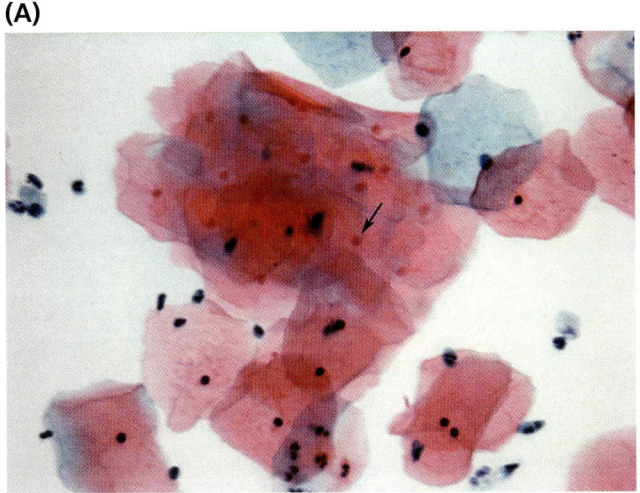

(B)

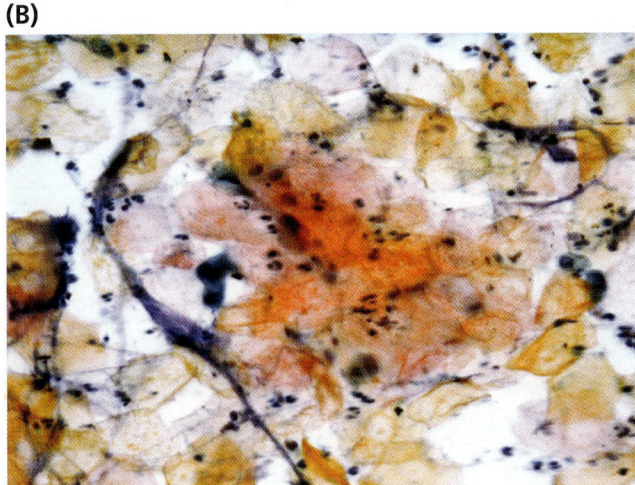

Figure 2.17 (A, B) Hyperkeratotic cells cervical smear. (A) notice the ghost nucleus (arrow). (B) fine needle aspiration intradermal inclusion cyst, vaginocervical. (A) direct smears; (B) Pap stain.

(A)

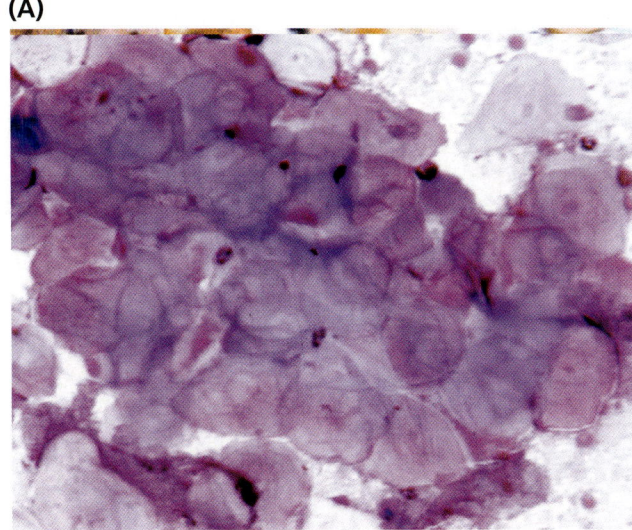

(B)

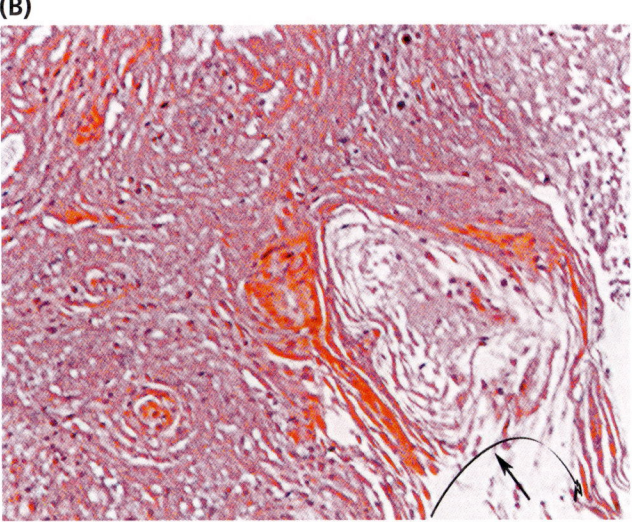

Figure 2.18 (A, B) Hyperkeratotic squamous cells, cavitary lung lesion. (A) fine needle aspiration, Diff-Quik stain. (B) hyperkeratosis overlying squamous cell carcinoma lung (arrow), tissue section, H/E stain.

Superficial

Cells occur most often in the cervical/vaginal, oropharyngeal, esophageal, and sometimes lower urinary tract samples. They are usually polygonal in shape with a well-defined angular margin and cell borders, and the cytoplasm is spread evenly from the center and tends to thin out at cell edges. In certain situations the cytoplasmic edges may merge imperceptively with the surroundings. The nucleus is usually pyknotic. In the healthy state, these cells almost always occur singly. The Papanicolaou stain may sometimes reveal staining and tinctorial variations among these cells and they may appear cyanophilic (Figure 2.19).

Intermediate

These are located under the superficial cells and reveal a less mature phase in the differentiation of squamous epithelium. These cells, in contrast to the superficial cells described before, have a vesicular nucleus, i.e. a nucleus in which nuclear details (chromatin pattern, parachromatin, and nuclear envelopes) can be observed. A sex chromatin (Barr body) can also sometimes be recognized attached to the nuclear margin (Figure 2.20). The cytoplasm in these cells also tends to thin out toward the edge. They generally stain cyanophilic by the polychromatic Papanicolaou stain.

Intermediate cells are metabolically active and may contain glycogen or similar material often seen in physiological and pathological hormonal effects (Figures 2.21 and 2.22). The glycogen may serve as a nutrient for the growth of fungal organisms (*Candida*) and support the growth of lactobacilli. The individual cells generally occur with soft

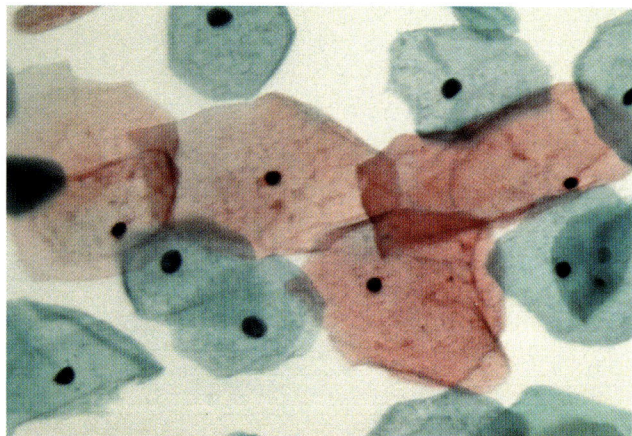

Figure 2.19 Superficial squamous cells. Notice the pyknotic nuclei. Similar cells may occur in oropharyngeal and anal specimen. Cervical smear, Pap stain.

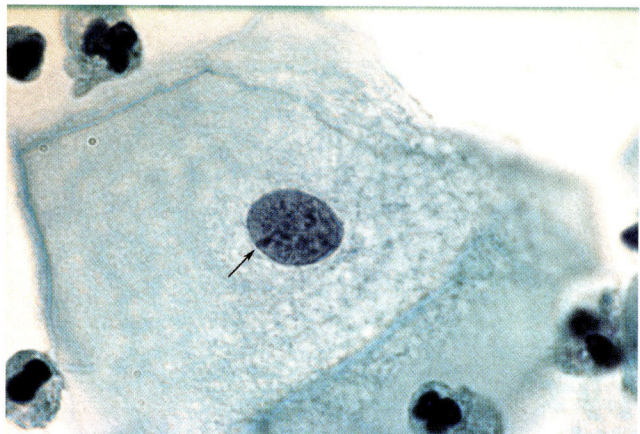

Figure 2.20 Intermediate squamous cell with vesicular nucleus and fine nuclear chromatin. Sex chromatin (Barr body) is seen at the nuclear margin (arrow). Pap stain.

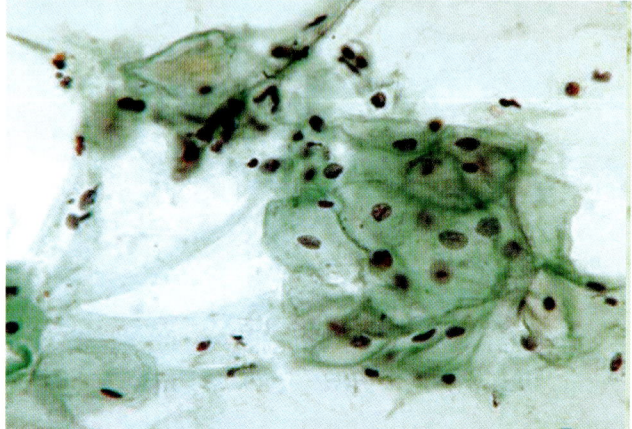

Figure 2.21 Intermediate cells with folded nuclear edges – navicular cells. These changes occur under hormonal influence in pregnancy and the late luteal phase in the menstrual cycle. Vaginocervical smear, Pap stain.

(A)

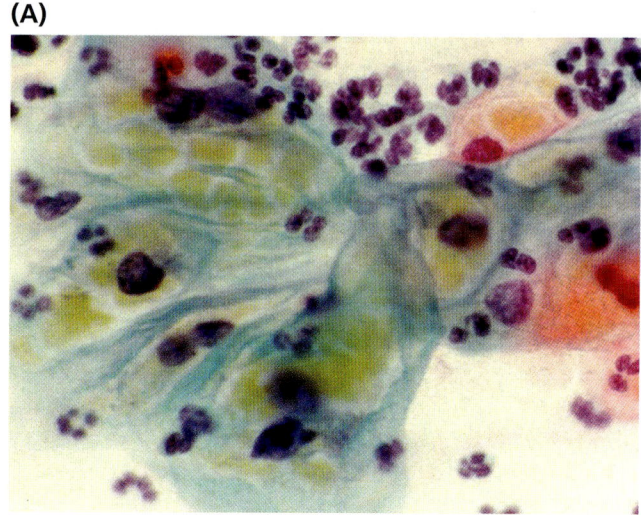

(B) **(C)**

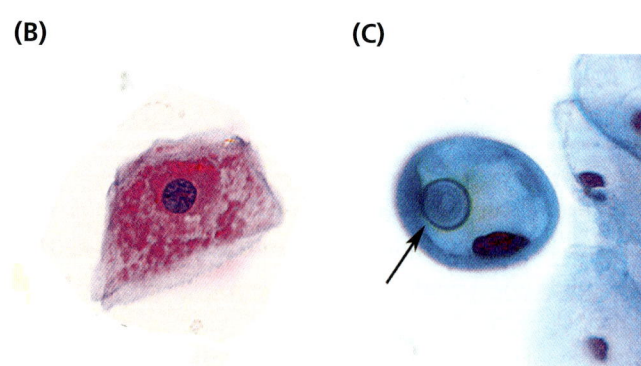

Figure 2.22 (A) Intracytoplasmic golden yellow glycogen in intermediate cells, Pap stain. (B) PAS positivity of glycogen in an intermediate cell. (C) Intracytoplasmic glycogen inclusion (arrow). Cervical specimen, LBP.

edges and somewhat blurred margins. They may show cytoplasmic folds similar to the curling of "rose petals" (Figure 2.21).

Glycogen appears as a golden brown pigment by Papanicolaou stain. It is water-soluble and generally not readily displayed. Glycogen may also appear as intracytoplasmic inclusions.

Parabasal

In the fully mature intact epithelium, parabasal cells are seen in the prickle cell layer (Malpighi) between the germinal cells and the overlying intermediate squamous cells. They rarely exfoliate in the normal physiological states; however, they can be observed in the premenarcheal age group as well as in post-menopausal women. Immediately

after child birth, they continue to be shed in the vaginal pool material and are called post-partum (PP) cells. PP cells contain glycogen-type intracytoplasmic secretions. Their occurrence in gynecological specimens may reflect a

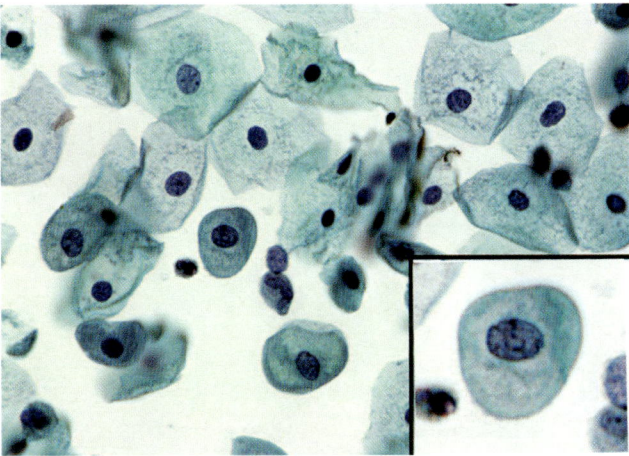

Figure 2.23 Parabasal cells. Notice the thick cytoplasm among round and oval cells. Nuclei are vesicular (insert). Cervical specimen, LBP, Pap stain.

(A)

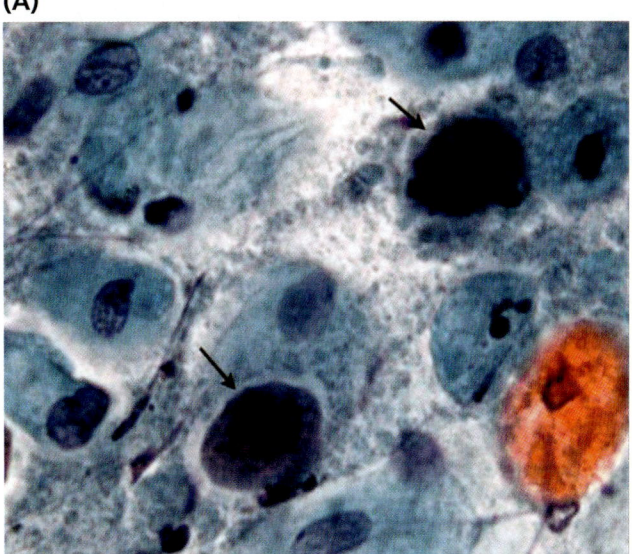

(B)

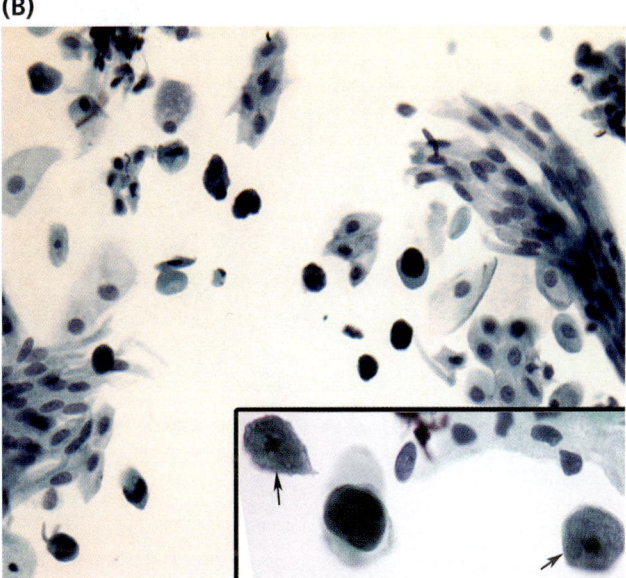

Figure 2.25 Blue blobs in atrophic smears. (A) Conventional smear (arrow); (B) liquid-based preparation, arrows. Insert with nucleoli (arrows) and scant cytoplasm. Pap stain.

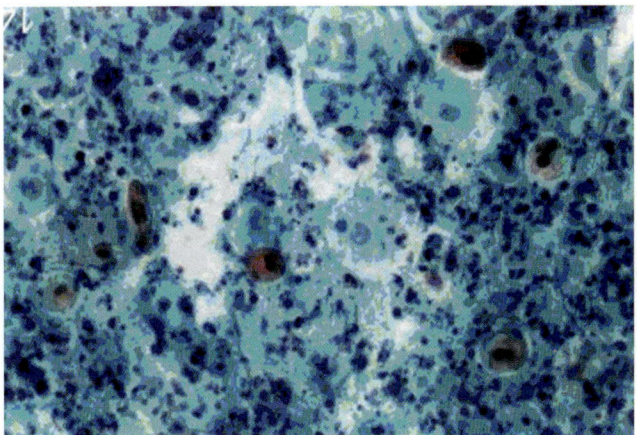

Figure 2.24 Atrophic smear with parabasal cells and inflammation. Vaginocervical smear, Pap stain.

state of arrested or low maturation, such as hormonal changes or imbalance, lack of estrogens, atrophy, healing, and repair. Unlike other squamous cells, parabasal cells are round or oval in shape, lack angulations, and the cytoplasm is thick and does not display typical cytoplasmic thinning. The nuclei of most of the parabasal cells are usually vesicular but can be pyknotic (Figs 2.23–2.26).

Parabasal cells in the basal type of atrophic vaginal smears can be extremely degenerated, hyperchromatic and appear "atypical" (Figures 2.23–2.25). They can acquire altered N:C ratio and appear dysplastic or high-grade intraepithelial lesion; such cells are referred to as "blue blobs." Besides being parabasal, they may be endocervical in origin and may contain inspissated mucus (Figure 2.24). Parabasal cells should not be confused with metaplastic and dysplastic type cells.

Metaplastic cells

Epithelial metaplastic change is invariably reversion to a more primitive epithelium, such as to squamous from glandular or ciliated types. This change occurs most commonly under chronic irritation, following an injury or hormonal effect. Metaplastic cells tend to occur in groups with thick cytoplasm and altered N:C ratios. They generally have nucleoli and finely granular chromatin. Proper identification of squamous metaplastic cells can be extremely difficult. Metaplastic cells are often similar to parabasal cells in appearance (Figures 2.23, 2.26–2.28).

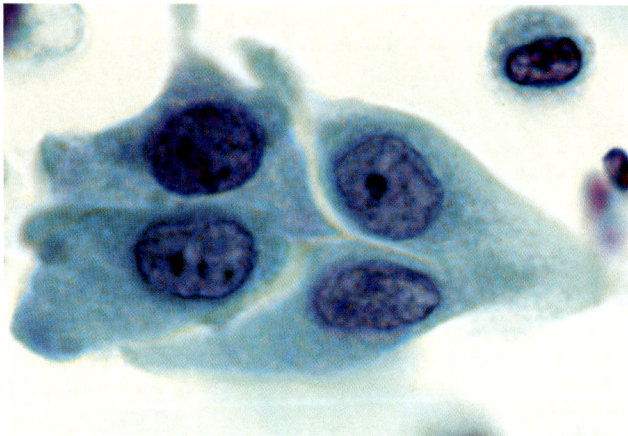

Figure 2.26 Metaplastic cells. Notice the granular chromatin and nucleoli. Cervical specimen, LBP, Pap stain.

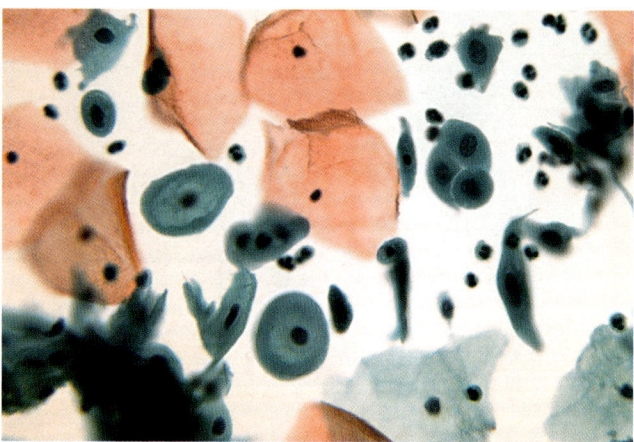

Figure 2.27 Metaplastic cells showing variable shapes. Cervical specimen, LBP, Pap stain.

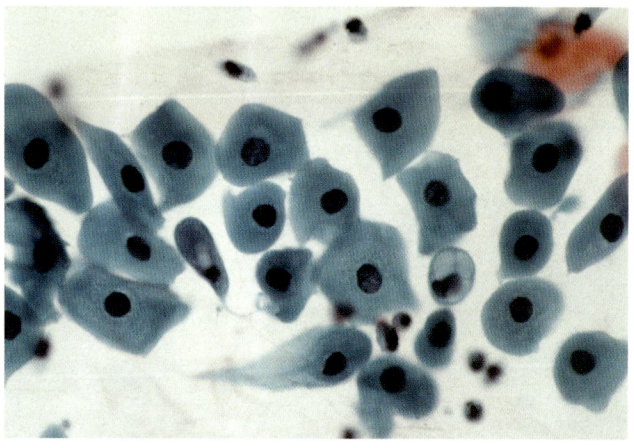

Figure 2.28 Metaplastic cells depicting morphologic features from mature squamous to columnar forms. Cervical specimen, LBP, Pap stain.

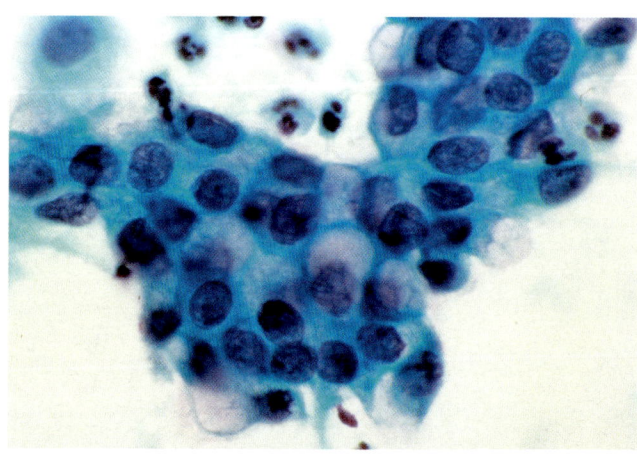

Figure 2.29 Metaplastic changes, columnar epithelial cells (ARC I, Patten). Notice the mucus-bearing cells intermixed with undifferentiated forms. Conventional cervical smear, Pap stain.

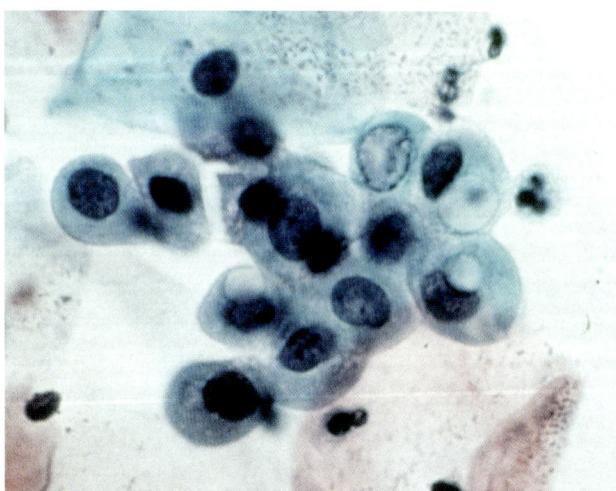

Figure 2.30 Metaplastic changes (ARC II, Patten). Notice the thick cytoplasm and nuclear features. Conventional cervical smear, Pap stain.

The shape of the metaplastic cells may be columnar to squamoid; when recognizable, intercellular bridges are a good criterion for squamous differentiation (Figures 2.26–2.32).

Ciliated cell metaplasia may occur in the columnar epithelium, especially under the effect of persistent inflammation as in chronic cervicitis and reactive processes resulting in tubal metaplasia (Figure 2.33). Extremely rarely, ciliated metaplasia may be seen in malignant ovarian, and endometrial or endocervical tumors.

While oncocytic metaplasia occurs commonly in epithelial cystic lesions such as breast (apocrine) and thyroid (Hurthle) (Figure 2.34), keratinizing metaplasia may occur in mesothelial cells in the presence of chronic inflammation, irritation or therapy (Figure 2.35).

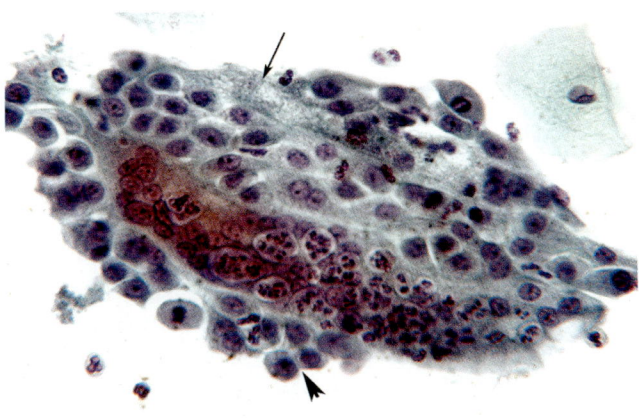

Figure 2.31 Squamous metaplasia. Notice the large undifferentiated appearance of the cells. Intercellular bridges are visible among the cells (arrow). Arrowhead points to the small cuboidal undifferentiated cells. Vaginocervical conventional smear, Pap stain.

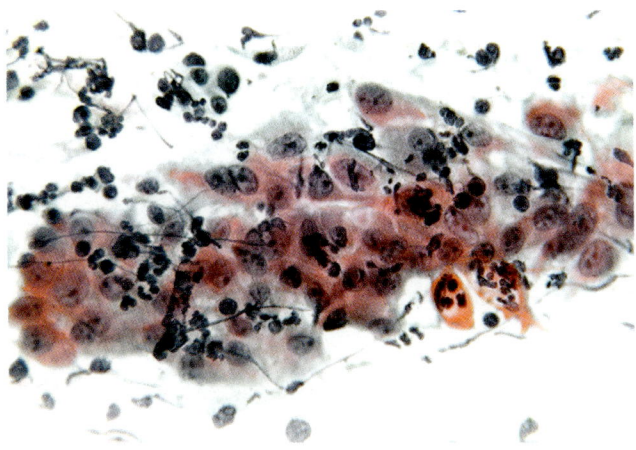

Figure 2.32 Squamous metaplasia (ARC III Patten). Notice the extensive keratinization and well-differentiated squamous feature. Such cells can be mistaken for squamous cell carcinoma. Vaginocervical conventional smear, Pap stain.

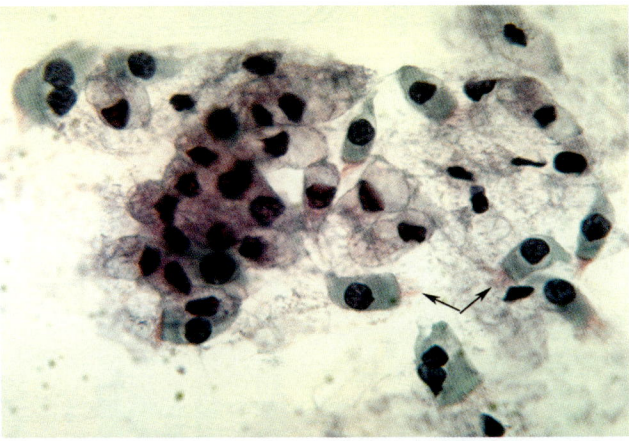

Figure 2.33 Tubal metaplasia, cervix. Ciliated cells (arrows) are mixed with mucus-containing goblet cells. Vaginocervical conventional smear, Pap stain.

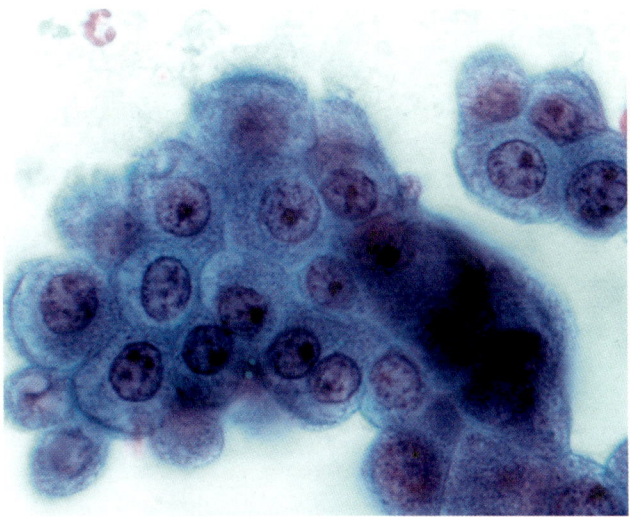

Figure 2.34 Apocrine metaplasia, breast cyst aspiration. Notice the large polygonal cells with prominent nuclei. Millipore filter, Pap stain.

Uncommonly, mucoid metaplasia may occur in post-menopausal atrophic vaginal smears or following hysterectomy (Figure 2.36).

Another type of cell often mistaken for squamous or metaplastic in nature is the dysplastic cells and decidual cells. Dysplastic cells generally exhibit nuclear membrane and chromatin pattern changes. There can be a substantial morphological overlap between the parabasal, metaplastic and the atypical squamous cells suspect high grade (ASC-H) (The Bethesda System, TBS) terminology. Para-basal cells can resemble the decidual cells, which may be seen in the cervical specimen obtained during pregnancy (Figure 2.37). These cells are often few in number (less than 10 per slide), cuboidal or columnar in appearance and

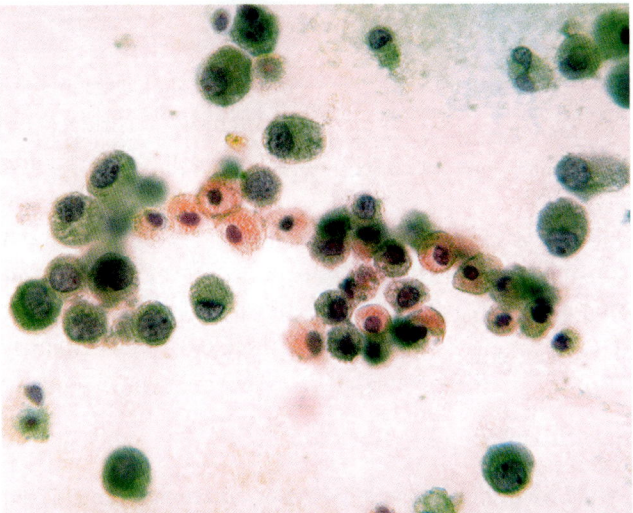

Figure 2.35 Mesothelial cells with squamous metaplastic cells, pleural effusion. Patient with breast adenocarcinoma under chemotherapy. Cytospin slide, Pap stain.

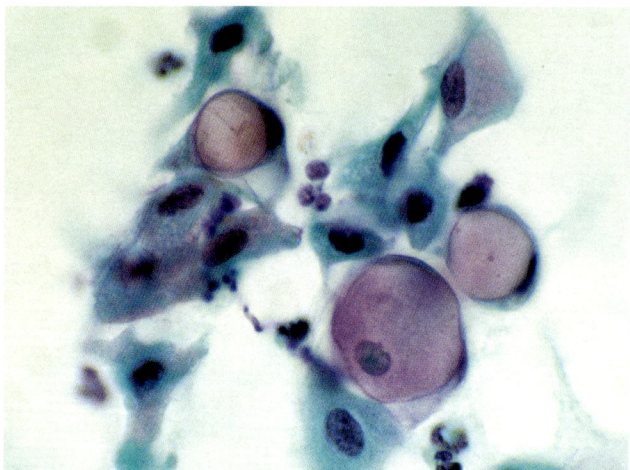

Figure 2.36 Goblet cell or mucoid metaplasia. These changes are considered true in nature and are a result of epithelial cells implantation after surgery, proliferation of mucus-producing cells, or differentiation from pleuripotential cells. Vaginal smear, Pap stain.

(A)

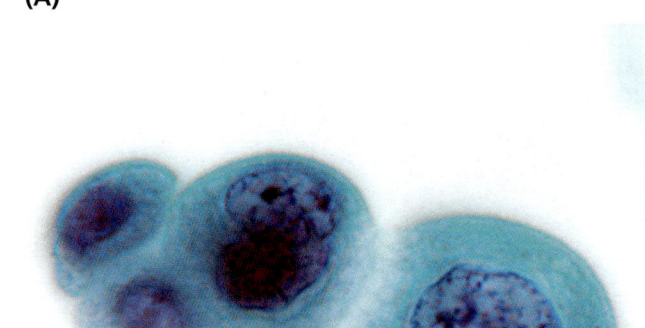

(B)

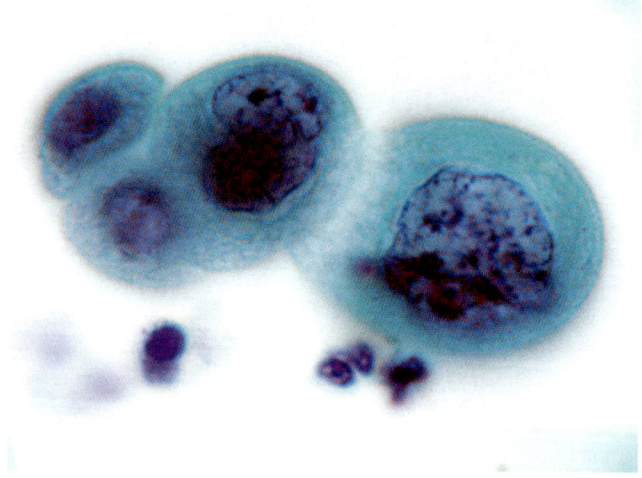

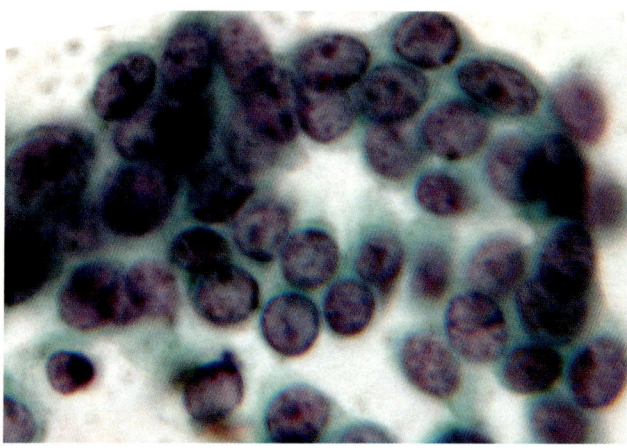

Figure 2.38 Reserve cells, ureteric brush. Note the high N:C ratio and prominent nucleoli. Conventional smear, Pap stain.

occur in small groups. They contain basophilic cytoplasm with or without fine vacuoles, and hyperchromatic nuclei containing granular chromatin with one or two prominent nucleoli.

Germinal basal or reserve cells

These have a high N:C ratio, are attached to the underlying tissues, and generally do not exfoliate; therefore, they are not usually encountered in routine specimens. Reserve cells, however, can be forcibly dislodged with scraping or brushing of the surface epithelium. They are a common occurrence in bronchial and urothelial brushings and bile duct specimens, and can be common cause of diagnostic errors (Figure 2.27). These cells usually appear as small and uniform, occurring singly or in small groups with or

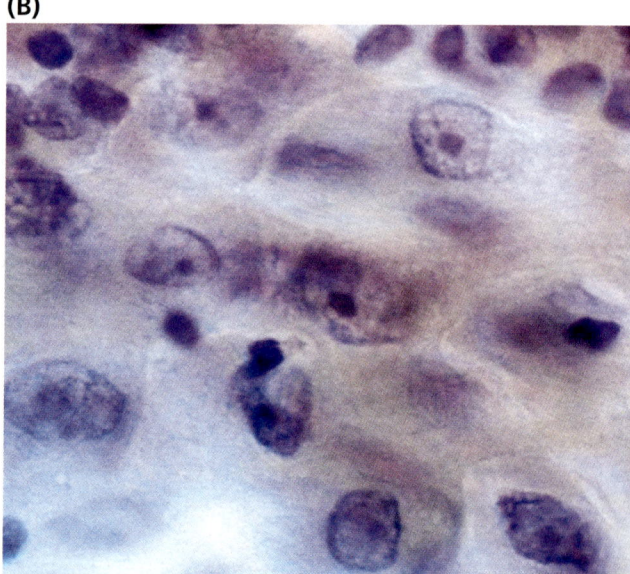

Figure 2.37 (A, B) Decidual cells cervical smear. Cells appear to be undifferentiated resembling (A) ARC II, and (B) ARC III. They have abundant cytoplasm and prominent nucleoli. (A) Vaginocervical conventional smear; (B) Cervical specimen, LBP, Pap stain.

without associated nucleoli (Figures 2.38–2.40). If not carefully examined, basal/reserve cells can be mistaken for an undifferentiated malignant epithelial neoplasm, neuroendocrine tumors, or hematopoietic cells.

Sex chromocenter (Barr body)

While identification and reporting of chromocenter–Barr body in cytopathology material is of historical importance, it has limited diagnostic value. Well-preserved resting epithelial cells with an XX chromosome pair usually show the

(A)

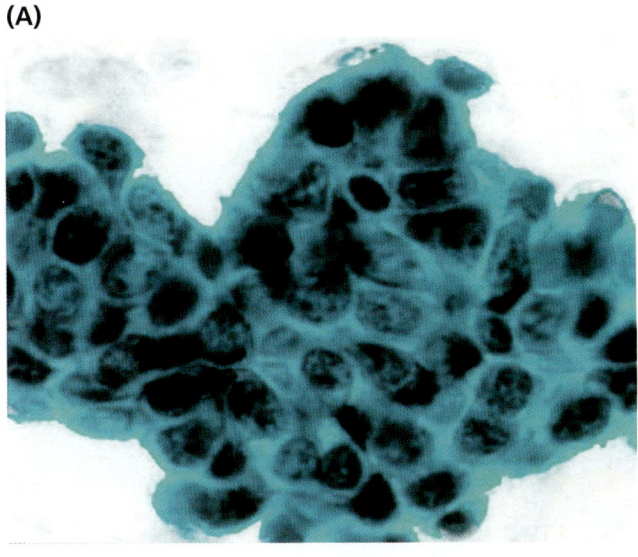

(B)

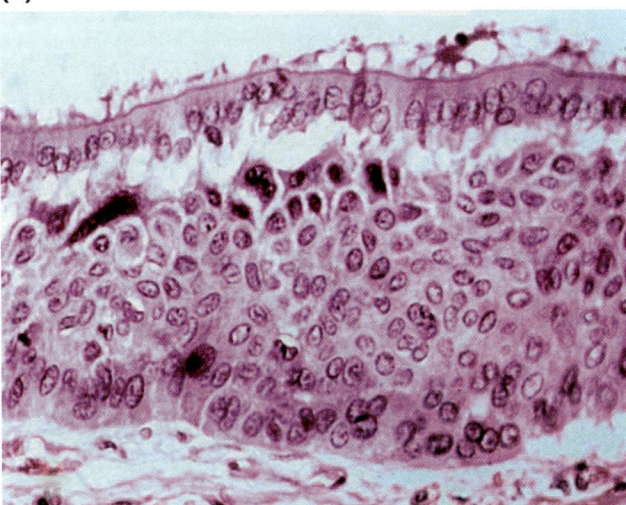

Figure 2.39 (A) Reserve cells bronchial brush, and (B) corresponding bronchial biopsy, depicting similar cells in the sub surface region. Early Lung Cancer Project, Millipore filter, Pap stain (A), H/E (B).

(A)

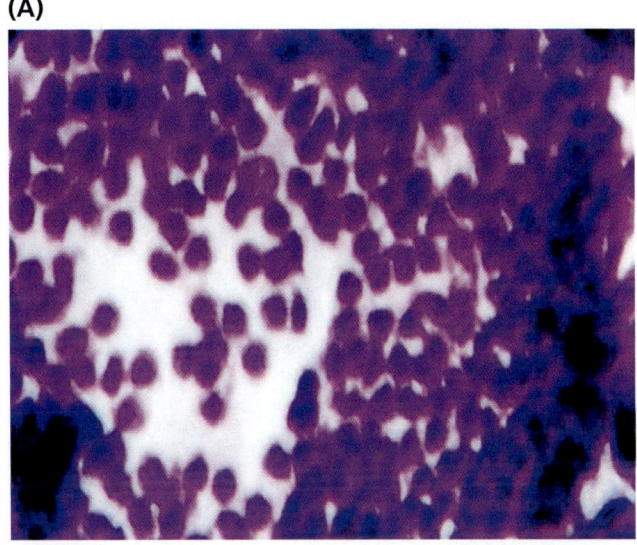

(B)

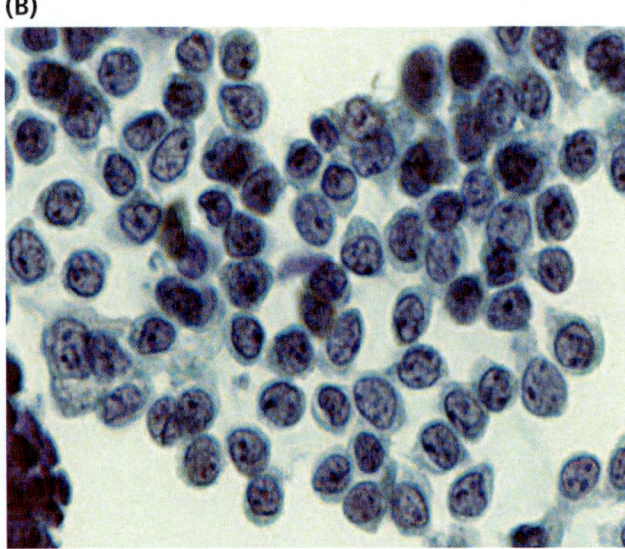

Figure 2.40 Bronchial reserve cells. Notice the high N:C ratios and resemblance to small cell neuroendocrine tumor. (A) Direct smear, Diff-Quik stain. (B) Direct smear, Pap stain.

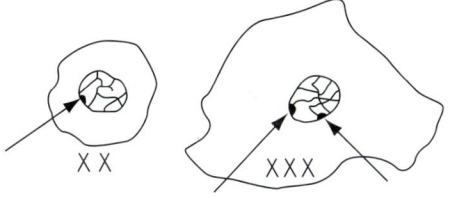

Figure 2.41 Line diagram depicting location of sex chromatin–Barr Body along the nuclear membrane in well preserved vesicular nuclei. Extra Barr bodies may be observed following radiation and in some malignancies (see Figure 2.42).

Barr body as having heterochromatin with a chromatin mass measuring approximately one micron in diameter on the nuclear membrane (Figures 2.41 and 2.42). To be diagnostic, the sex chromatin center must be a part of the nuclear membrane, melting imperceptibly when examined under high-magnification oil emersion. It is usually identifiable in approximately 20–40% of well-preserved normal female epithelial cell nuclei in the vaginal specimens. With strict morphological diagnostic criteria one does not find a similar-appearing Barr body in the XY nuclei. Occasionally it appears with large or small apparently normal XX chromosome; double or paired or triple Barr bodies have been formed in cases of XXX or XXXX, respectively.

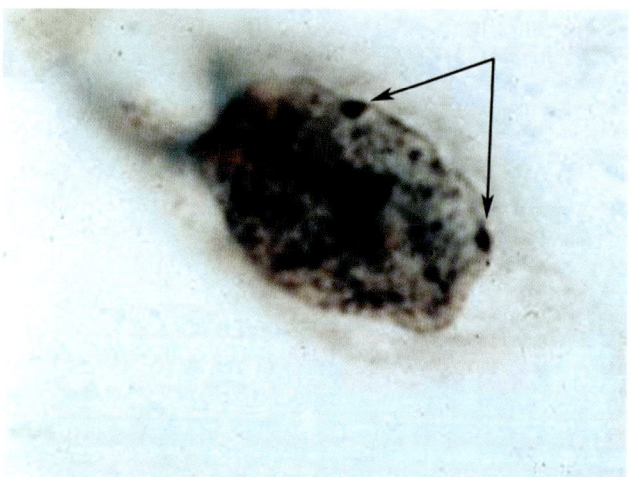

Figure 2.42 Two Barr bodies (arrows) in an irradiated squamous cell carcinoma cell. Cervicovaginal smear, Pap stain.

Hormonal evaluation

Hormonal evaluation of cytology specimens is rarely utilized nowadays. The excessive estrogen effect as seen by the increased number of superficial cells in post-menopausal and women not using hormones can have clinical significance. The upper third of the vaginal wall as well as the trigone region in the urinary bladder and other tissues in the body respond predictably to sex hormone changes in the body.

Under the influence of steroidal hormones, glandular (endocervical) cells may develop small nuclear protrusions (Figure 2.43). Although these have been considered to represent smearing artifacts, they can be seen in liquid-based gynecologic preparations that do not have any smearing effects.

Endocervical cells under non-physiological and peri-menopausal states can exhibit extremely bizarre nuclear and cytoplasmic changes. These can be easily misinterpreted as neoplastic and are often reported as "atypical" (Figure 2.44). Cells may occur as a part of an endocervical tissue fragment or, uncommonly, singly.

In Papanicolaou smears from patients on Tamoxifen or similar hormonal treatment for breast, ovarian or endometrial cancer, the hormonal pattern may reveal three types of cells: superficial, intermediate, and parabasal. These cells have unpredictable cytoplasmic changes and bizarre nuclear changes with or without glycogenation of the parabasal cells (Figure 2.45).

Decidual cells

These appear as metaplastic forms with dense cytoplasm, hyperchromasia and prominent nucleoli.

(A)

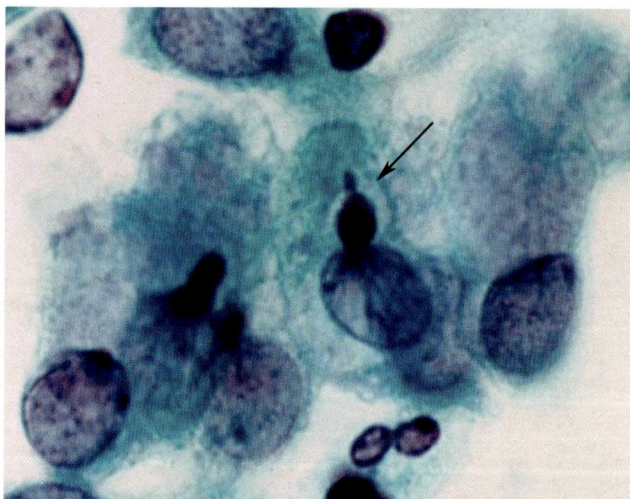

(B)

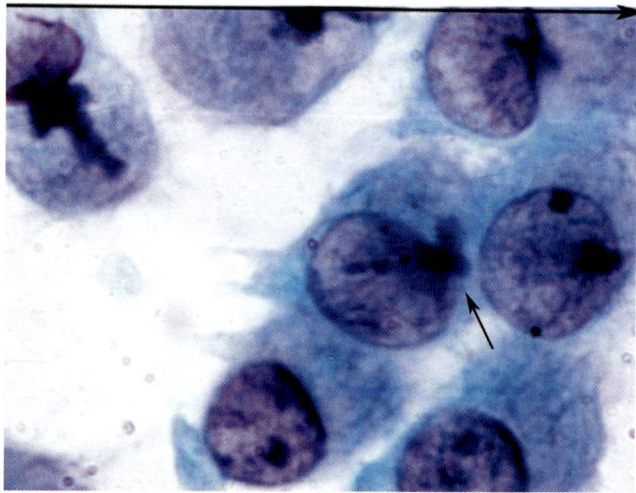

Figure 2.43 Nuclear protrusions, endocervical cells (arrow). These are generally considered to be hormone-dependent. (A) Conventional smear; (B) SurePath, Pap stain.

Trophoblastic cells

In addition to the decidual cells, trophoblastic cells can sometimes be seen in vaginal smears (Figure 2.46). These multinucleated cells may have prominent nucleoli and can be correctly identified by specific staining with human chorionic gonadotropin (HCG) antibodies (Figure 2.47). Multinucleate giant cells can occur in vaginal smears, most commonly after surgical intervention, radiation or in association with atrophy or chronic inflammation, and become hyperchromatic and atypical. They can occur singly or as a part of a small tissue fragment (Figure 2.46).

"Pearl" formation

The most frequent cause for "pearl" or "pearly body" formation is collection of stratified squamous cells in a

(A)

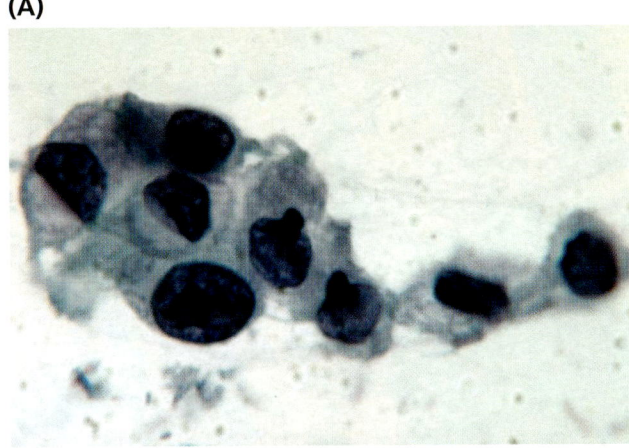

(B)

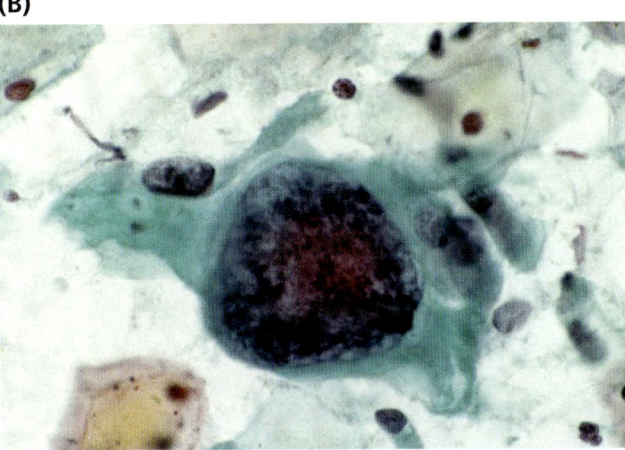

Figure 2.44 (A, B) Hormonal changes in endocervical cells. (A) Tissue fragment with nuclear protrusion and atypia. (B) Single endocervical cell showing pronounced nuclear atypia. (A) Vaginocervical smear; (B) LBP, Pap stain.

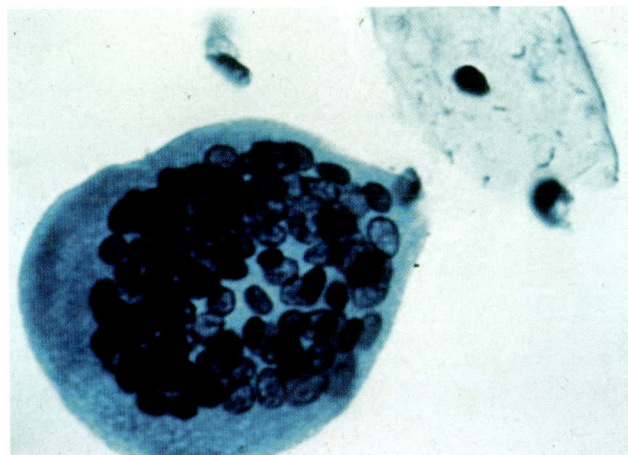

Figure 2.46 Multinucleated syncytiotrophoblast. This may be seen in late pregnancy or in association with trophoblastic disease. Vaginocervical smear, Pap stain.

(A)

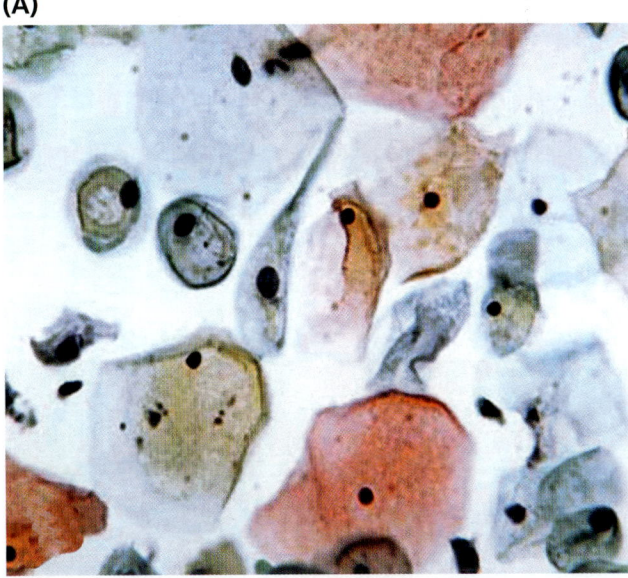

(B)

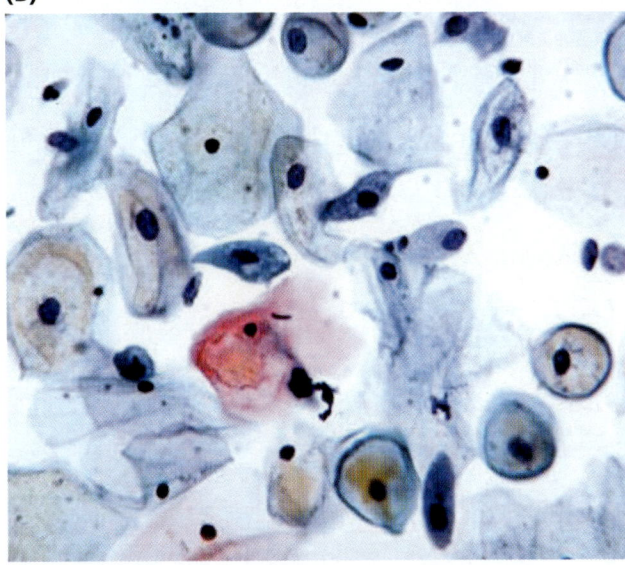

Figure 2.45 Tamoxifen changes. Although not specific, these often reveal bizarre cell forms: an unevenly distributed hormonal pattern (A) and a spread hormonal pattern (B). Cervical specimen, LBP, Pap stain.

pit on the epithelial surface between the surrounding acanthotic epithelium. This leads to the development of a squamous plug or core (Figures 2.48 and 2.49). When shed, the cells may appear to be embracing each other concentrically; however, on closer inspection, they are usually found stacked on top of each other in swirled fashion.

At times, however, the peripheral epithelial cells wrap around each other in true concentric fashion. Pearls occur in benign as well as malignant conditions. The nuclei of the various cells in a pearl tend to be uniform and predictable,

(A)

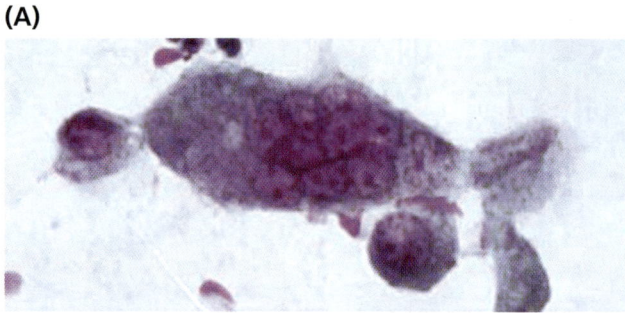

(B)

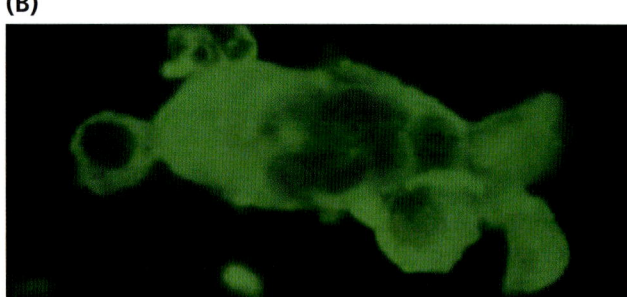

Figure 2.47 (A) Syncytiotrophoblast; (B) specific cytoplasmic immunofluorescence using HCG antibodies. Vaginocervical smear.

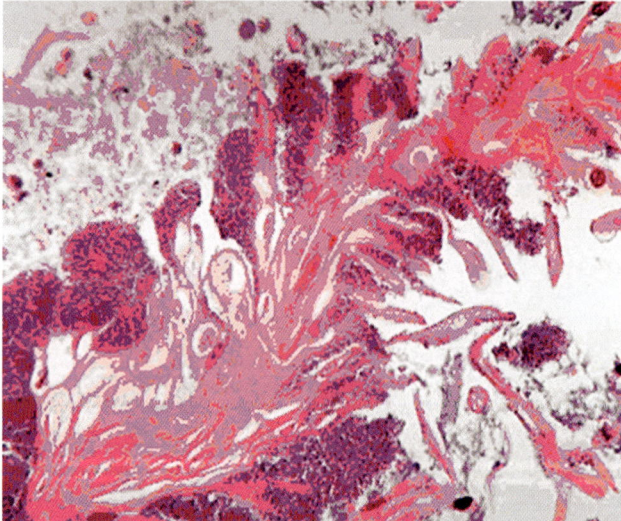

Figure 2.49 Squamous pearl. Notice the central core of anucleate cells. Sputum specimen cell block section. H/E stain.

whereas they show features such as variation, chromatin clearing and nuclear membrane changes when occurring as part of a malignant transformation (Figures 2.50 and 2.51). Pearls can occur in benign as well as malignant conditions (Figures 2.51 and 2.52).

Cannibalization

Cell-to-cell cannibalism in cytologic preparations is noted as two cells giving rise to an "owl-eyed" structure, also

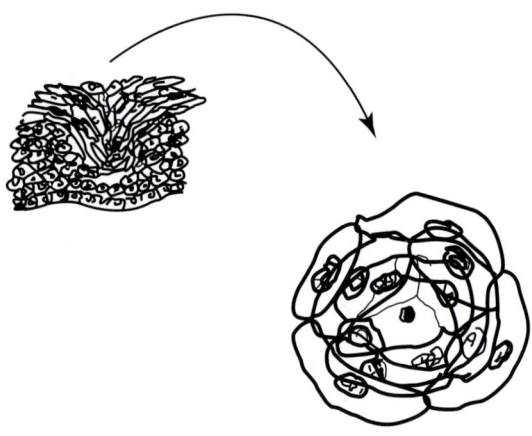

Figure 2.48 Line drawing depicting the formation of a squamous epithelial pearl. Notice the concentric cell arrangement.

(A)

(B)

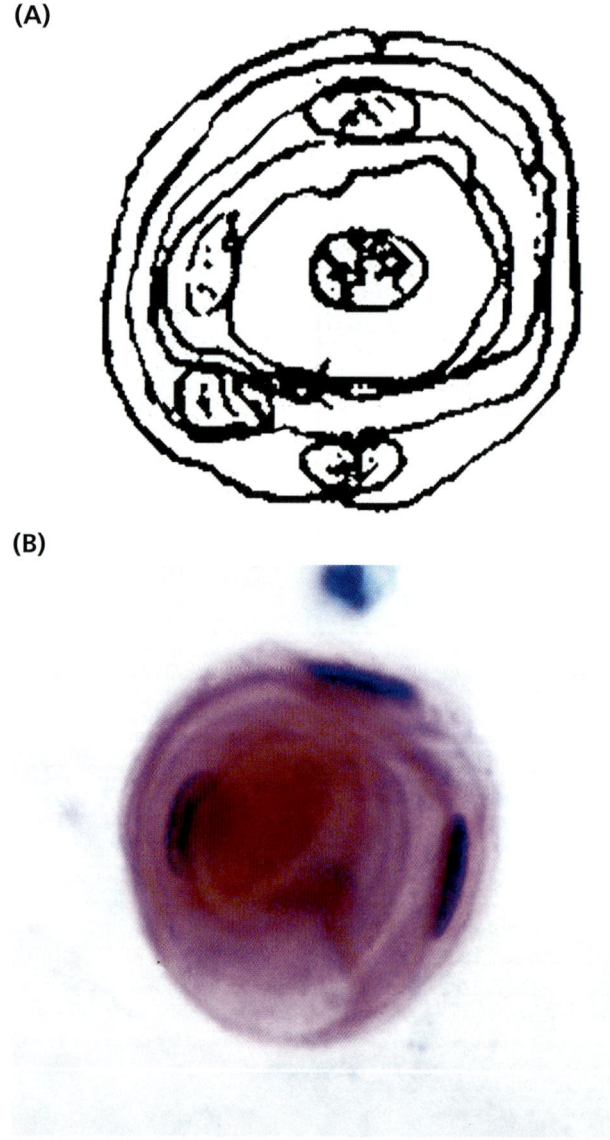

Figure 2.50 (A) Line drawing depicting the wrapping of the benign squamous cells to produce a pearl. (B) Sputum specimen with a benign pearl. Notice the enclosing of stretched squamous cells around the central keratin plug. Bronchial brush, Early Lung Cancer Project, Pap stain.

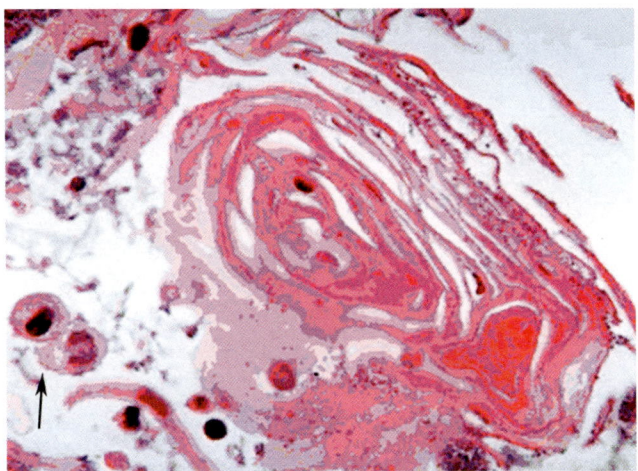

Figure 2.51 Notice the nuclear features in this malignant pearl with an atypical form of functional differentiation. Dysplastic squamous cells are present around it (arrow). Fine needle aspiration, neck lymph node, cell block. H/E stain.

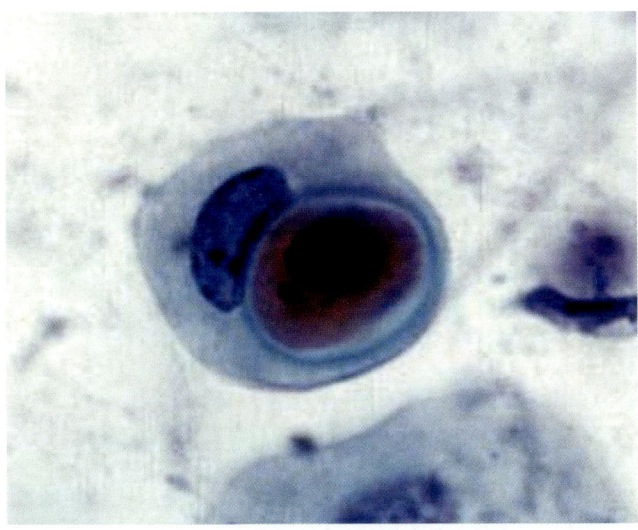

Figure 2.53 Cell-in-cell arrangement, squamous cell carcinoma cervix, cervicovaginal smear. Pap stain.

(A)

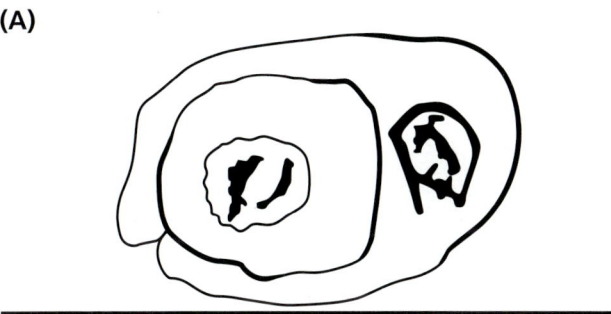

(B)

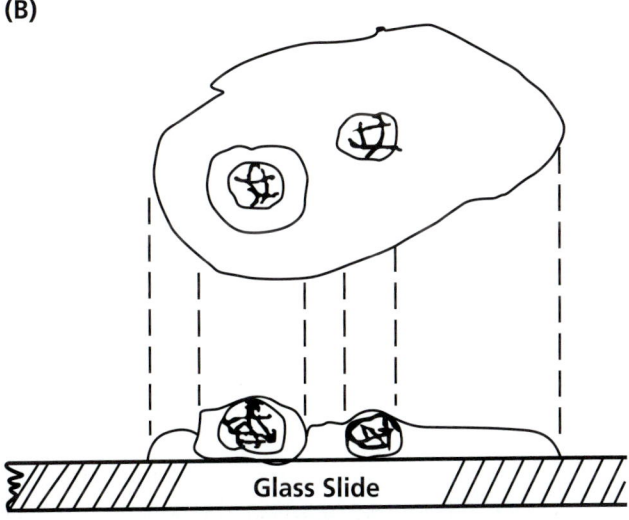

Glass Slide

Figure 2.52 (A, B) Line drawings of cell-in-cell appearance (A). How they can be examined in a slide (B).

COLUMNAR EPITHELIAL CELLS

General features

Columnar epithelium ranges from extremely thick (pseudostratified columnar) to markedly thin simple "squamous" cells. The actual epithelial cell form depends upon its functions (defense, secretion, absorption, transportation) and physiological demands. These cells, whether tall columnar, cuboidal, and stratified or the thinnest single layer (pulmonary alveoli, renal glomeruli), orient perpendicularly to the basement membrane. They mature individually and may demonstrate secretion, a brush border or cilia (Figures 2.57 and 2.58).

When exfoliated and viewed in profile, columnar cells display symmetry along one axis (the long axis). The nucleus rests at the basal end of this axis with scanty cytoplasm, usually in the form of a thin tail, while abundant cytoplasm lies along the opposite (luminal) end of the axis. This nucleo-cytoplasmic orientation is an important feature for identifying columnar

known as "cannibalization." This formation is not exclusive to malignancy, and can be seen in reactive bronchial, mesothelial as well as in squamous cells. A number of epithelial tumors such as breast, small cell carcinoma of the lung, melanoma, and gastric carcinoma can show cannibalization (Figures 2.52–2.56) with degeneration or dyskaryotic changes due to reactive change or repair, which may be mistaken for malignancy.

When one cell is lying in a depression on the surface of the other it may appear as "cannibalization;" this situation is readily discernible by focusing the microscope up and down (Figures 2.54–2.56).

(A)

(B)

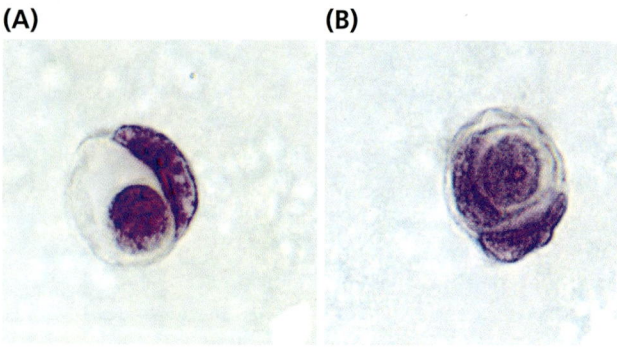

(C)

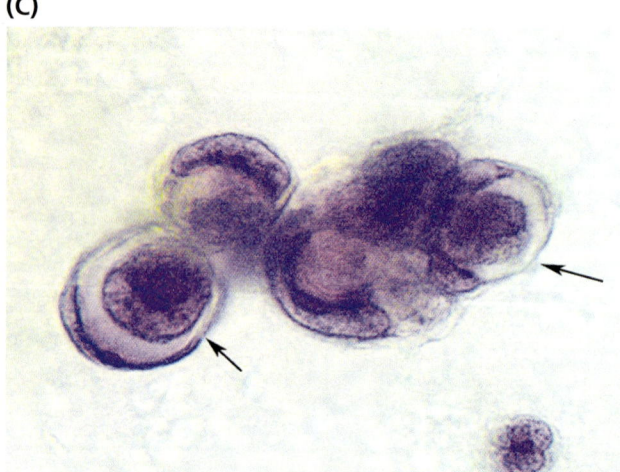

Figure 2.54 (A–C) Cell-in-cell pattern. Two cells (A), three cells (B), and tissue fragment of multiple cells (C). Notice the thin, stretched-out cytoplasm (arrows). Small-cell carcinoma lung. Cytoplasmic vacuolation represents degeneration and not secretions. Cerebrospinal fluid, Millipore filters, Pap stain.

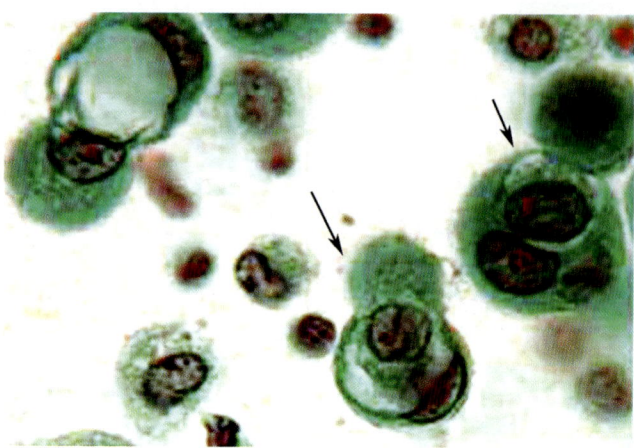

Figure 2.55 Cannibalism (arrows), malignant cells, pleural fluid. Such formations can be resolved by focusing cells up and down under higher magnification of the microscope. Breast adenocarcinoma, pleural fluid. Pap stain.

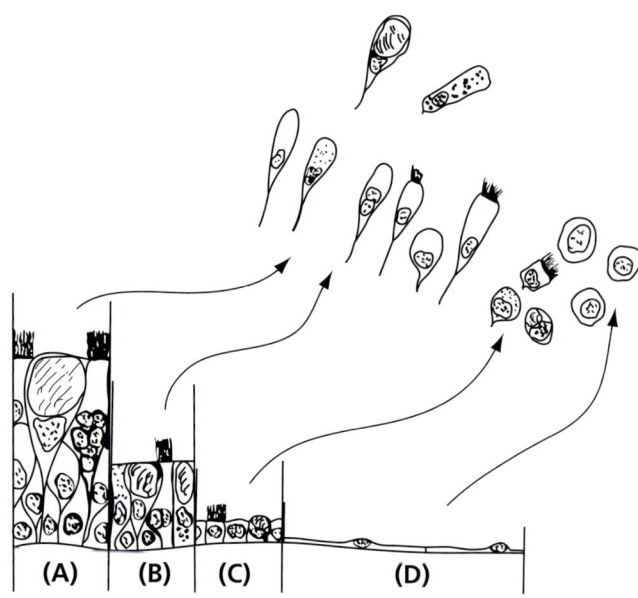

(A) **(B)** **(C)** **(D)**

Figure 2.57 Line drawings depicting the various forms of columnar cells and their exfoliation. Cells have columnar appearance with non-ciliated cells extending to the basement membrane (A). Cells are columnar to low columnar with multinucleation (B). Cells are cuboidal with or without cilia (C); they are flat and squamoid (D).

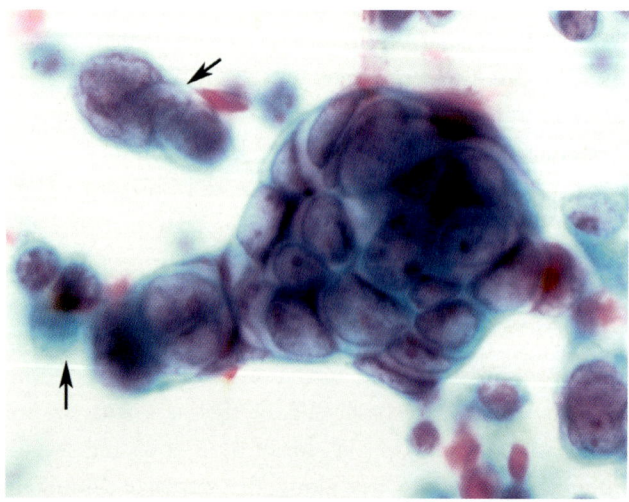

Figure 2.56 Small-cell carcinoma showing cell cannibalism (arrows), pleural fluid. Direct smear, Pap stain.

epithelium (Figures 2.59 and 2.60). When viewed *en face*, these cells appear cuboidal or polygonal arranged in a honeycomb arrangement (Figure 2.60). Simple flat mesothelial cells tend to be round and appear as two-dimensional structures (Figure 2.61). Columnar cells can be variable and appear in pleomorphic forms especially under situations of stimulation, inflammation, and degeneration (Figure 2.62).

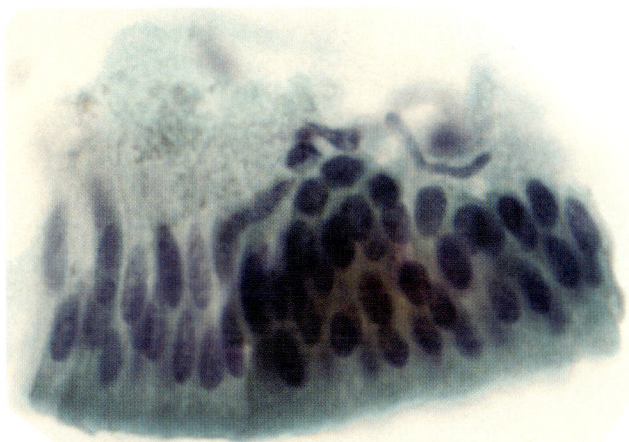

Figure 2.58 Pseudostratified columnar cells. Bronchial brush specimen. LBP, Pap stain.

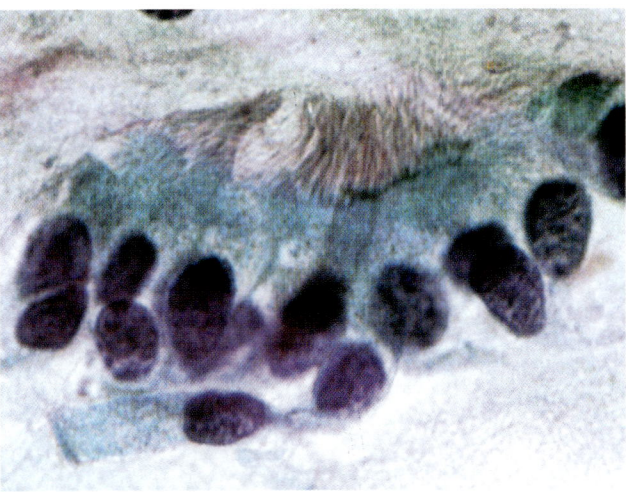

Figure 2.59 Groups of columnar cells with nuclear orientation and terminal cilia. Note the uniformity, right angle attachment and periodicity, features critical for their diagnosis. Bronchial brush, direct smear, Pap stain.

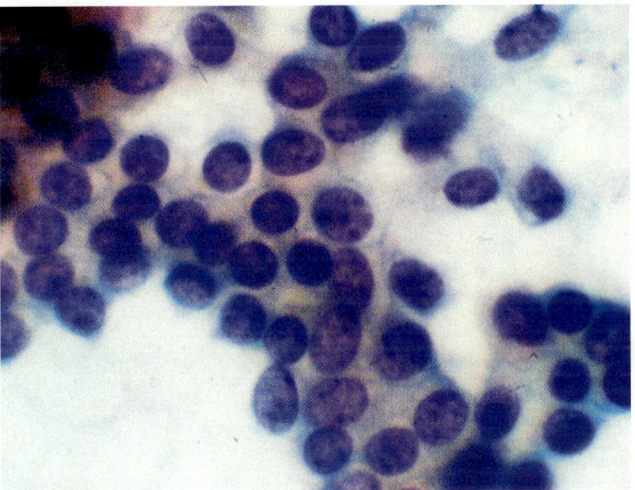

Figure 2.60 Columnar cells with cuboidal forms. Bile duct brush specimen. Cells are seen en face and appear polygonal with well-defined margins. Direct smear, Pap stain.

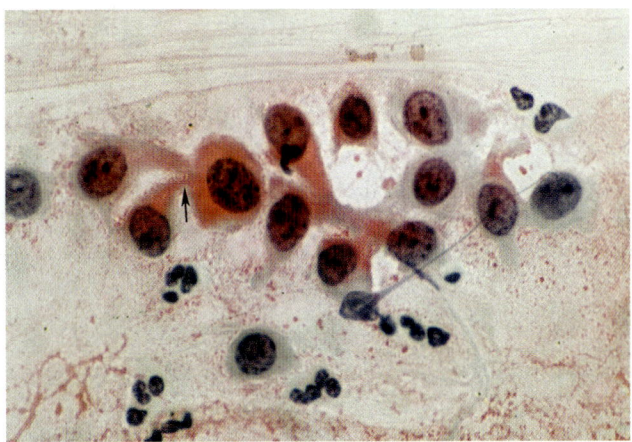

Figure 2.61 Mesothelial cells displaying varying cytomorphology – columnar/elongated (arrow), cuboidal shaped and with orangophilic cytoplasm (mimicking squamous change). Lung apical mass, FNA, direct smear, Pap stain.

Unicellular maturation (differentiation)

"Non-secretory"

The so-called "non-secretory" columnar cell can have either abundant or scanty cytoplasm, which appears clear, amorphous, foamy, or with minute red granules. It does not, however, contain obviously secretory vacuoles (Figures 2.63–2.66).

Secretory

The secretory columnar cell contains cytoplasm that varies from being foamy to vacuolated. The vacuoles can be multiple or coalesce to form large, single vacuoles. The

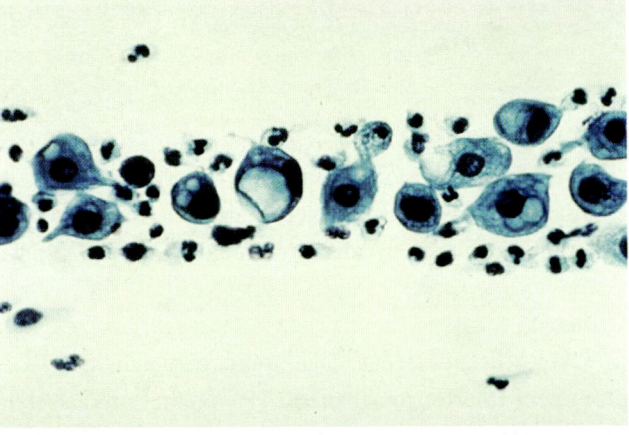

Figure 2.62 Columnar cells: notice the columnar shapes, cilia, and degenerative changes. While ciliocytophthoria is typically seen in specimens from viral infections of the respiratory tract, metaplastic changes of varying degree occur in chronic irritations, such as smoking and respiratory tract infections. Bronchial wash specimen, conventional smear, Pap stain.

27

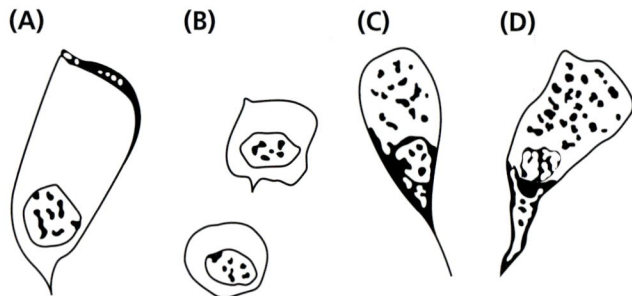

Figure 2.63 Line drawings depicting the non-secretory cells. Typical non-secretory columnar cell (A); cuboidal form (B); intracytoplasmic granules (C); and cell with terminal nucleus (D).

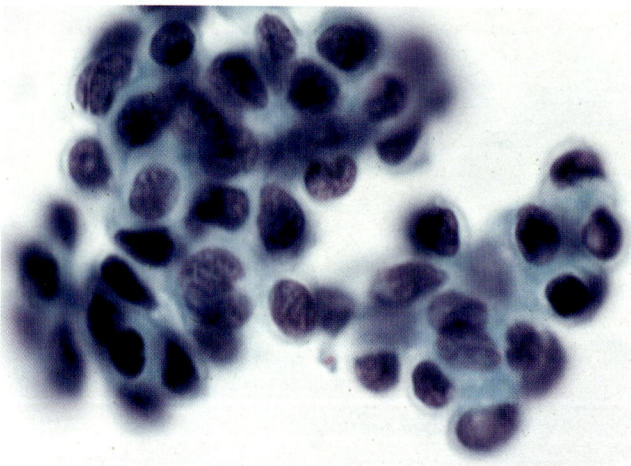

Figure 2.64 Cuboidal "non-secretory" columnar cells. Breast fine needle aspiration, direct smear, Pap stain.

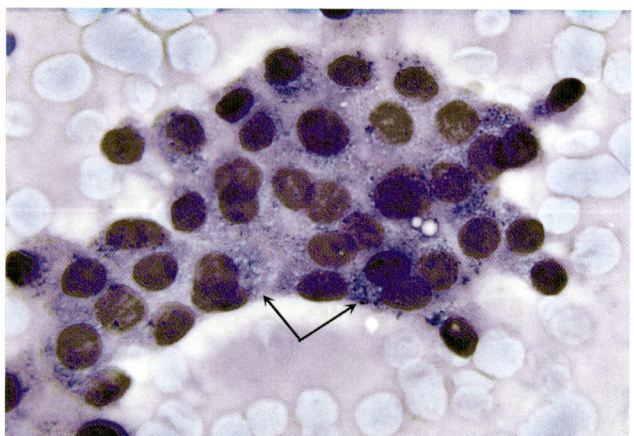

Figure 2.65 Intracytoplasmic granules of lysosome origin, thyroid follicular cells. Fine needle aspiration, direct smear, Diff-Quik stain.

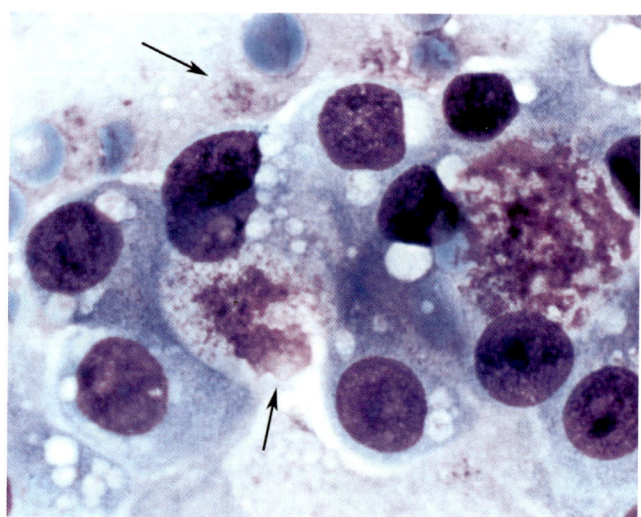

Figure 2.66 "Non-secretory" columnar form cells with intracytoplasmic zymogen granules. Salivary gland (arrows). Fine needle aspiration, direct smear, Diff-Quik stain.

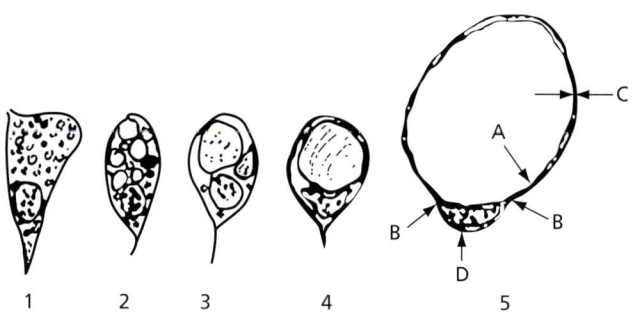

Figure 2.67 In the hyperdistended cell (5), there is "pouching out" of the vacuole A, loss of cytoplasm at the "nucleovacuolar angle" B, extreme cytoplasmic thinning C, and a demilune compression of the nucleus D.

abnormal hormonal states (endometrial hyperplasia), and neoplasia (adenocarcinoma).

"Signet" cell formation in body cavity specimens is common, and generally indicates degeneration and not secretion, neoplasm, or adenocarcinoma (Figure 2.72).

Ciliated

In these cells numerous cilia occur, perpendicular to a prominent line (terminal plate, TP), at the luminal end. The cilia generally acquire a red or lavender coloration when treated with Papanicolaou procedures. Seen commonly in bronchial, nasopharyngeal, and endocervical tissue fragments, cilia are frequently the first structure to be lost with degeneration (Figures 2.73–2.75). It is

large single vacuole is characteristic of cytoplasmic secretion, except in watery fluids (such as pleural, abdominal and pericardial) where the cells may imbibe fluid, mimicking cytoplasmic secretion (Figures 2.67–2.72). Such hyperdistended secretory vacuoles are noted in chronic inflammatory conditions (cervicitis, gastritis, asthma),

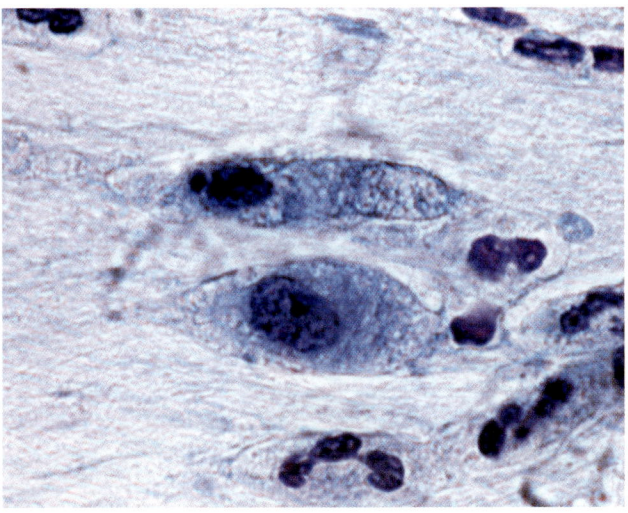

Figure 2.68 Finely vacuolated foamy intracytoplasmic secretions. Bronchial columnar cells, direct smear, Pap stain.

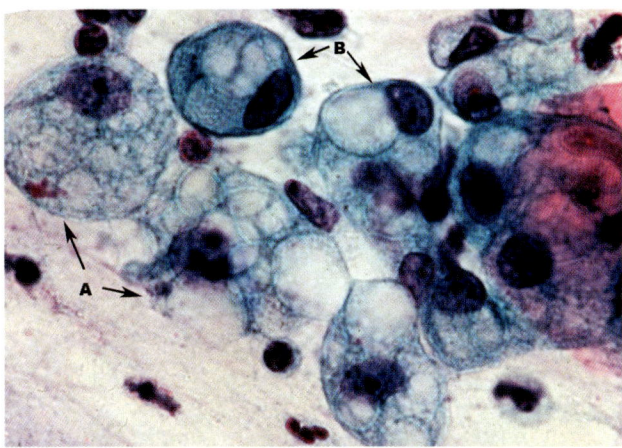

Figure 2.69 Secretory type cells. Multiple vacuoles (A), coalesced cytoplasmic vacuoles (B). Gastric brush specimen, direct smear, Pap stain.

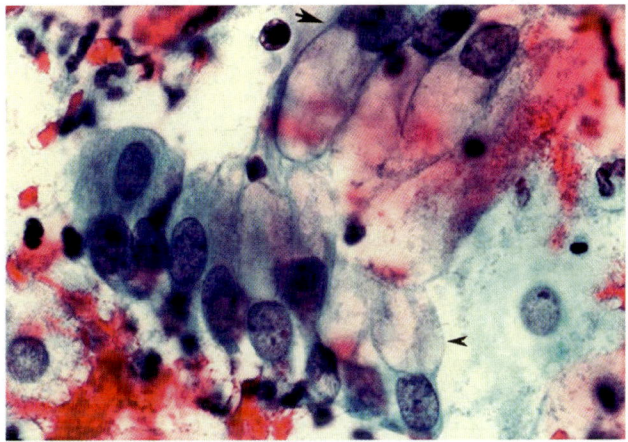

Figure 2.70 Large single intracytoplasmic vacuole. Loss of nucleocytoplasmic angle (large arrowhead), thin cytoplasm (small arrowhead). Pulmonary specimen, direct smear, Pap stain.

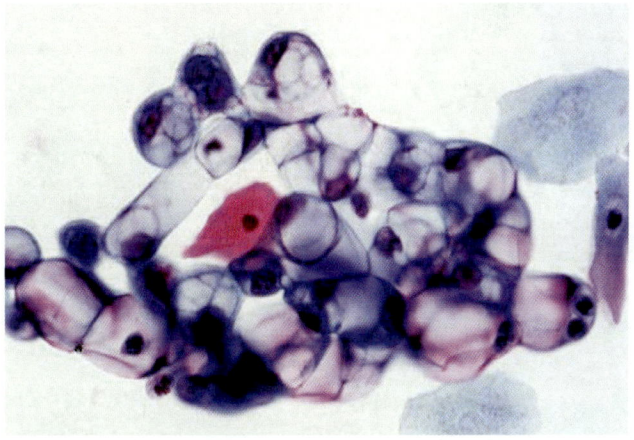

Figure 2.71 Intracytoplasmic hyperdistended vacuoles, endocervical cells, oral contraceptive user. Vaginocervical smear, Pap stain.

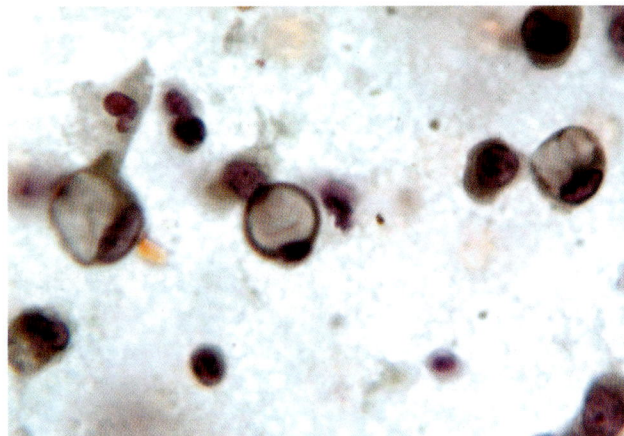

Figure 2.72 Signet cells pleural fluid; metastatic gastric adenocarcinoma. Millipore filter, Pap stain.

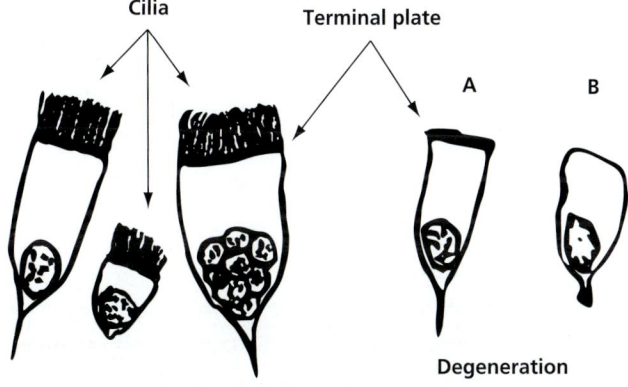

Figure 2.73 Line drawings depicting the cilia, terminal plates, and ciliated cell degeneration. In the early stage, the terminal plate is visible and generally prominent (A); in late degeneration both the cilia and the terminal plates are lost (B).

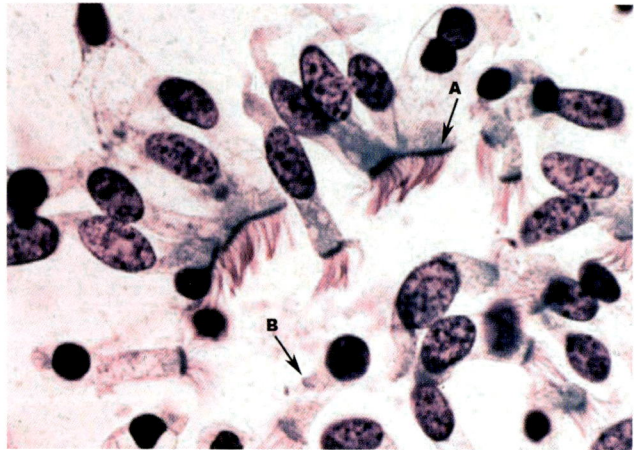

Figure 2.74 Ciliated columnar cells with prominent terminal plate (A) and early degeneration (B). Bronchial wash, direct smear, Pap stain.

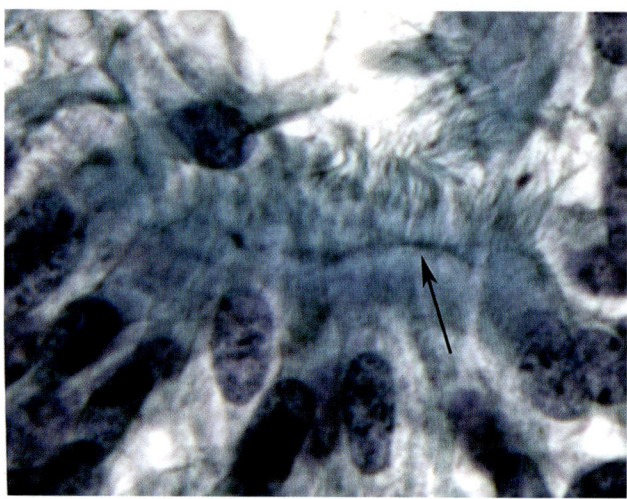

Figure 2.75 Retained terminal plate (arrow) with early ciliary degeneration. Bronchial brush, direct smear, Pap stain.

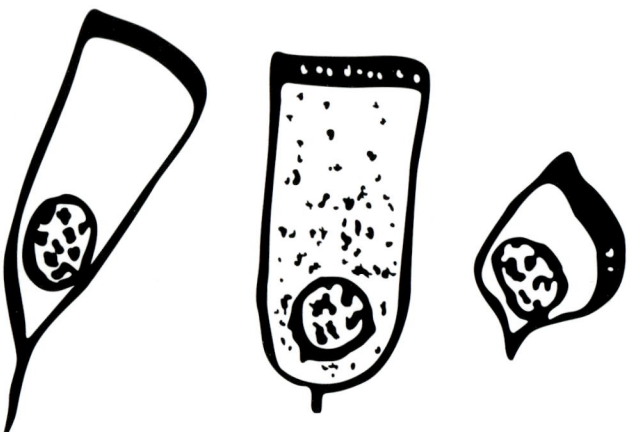

Figure 2.76 Drawings depicting the brush border columnar cells.

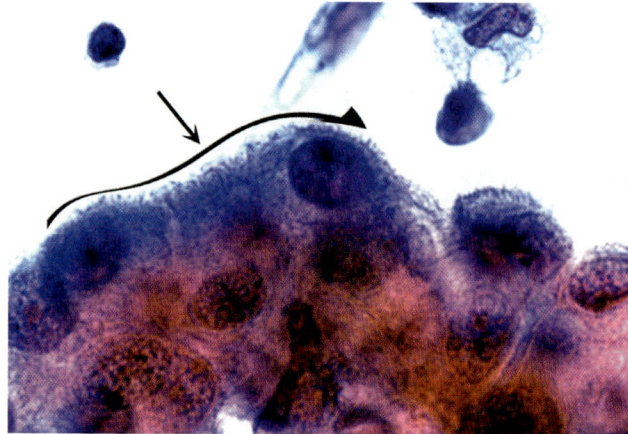

Figure 2.77 Brush border columnar cells (arrow). Notice the variable length, loss of periodicity, and terminal plate. Gastric brush, direct smear, Pap stain.

important to correctly identify true cilia; they are multiple, uniformly thin, parallel to each other, of a uniform length, with uniform periodicity, and with their ciliary rootlets extending into the cytoplasm at the TP. At times, cytoplasmic vacuoles and intercellular bridges can be mistaken for cilia (Figure 2.47). The identification of cilia is diagnostic of benignancy along with uniform chromatin and nucleolar pattern.

Brush border cell

Certain exfoliated columnar cells, mainly intestinal, may have a thick luminal margin which stains deeply. At times this appears to have perpendicular lines throughout, and the cells are arranged so closely that they give rise to a brush-edge appearance. They are not as long as cilia and do not wave freely (Figures 2.76 and 2.77).

Multicellular tissue formations

Sheets

When occurring as a sheet and viewed on end (*en face*), columnar cells have symmetry similar to squamous cells, with the nucleus lying symmetrically in the center of the cytoplasm. However, the cytoplasmic borders are sharp and uniformly hexagonal, displaying a characteristic honeycomb appearance (Figures 2.78 and 2.79). Around the edge of such a sheet, one should look for cells lying upon their sides (edge on), where their columnar shape can be easily recognized (Figure 2.79). Frequently, histiocytes appear in sheet formations. This may be observed in thyroid fine needle aspirations and in specimens prepared by liquid-based techniques (Figure 2.80). Immunocytochemical studies are often helpful in such cases.

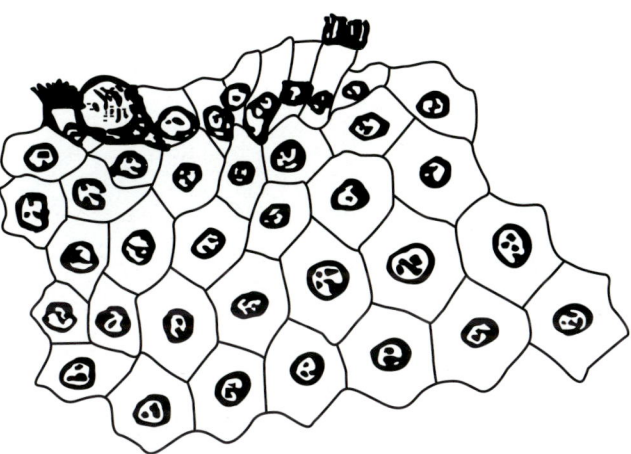

Figure 2.78 Line drawing depicting features of a columnar cell sheet of endocervical origin.

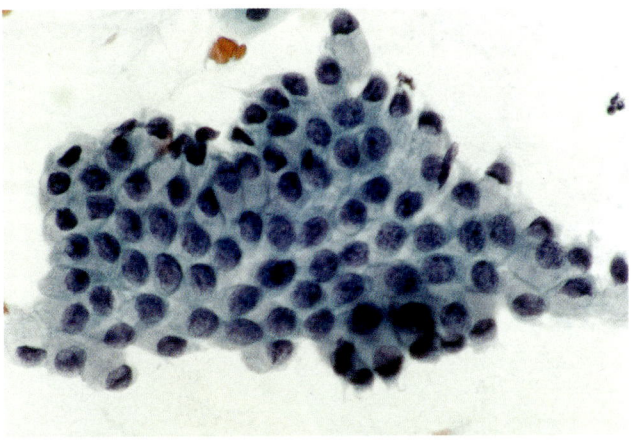

Figure 2.79 Sheet of endocervical cells. There is a honeycomb pattern in the center and columnar cells at the free edge. Vaginocervical smear, Pap stain.

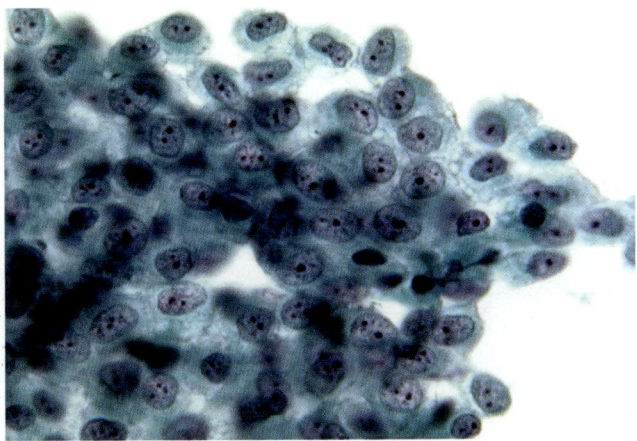

Figure 2.80 Group of macrophage cells in a sheet formation. An examination of the free edge helps determine the nature of the cells. Thyroid fine needle aspiration, direct smear, Pap stain.

Acini (polypoid or papillary fragments)

These represent three-dimensional exfoliation of epithelial cells derived from the same clone. These cells may grow together and appear as a "tennis ball" or "morula" formation. They usually have three distinct planes of interwoven epithelial cells. Although these may appear multilayered and imperfectly formed, it must be appreciated that the three-dimensional structure is not a cluster, clump, aggregate, group, or bunch; similar terms should be avoided to classify acini or polypoid and papillary fragments.

When the acinus of a gland is shed, the columnar cells are in a three-dimensional (i.e. "tennis ball" or morula) arrangement. One can appreciate and recognize this frequently important diagnostic feature by moving a microscope high-power plane of focus up and down to scan through the structure (Figures 2.81 and 2.82).

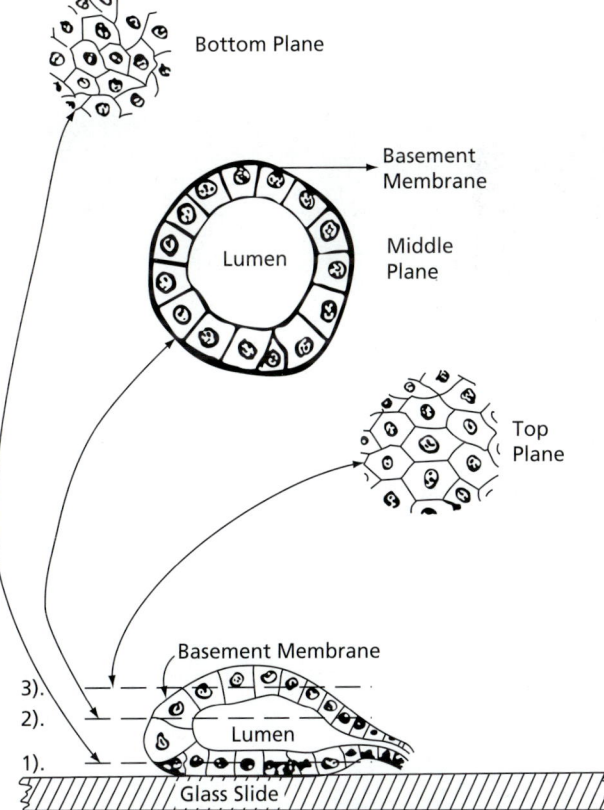

Figure 2.81 Schematic representation of an acinus as seen in cytology specimens. It should be appreciated that these represent planes of cells occurring in an acinus. Each plane may have a variable number of cell thickness and they are often not vertically oriented and situated on top of each other. Also, they represent clonal proliferation and are diagnostically critical for accurate interpretation of cells in body cavity fluids and some fine needle aspiration specimens.

(A)

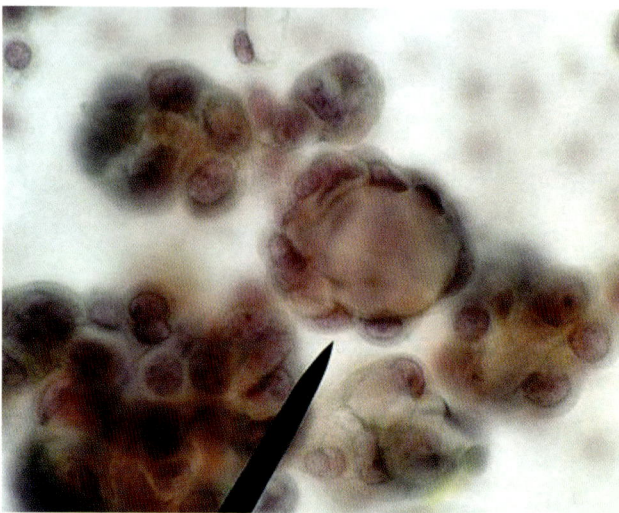

(B)

(C)

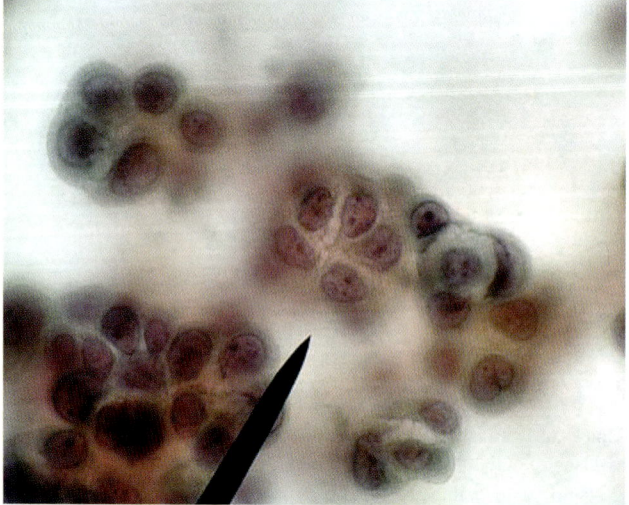

Figure 2.82 Acinic formations of malignant cells in an effusion representing breast adenocarcinoma. Notice the three planes, (A) the deepest, (B) the middle with luminal border, and the top layer (C) giving a honeycomb appearance. Pleural effusion, Millipore filter, Pap stain.

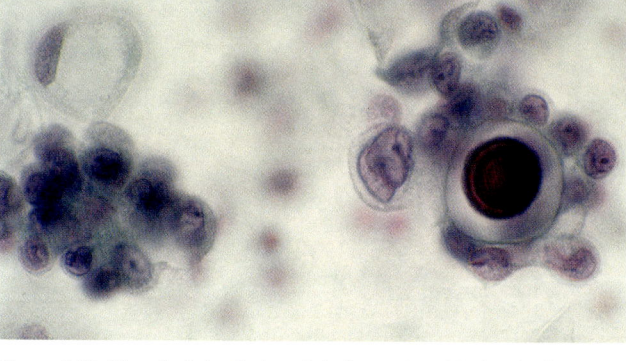

Figure 2.83 Mesothelial cells in acinic formation. Notice the loop-to-loop arrangement of outer cells and intraluminal psammoma body. The second group shows acinic lumen. Pelvic wash, Millipore filter, Pap stain. Such changes can be observed in rectovaginal pouch aspiration specimens obtained from healthy women.

(1) Beginning on the glass slide, the lower wall of the acinus is viewed as an *en face* sheet of cells.

(2) Moving up, the equatorial rim of the sides is viewed as a ring, with the nuclei on the outer end of the cell near the basement membrane; the bulk of the cytoplasm, with or without secretion, lies on the inside end of the cells near the lumen.

(3) Upon reaching the top of the acinus, the upper wall appears, again as an *en face* sheet of cells, as with (1), but it is a different sheet from (1).

These three key planes are identifiable and, while focusing up and down, blend into the total shell-like, three-dimensional structure.

For diagnostic true tissue fragment (DTTF) in an acinic formation, notice the three distinct, identifiable plans of the fragment. Rarely, true tissue fragments can occur in non-neoplastic conditions (radiation, autoimmune diseases, viral infection, infarct, local therapy) (Figures 2.83 and 2.84). Acinic and polypoidal structures can be observed in rectovaginal pouch aspirations among healthy women. However, malignant nuclear features must be recognized before rendering such a diagnosis. These tissue fragments most often have a smooth outer border. At times a loop-to-loop or scalloped outer margin can be seen. This pattern is, however, more common in papillary formations and is a common occurrence in pleural fluid specimens from cases of mesothelioma.

Often there may be more than one layer of cells in each plane; the configuration is similar to a slinky, and focusing the microscope up and down is generally helpful (Figure 2.85). The edges of mesothelial, urothelial and other cells in

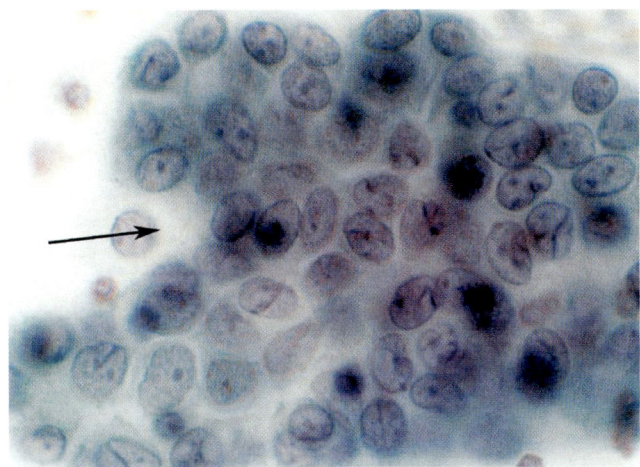

Figure 2.84 Mesothelial cells, abdominal washings. Notice the luminal structure (arrow), direct smear, Pap stain.

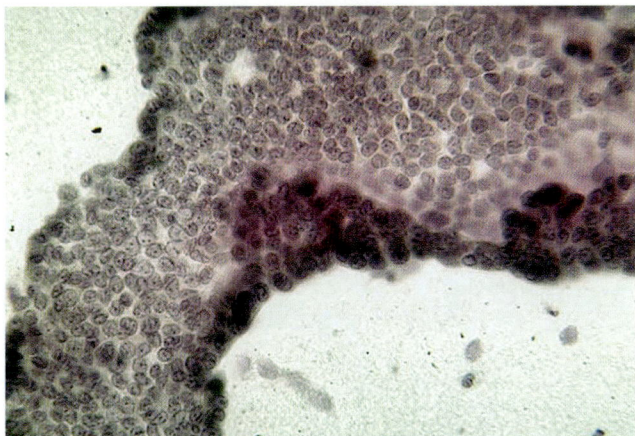

Figure 2.86 Urothelial cells in a ureteric brush specimen. Notice the rolling of the epithelial cells along the two free edges producing a luminal border and polypoidal formation. Millipore filter, Pap stain.

a liquid environment can sometimes roll at the edges and produce pseudo-papillary groups (Figure 2.86). Such structures are a common cause of false cancer diagnosis. Upon careful examination, rolled edge and a lack of cellular maturation is often a helpful diagnostic feature.

Cells suspended in body fluids by either collection or processing methods may appear to form "tissue fragments." These generally do not have a continuous outer margin (community border); the cells also lack molding and have interspersed clear spaces or "windows." Such pseudo-papillary formations are of limited diagnostic value (Figure 2.87).

Polyps

When a polyp, papillary frond, or inter-glandular villus is shed, one should be able to obtain the same three planes of

(A)

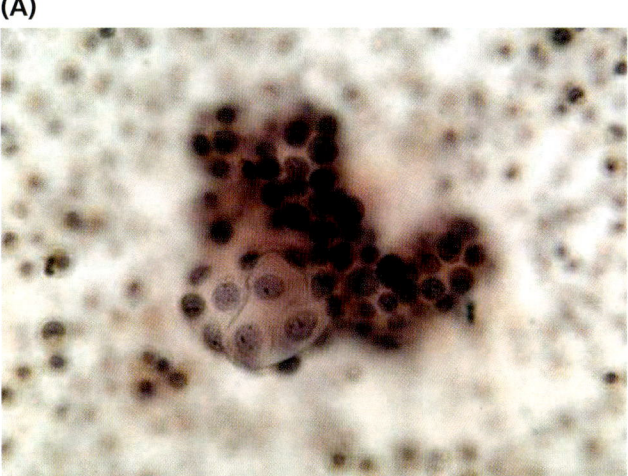

(B)

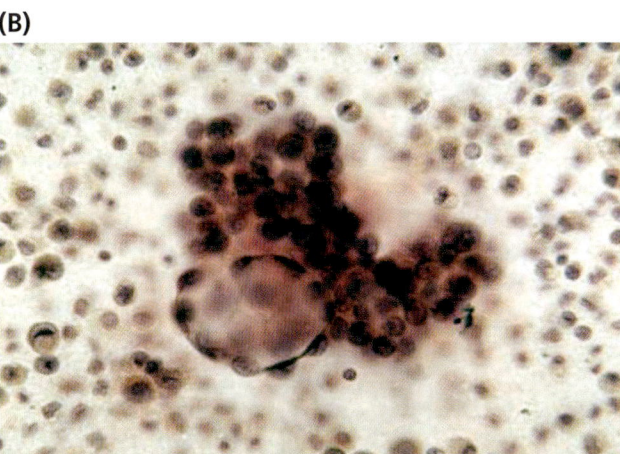

(C)

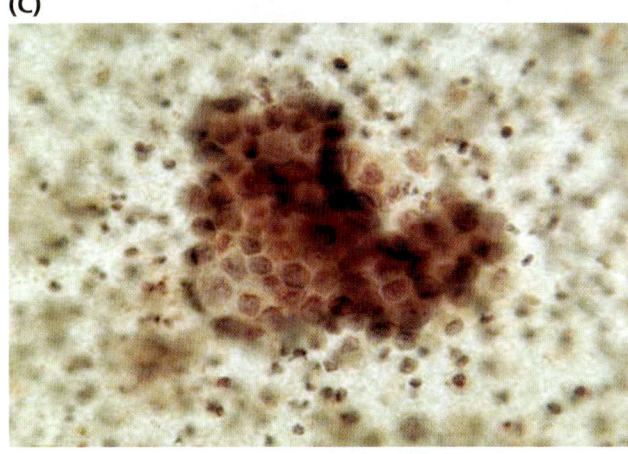

Figure 2.85 Acinic structure with uneven distribution of cells in various planes "The Slinky Effect" (A, B, C). Most of the cells have accumulated along the upper right side and in the bottom (A) and luminal planes (B). Abdominal fluid, Millipore filter, Pap stain.

focus as seen in acinic formations, but with the important difference that the position of the nucleus and the bulk of the cytoplasm change places in the mid-plane (2) so that the basement membrane and nucleus are near the inner

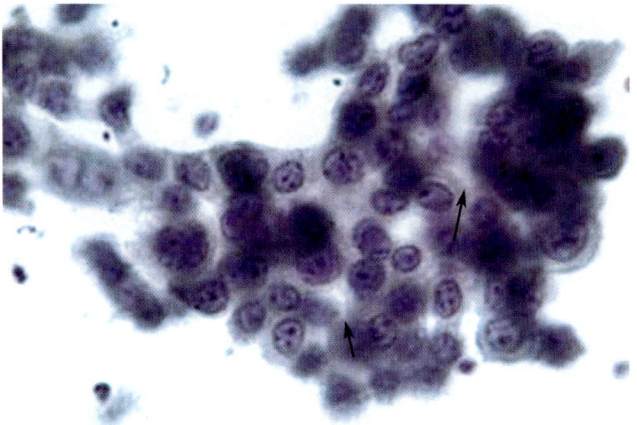

Figure 2.87 Pseudo acinic formation. This has a glandular appearance but with "windows" (arrows), suggesting a lack of clonal proliferation and an artificial amassing of mesothelial cells. Pleural fluid, Millipore filter, Pap stain.

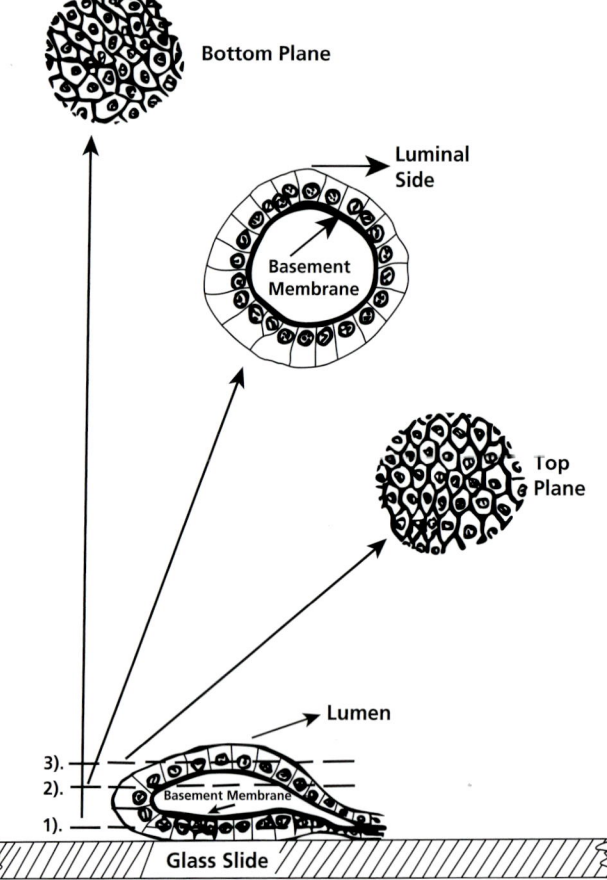

Figure 2.88 Schematic planes of a polyp as seen in a cytologic preparation. A polyp contains a central connective tissue core instead of the lumen as seen here. They are seen in papillary lesions. Care should be exercised in determining malignant features before rendering a diagnosis. The three-dimensional nature of a polyp is often better recognized in cell block slides.

(A)

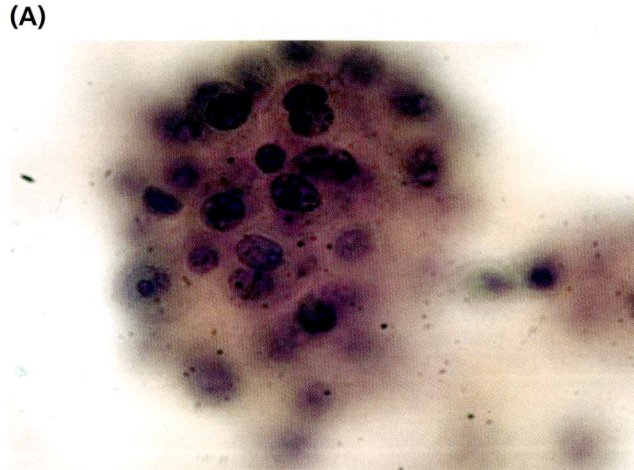

(B)

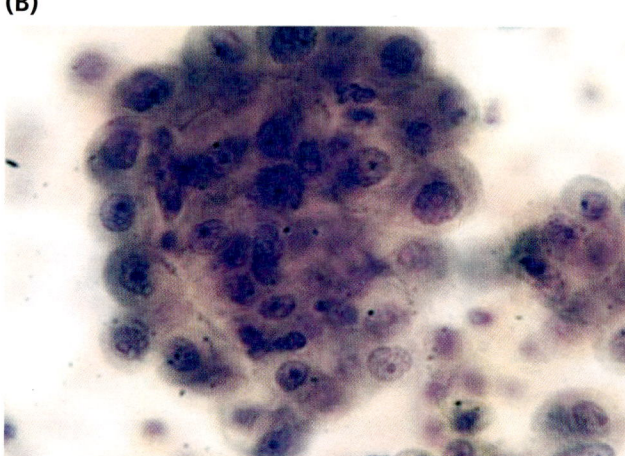

(C)

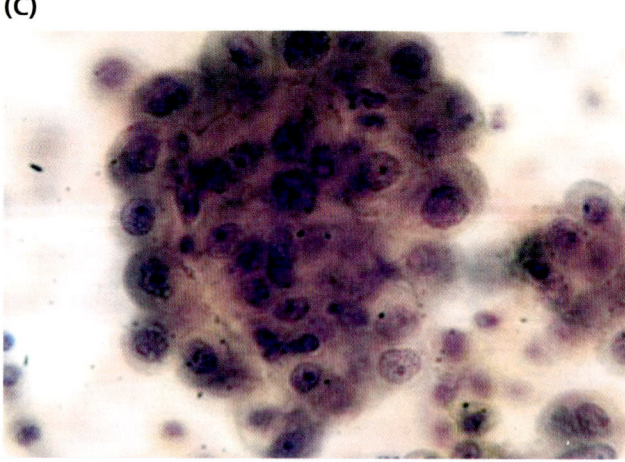

Figure 2.89 Three-dimensional features of a polyp. (A) is the deepest or bottom plane, notice the epithelial layer, (B) the middle plane with fibroconnective tissue core in the center, and (C) the top plane with a layer of epithelial cells. Pleural fluid, Millipore filter, Pap stain.

end of the cell, while the bulk of the cytoplasm faces the outer wall of the lumen (Figures 2.88 and 2.89).

A papillary fragment contains central connective tissue/ fibrovascular core instead of the lumen as seen here. They

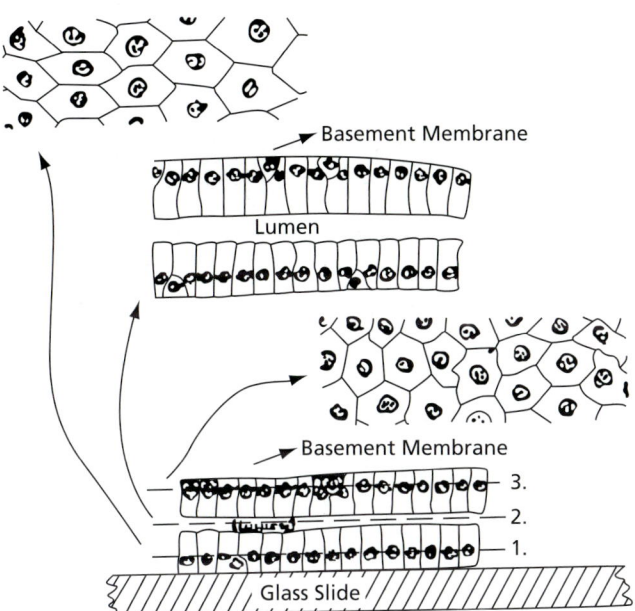

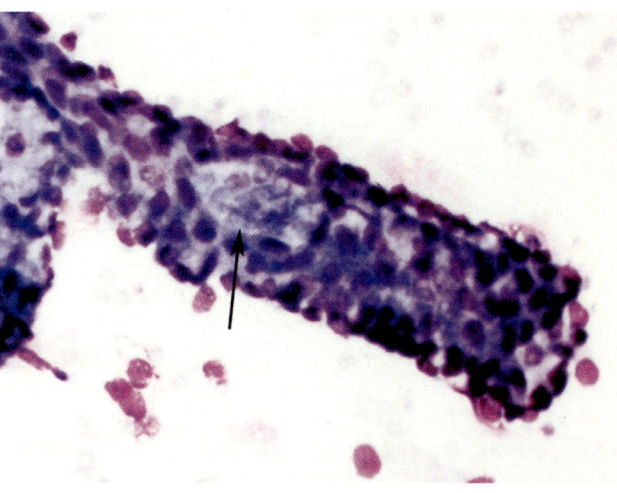

Figure 2.91 Fragment of pancreatic duct. Notice the lumen (arrow). The full thickness duct is visible to the right of the arrow. Pancreas fine needle aspiration. Direct smear, Diff-Quik stain.

Figure 2.90 Line drawings depicting the cytomorphologic features of a duct. Notice the three distinct planes of focus similar to seen in acinic and papillary formations.

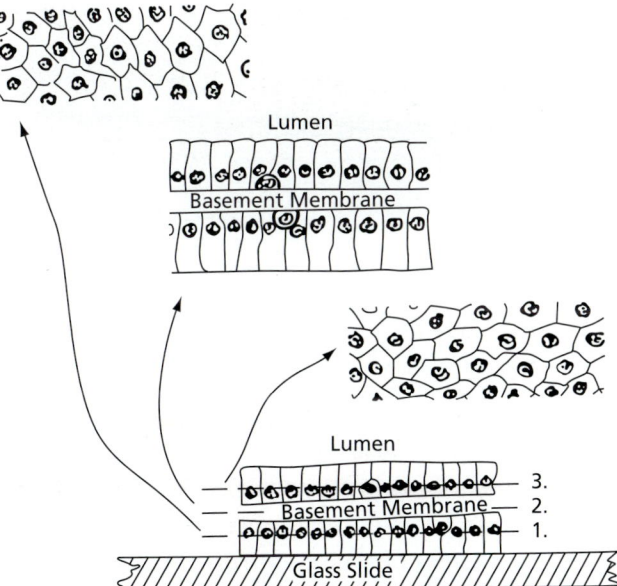

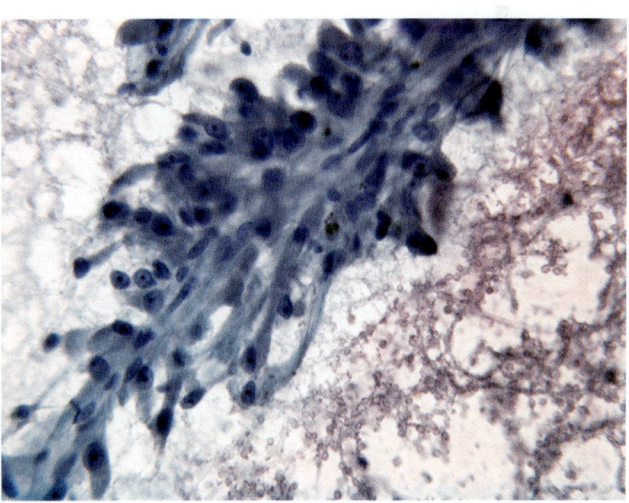

Figure 2.93 Papillary stalk, tissue fragment, renal cell carcinoma. Notice the fibroconnective tissue core in the center and the tumor cells on the outer sides. Fine needle aspiration renal mass, Pap stain.

Figure 2.92 Line diagram depicting the features of a stalk. It is similar to a duct, but the luminal surface is toward the outside and the central core contains the basement region and fibrovascular core.

Ducts and stalks

When a duct is shed, the appearance is that of an elongated, open-ended acinus with the nuclei in the mid-plane (2) near the outer end of the cells (Figures 2.90 and 2.91).

are seen in papillary lesions. Depending on the site and nature of the specimen, care should be exercised in determining malignant nuclear features before rendering a diagnosis of papillary carcinoma. Interventional studies and intra-cavitary treatment may cause papillary proliferation of the mesothelial cells. Occasional papillary fragments of choroid cells may occur after subdural implantation of a catheter or Ommaya reservoir.

When a stalk is shed, it has the appearance of an elongated polyp with the nuclei in the mid-plane (2) near the inner end of the cells. The lumen in such a formation is towards the outside (Figures 2.92 and 2.93).

Proper recognition of the DTTF is critical. Similar structures occur commonly, resulting from poor preservation, fixation, and preparation. Pseudo-papillary formations of urothelial cells are observed commonly in bladder wash and post-bladder wash urine specimens.

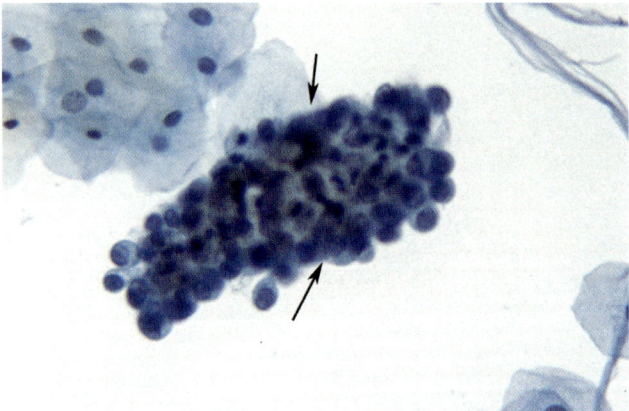

Figure 2.94 Pseudo papillary formation of urothelial cells. Notice the infolding of cells at the edges (arrows). Bladder wash, LBP, Pap stain.

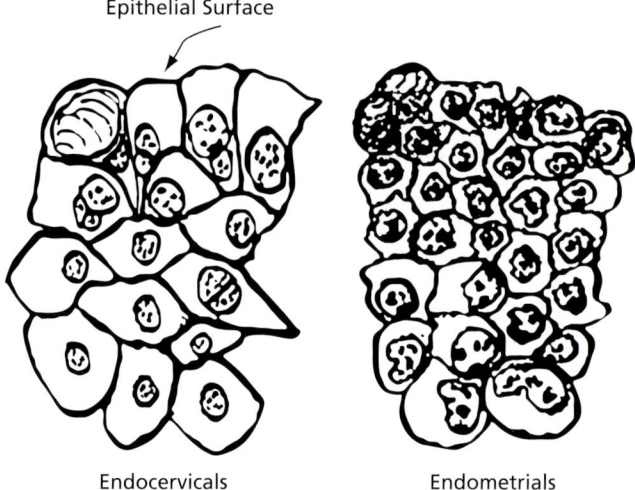

Epithelial Surface

Endocervicals   Endometrials

Figure 2.95 Line drawings depicting salient features of endocervical and endometrial cells.

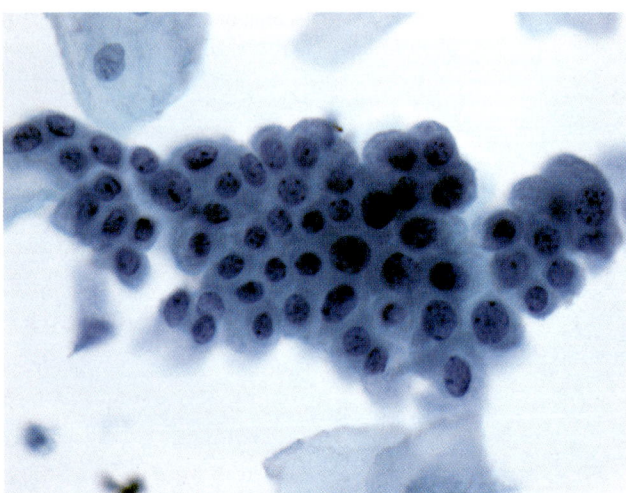

Figure 2.96 Sheet of endocervical cells. There is a honeycomb pattern in the center and columnar cells at the free edge. LBP, Pap stain.

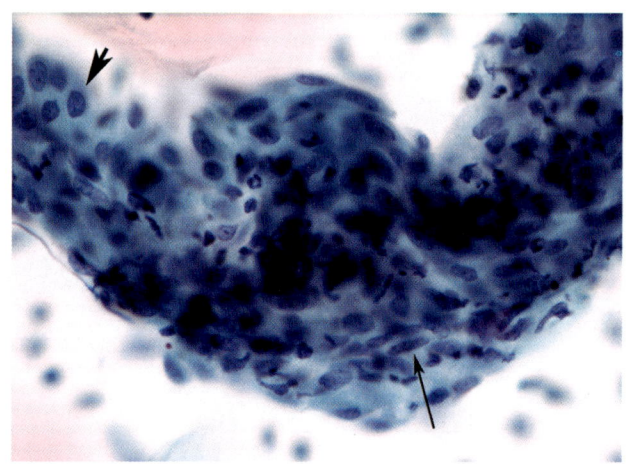

Figure 2.97 Endocervical cells (small arrow) and stromal cells (long arrow). Vaginocervical smear. LBP, Pap stain.

A smooth fold along the edge and epithelial cell maturation are helpful features (Figure 2.94).

Table 2.1 depicts some identifying criteria. These features may be altered considerably by fixation and processing of the specimens by monolayer techniques (ThinPrep® slides, SurePath®) and cytospins.

Body site-specific cell types

Endocervix

One of the most challenging tasks in gynecologic preparations is to differentiate between endocervical and endometrial cells. Diagnostic significance of glandular cells in post-menopausal gynecologic specimens and the occurrence of endometrial cells among women over 40 and out of menstrual cycle have been emphasized. However, the correct identification of these cells can be difficult. Also, hormonal and reactive changes generally produce atypical and non-reproducible alterations. At times, reserve, parabasal, metaplastic, fragments of lower uterine segment, high-grade squamous dysplasia, hematopoietic, and histiocytic cells can all mimic endometrial/endocervical cells. Uncommon causes of similar-appearing cells in the gynecologic preparation include atrophic changes, fallopian tube cells, goblet cells, vaginal adenosis, mesonephric remnants, Bartholin glands, and rectovaginal fistula. The correct identification of endocervical and endometrial cells can also be difficult due to cyclic regenerative and degenerative changes and cellular changes due to contraceptives and intrauterine devices (IUD).

The salient cytomorphologic characteristics depicted in Table 2.2 can be helpful in distinguishing endometrial from endocervical cells. Often, it is not possible to correctly identify the endometrial cells with certainty, and it is preferable to report them as "endometrial-type" cells (Figures 2.95–2.98).

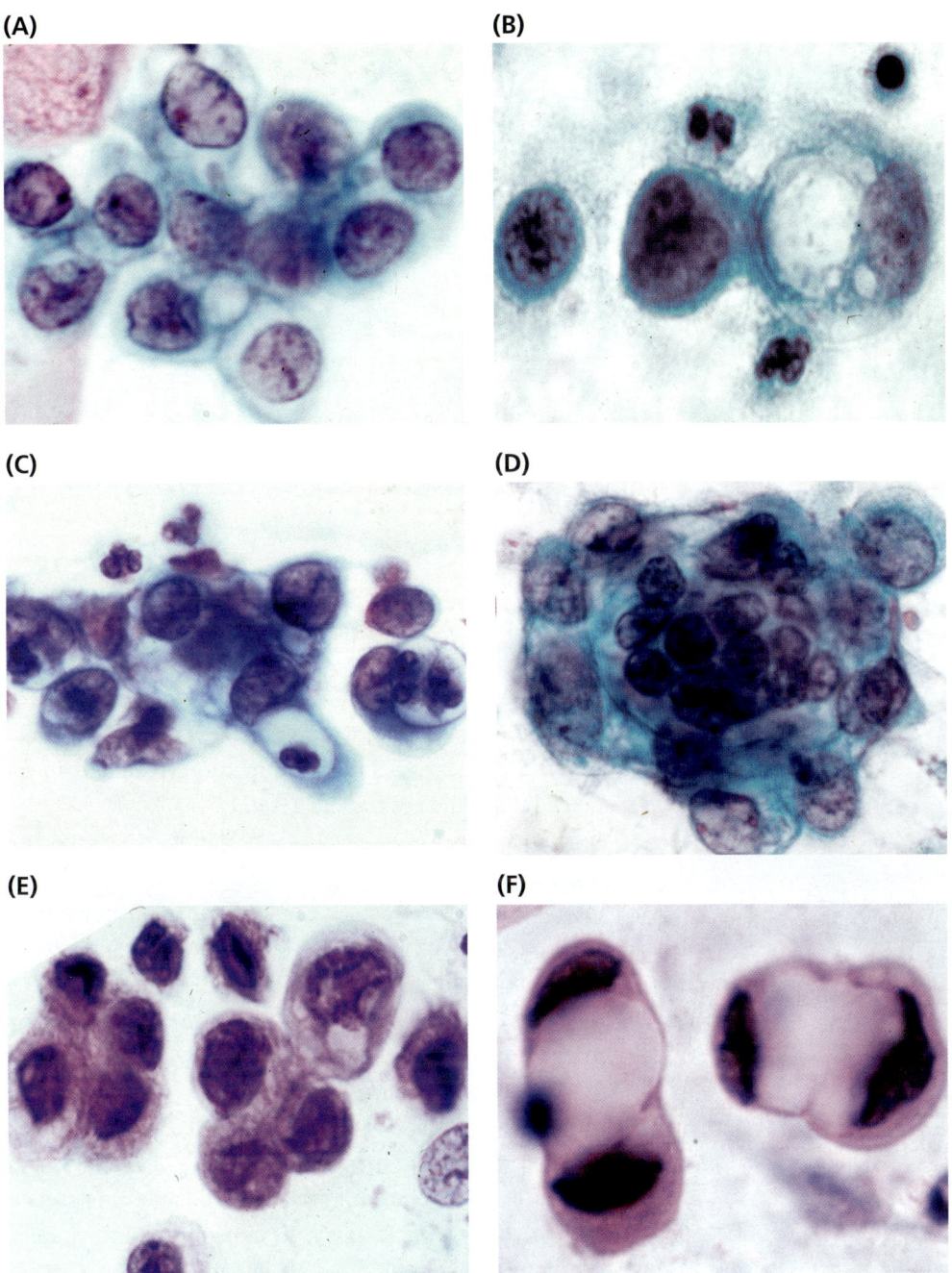

Figure 2.98 (A–F) Endocervical cells, glandular proliferation (A). Squamous metaplasia (B). Resembling endometrial cells (C). Multinucleation (D). Poor preservation (E). Signet cell change (F). IUD users (A) and (C). SurePath, remaining conventional vaginocervical smears. Pap stain.

Endometrium

Normal endometrial cells exfoliate naturally and only appear in the cervicovaginal specimens during the shedding phase of menstruation. In endometrial aspirates they are better preserved, and normal cells can appear differently than outlined above according to their phase of proliferation and secretion (Figures 2.99–2.101).

Endometrial cells can appear extremely atypical and bizarre. They can often be confused with neoplastic changes (Figure 2.102). Such alterations represent reactive and degenerative among epithelial and stromal cells and often follow surgical intervention, and post-partum (Figure 2.103).

Respiratory

Varying from tall columnar (with or without intracytoplasmic mucus and goblet cell changes), to low cuboidal, respiratory cells can appear darkly stained and crowded,

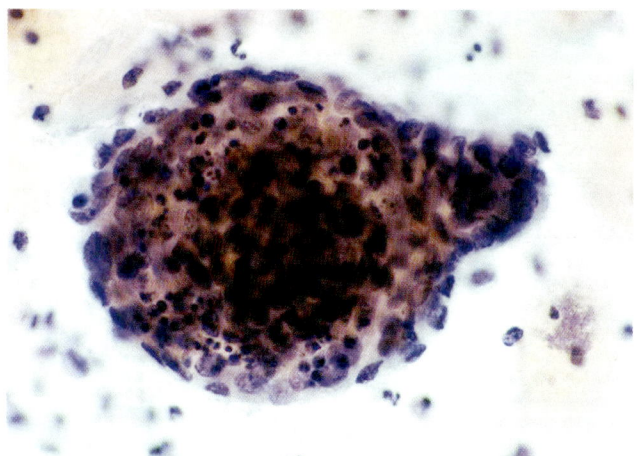

Figure 2.99 Endometrial cells during menses; morula formation with numerous inflammatory and histiocytic cells. Vaginocervical smear, Pap stain.

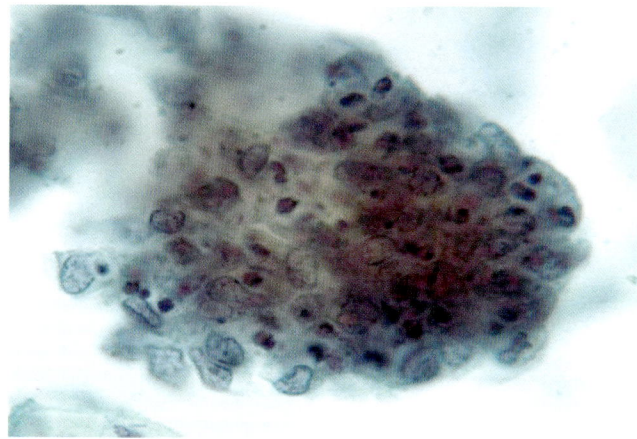

Figure 2.100 Endometrial cells during menses, high power. Notice the degeneration and intermixed inflammatory cells. LBP, Pap stain.

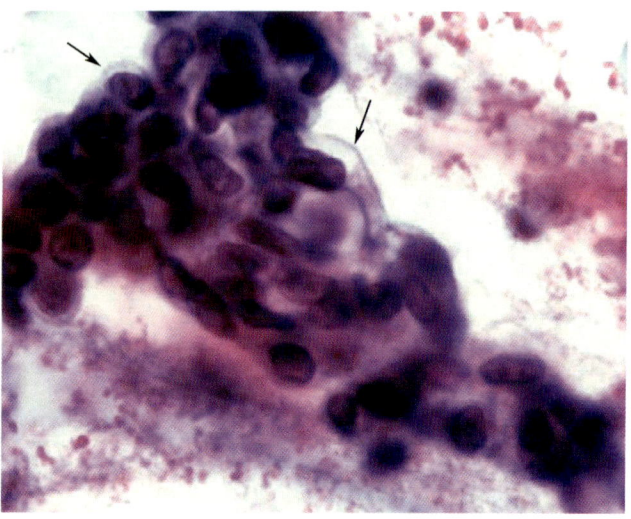

Figure 2.101 Endometrial cells, second half of the menstrual cycle. Notice cellular preservation, distinct cytoplasm with secretory changes (arrows). Vaginocervical smear, Pap stain.

leading to difficulties in their correct identification. Clumps of columnar cells can ball-up into "pseudo-pearls" or "Creola bodies," originally described as Epithelialzellballen by Vierodt (1883). The term Creola body was introduced by Naylor (1962) in recognition of the first patient reported from the United States with these changes. In some instances, the cells within the Creola body may show pronounced nuclear size change intercellular molding, which can be alarming and mistaken for malignancy (Figures 2.104 and 2.105).

The presence of Creola bodies can be of diagnostic significance in the estimation of airway hyper-responsiveness among patients with asthma. Occasionally, elongated Charcot-laden crystals (Figure 2.106) may be

associated with Creloa bodies supporting an eosinophilic response in an allergic reaction. These crystals are water-soluble and generally not seen in routine specimens.

In some cases, inspissated mucus in the bronchial tree may occur as Curshman's spiral, the strand being surrounded by heavy acute inflammatory excaudate intermixed with some eosinophils (Figure 2.107).

Creola bodies may sometimes be dominated by mucus-producing goblet cells (Figures 2.108 and 2.109). Cilia, if not identified in such cases, can lead to diagnostic error. It is critical to identify cilia in bronchial cells; their presence almost always denotes benignity. At times cilia may be present on the cell surface and can only be visualized by up and down focusing of the cells (Figure 2.110).

Intranuclear and intracytoplasmic inclusion bodies, found in early phases of some viral infections, are basophilic or acidophilic masses and may be observed in the infected bronchial cells. Chromatin in these cells is usually smudged; much of it concentrates around the nuclear membrane leaving a cleared "halo" around the inclusion body. Cytoplasmic destruction and degeneration leading to detachment of ciliary tufts (ciliocytophthoria (CCP)) as described by George Papanicolaou may also be observed (Figures 2.111–2.113).

Gastric

The presence of gastric epithelial cells is a common occurrence in endoscopic ultrasound (EUS)-guided procedures of the upper alimentary tract and gastric brush specimens. They can pose considerable diagnostic problems. Single gastric epithelial cells can exfoliate but are uncommon in cytologic specimens. A few mucus-producing columnar

(A)

(B)

(C)

(D)

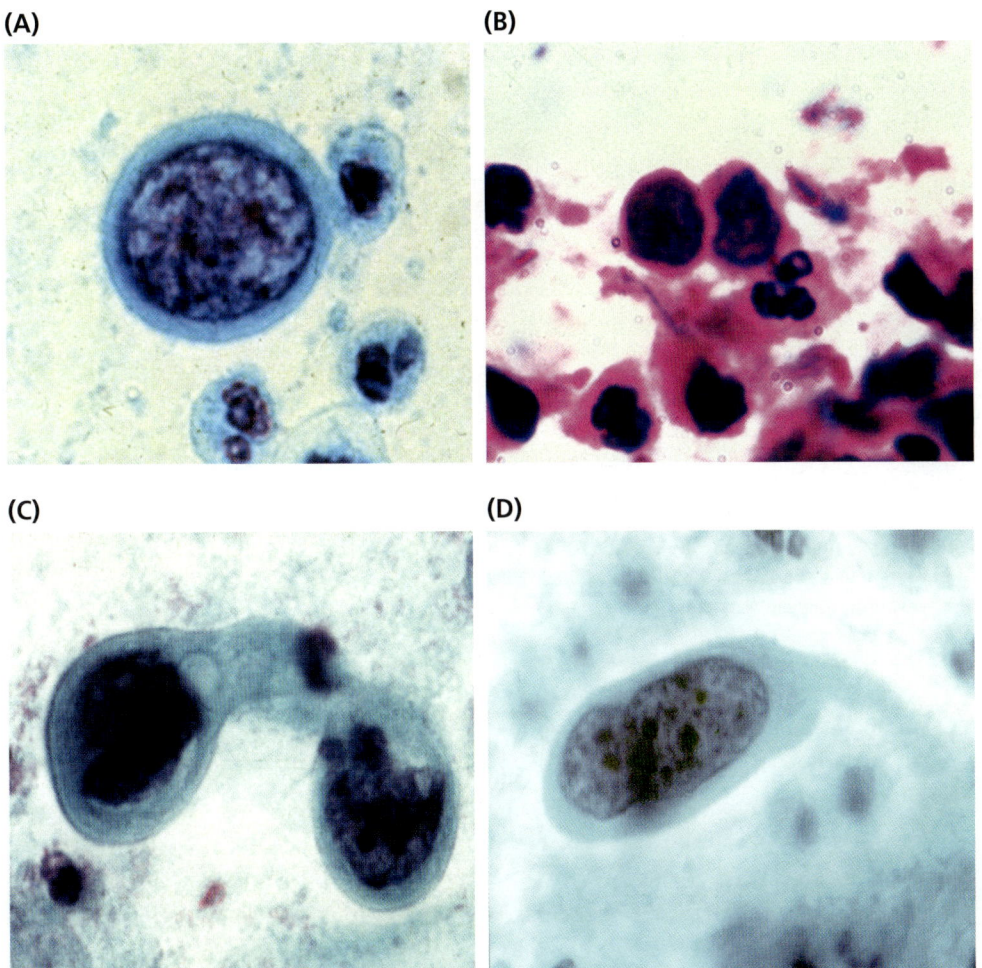

Figure 2.102 Endometrial cells seen with IUD usage. High N:C ratio endometrial cell (A), endometrial surface cells (B). Degenerated stromal cells mimicking malignancy (C, D). Vaginocervical smears, Pap stain.

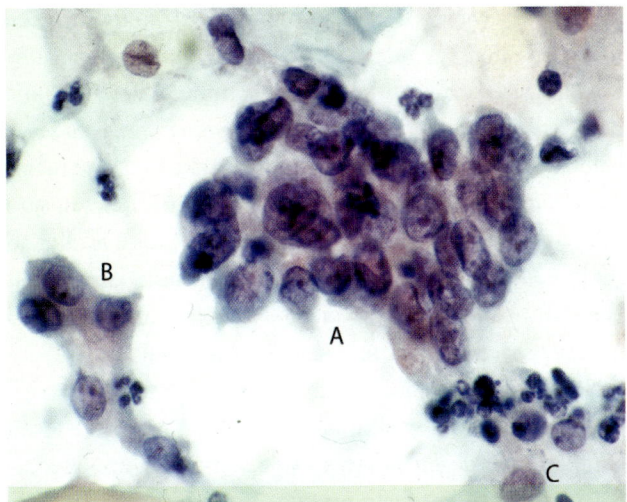

Figure 2.103 Endometrial cells following dilation and curettage (D&C) procedure. Nuclear details in reactive cell scan mimic malignant changes: prominent nucleoli and chromatin clearing (A), squamous metaplasia (B), apoptosis and nuclear degeneration (C). Vaginocervical smear, Pap stain.

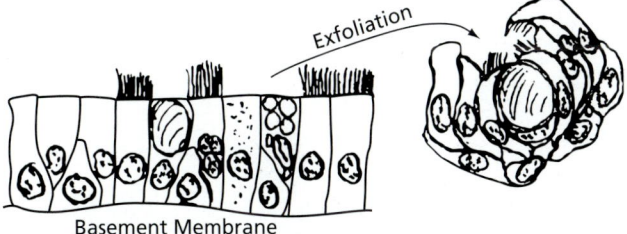

Figure 2.104 Line drawing depicting the intercellular molding and formation of a Creola body.

cells with abundant cytoplasm may be seen in association with gastric columnar cells, which in some instances may be indicative of intestinal metaplasia (Figures 2.114 and 2.115)

In the majority of cases, gastric columnar cells are shed in sheets with round to oval nuclei and abundant cytoplasm; however, proplastic changes can lead to marked variation in nuclear size, which causes diagnostic

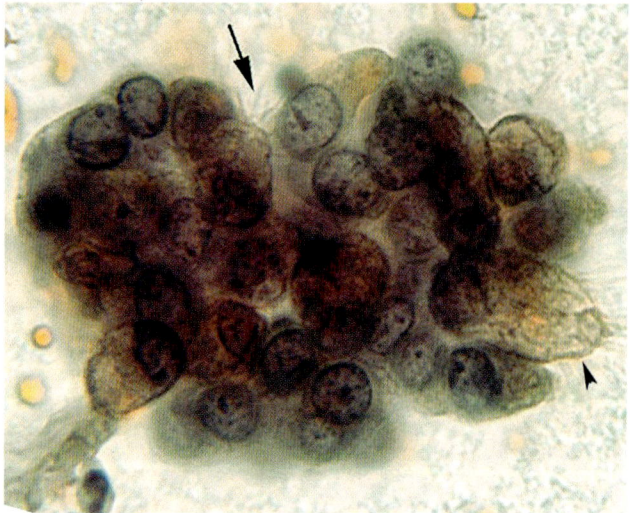

Figure 2.105 Creola body. Notice the cellular molding and the cilia (arrow) and mucus cells (arrowhead). Recognition of cilia is critical for accurate interpretation of these cells. Bronchial brush specimen, Pap stain.

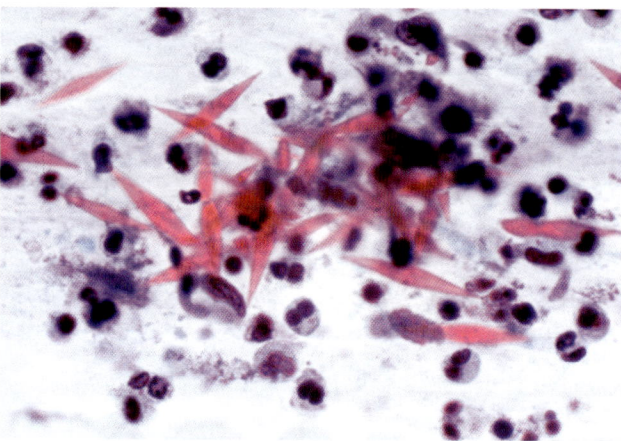

Figure 2.106 Charcot-laden crystals in a case of bronchial asthma. Notice numerous eosinophils associated with the crystals. Spontaneous sputum, direct smear, Pap stain.

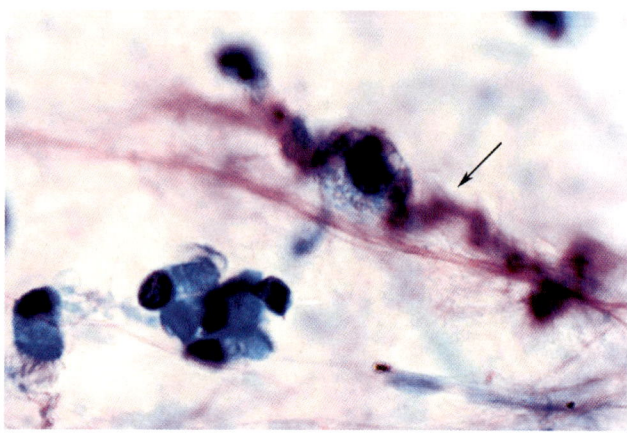

Figure 2.107 Curshman's spiral (arrow) in a case of bronchial asthma. Inflammatory cells and eosinophils may occur with the mucus spiral. Induced sputum, direct smear, Pap stain.

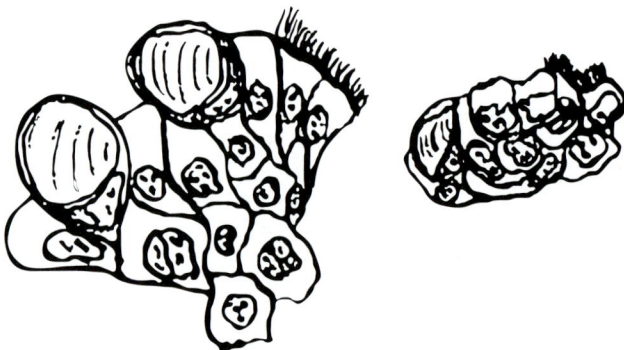

Figure 2.108 Line drawings depicting formation of Creola body with predominant goblet cells.

difficulties. In such instances, uniformity of both chromatin and nucleolar patterns among nuclei contained in the tissue fragment, an adequate "cushion" of cytoplasm uniformly placed around the nucleus, prominent cytoplasmic borders and "honeycombing" when seen *en face* is of great help in determining their true biologic nature. Cilia are not seen in gastric columnars (but are present in nasopharyngeal cells either obtained from the nasal passage due to the passage of a gastric tube or post-nasal discharge). Hyperdistended secretory-type vacuoles are common in the chronic gastritis. Gastric columnar cells from patients with megaloblastic anemia may demonstrate large nuclei with areas of cleared parachromatin which, when coupled with degeneration or dyskaryotic changes due to reactive change or repair, may be mistaken for malignancy.

Intestinal

Vacuolated secretory columnar cells from both the small and more prominently from the large intestine frequently

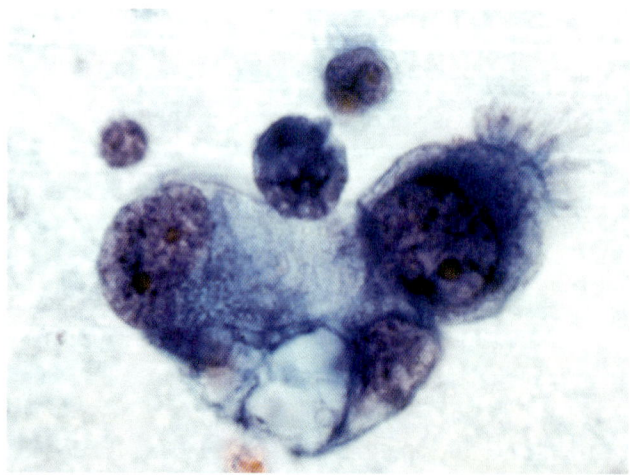

Figure 2.109 Fragment of bronchial cells predominantly containing goblet cells in a case of bronchial asthma. Bronchial brush, conventional smear. Pap stain.

(A)

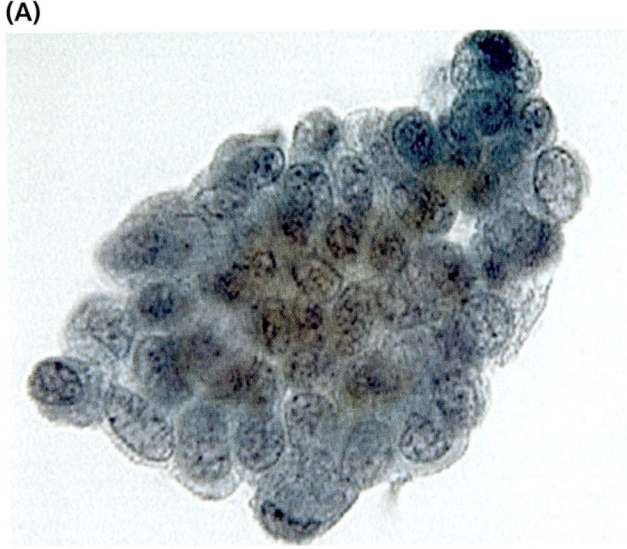

(B)

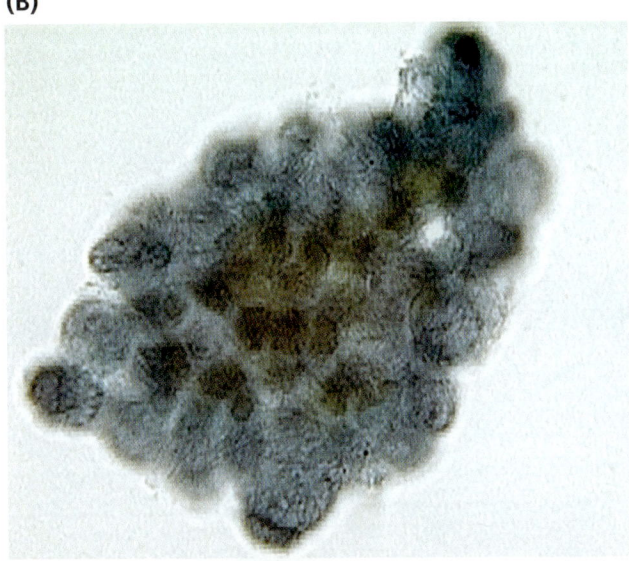

Figure 2.110 Ciliated bronchial cells without obvious cilia (A), cilia seen on the surface of bronchial epithelial cells (B). Bronchial brush, conventional smear. Pap stain.

have a single, typically secretory-type vacuole. At times the secretory vacuoles are hyper-distended, especially in chronic inflammatory conditions of the colon; they may contain intracytoplasmic neutrophils; brush-bordered cells are commonly encountered; as are sheets and *en face* configurations. The non-vacuolated columnar cell frequently contains golden-brown granules in its cytoplasm, apparently of a serous secretory nature.

Conduit

An ileal bladder or an ileal conduit is commonly employed after cystectomy. Sometimes, an Indiana pouch constructed from cecum may serve as an artificial urinary

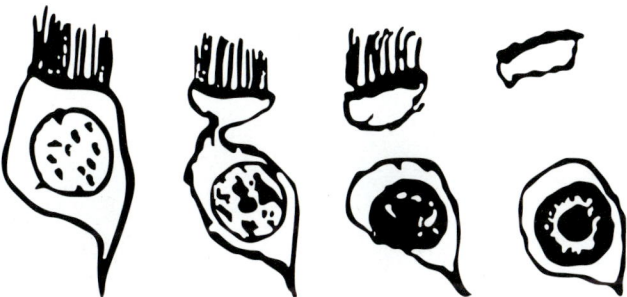

Figure 2.111 Line diagrams depicting the epithelial changes in viral infection.

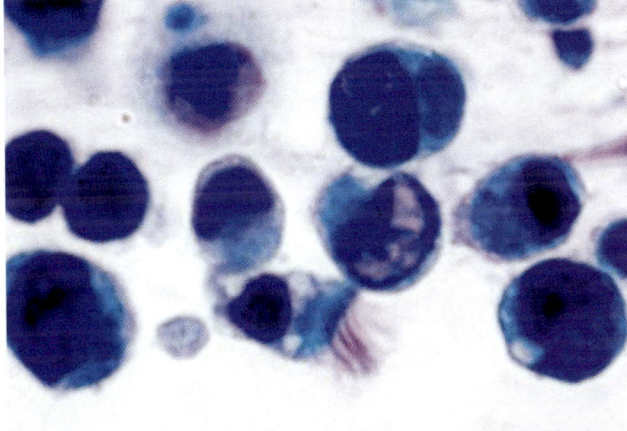

Figure 2.112 Bronchial cells showing various forms of viral infection. Bronchial wash, conventional smear. Pap stain.

bladder. Urine specimens are commonly examined for tumor surveillance and monitoring. Intestinal cells are generally poorly preserved. They occur as dark and pyknotic with intracytoplasmic inclusions. Rarely, well-preserved epithelial cells in small tissue fragments may be observed (Figures 2.116 and 2.117). Colonic cells in the Indiana Pouch specimen are extremely degenerated and as such not identifiable with any certainty.

Pancreatic acinic and ductal

Normal pancreatic acinar cells may be observed in aspirated material obtained by EUS or direct sampling procedures. These are uniform in size, cuboidal to low-columnar in shape, and occur in rosette formations. Rarely, cytoplasmic granules may be observed in these cells (Figures 2.118 and 2.119). Islet cells generally cannot be identified with certainty in cytologic specimens. They appear singly or in small groups resembling lymphoid cells with scant cytoplasm and eccentric vesicular nuclei (Figure 2.120). Ductal epithelial cells appear in small mono-layered tissue fragments as low cuboidal to columnar in appearance (Figures 2.121 and 2.122). Columnar forms are more common following an injury or reaction involving the ductal epithelium.

(A) 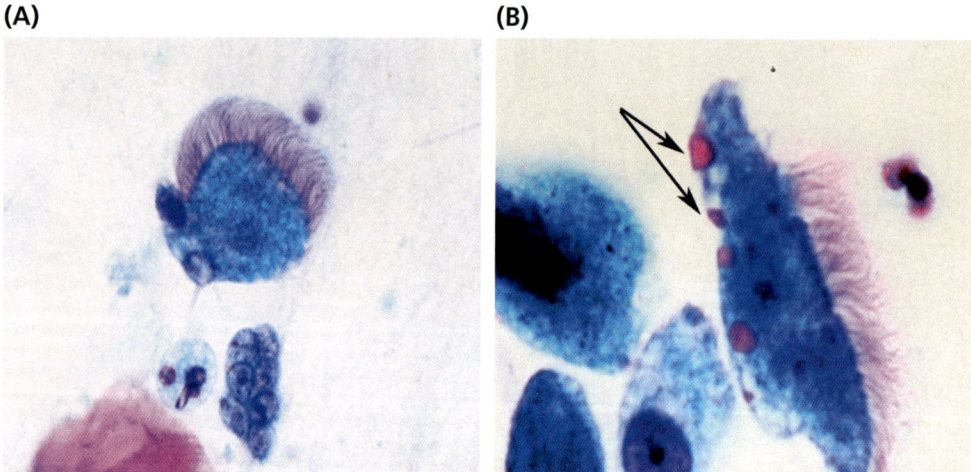 **(B)**

Figure 2.113 (A) Ciliocytophthoria and (B) intracytoplasmic eosinophilic inclusions. Bronchial washings specimen, conventional smear. Pap stain.

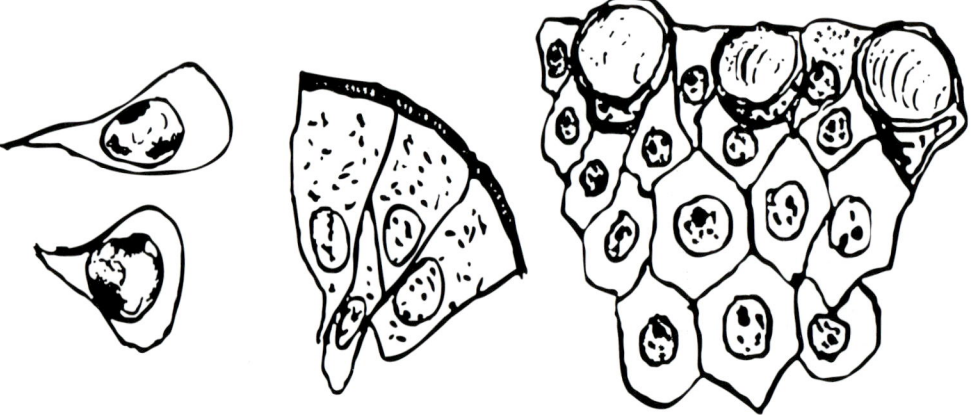

Figure 2.114 Gastric columnar cells as may occur, singly, metaplastic, and in sheets containing mucin and non-mucin producing types of cells.

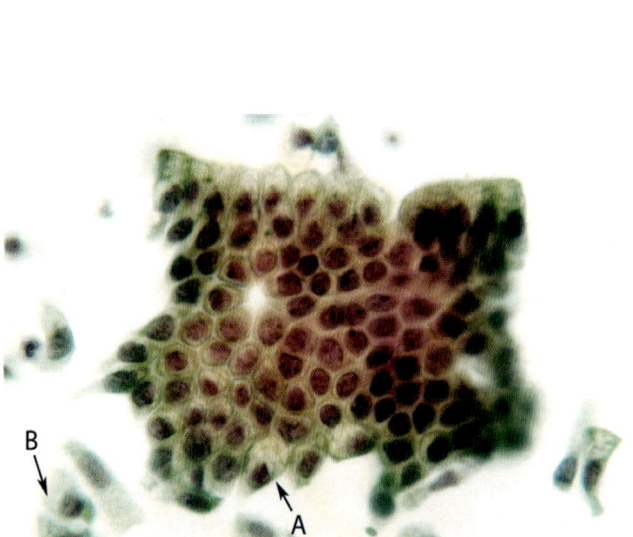

Figure 2.115 Gastric columnar cells. These are mixed with goblet cells (A) and intestinal metaplastic cells (B). EUS specimen, Pap stain.

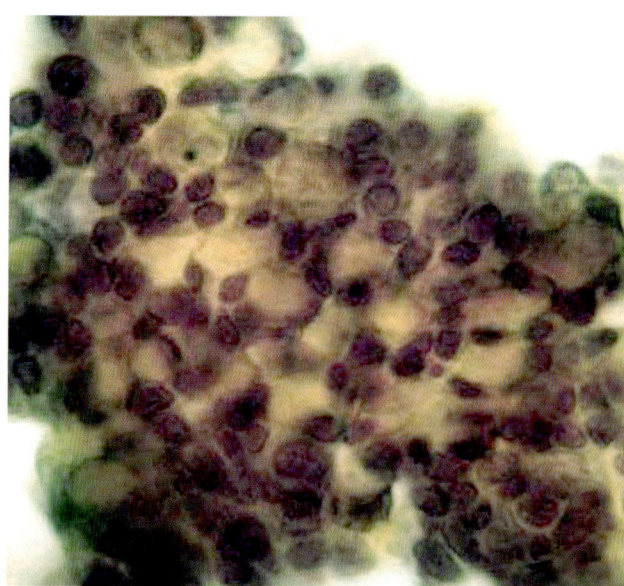

Figure 2.116 Group of colonic epithelial cells. Note the prominent mucus-containing goblet cells. Cells generally occur in sheets and may show folding at the edges. Colonic brush, conventional smear, Pap stain.

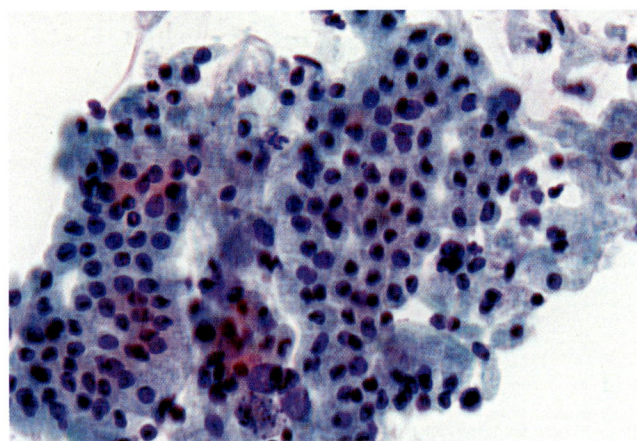

Figure 2.117 Group of colonic epithelial cells. Note the cellular degeneration, conduit urine, cytospin, Pap stain.

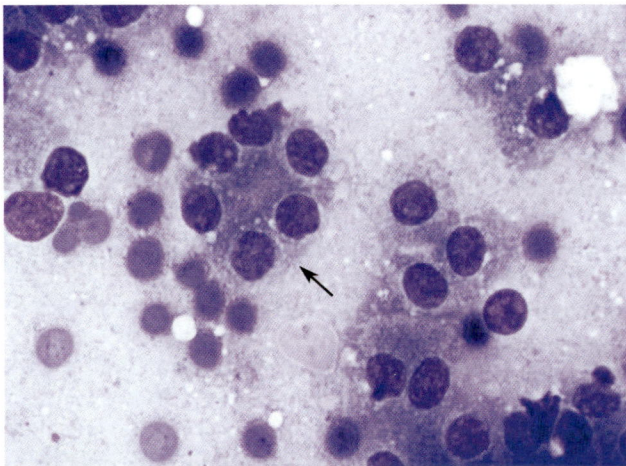

Figure 2.118 Acinic cells, pancreas. Note the acinic arrangement of epithelial cells (arrow). Intracytoplasmic granules are not very obvious in these cells. EUS specimen, direct smear, Diff-Quik stain.

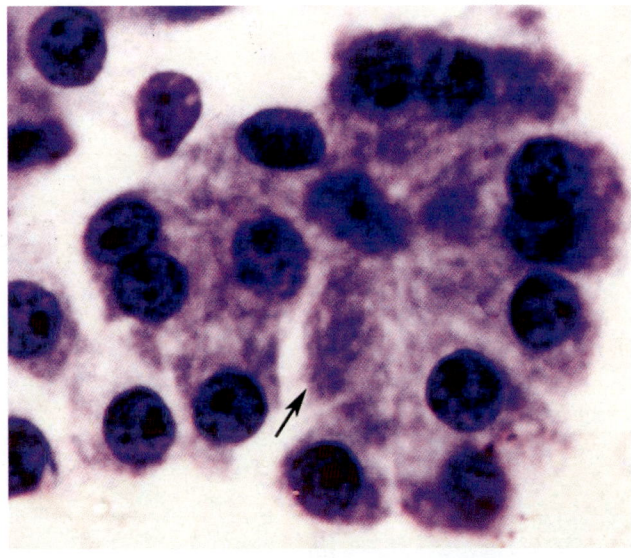

Figure 2.119 Acinic cells with intracytoplasmic granules (arrow). EUS specimen, direct smear, Diff-Quik stain.

PANCREATIC DUCT

These cells are low columnar to cuboidal in appearance. They appear in sheets, often as two-dimensional structures. When occurring singly, they can be difficult to recognize. In liquid-based preparations, cells tend to shrink and appear more rounded and cuboidal (Figure 2.121).

Bile duct

Columnar epithelial cells from the bile duct can vary from tall columnar to cuboidal in shape (Figure 2.122). These cells can be proliferative, extremely atypical, and bizarre, especially after irritation by a stent or a calculus.

Mammary

It is diagnostically important to clearly distinguish between two distinct types of columnar cells in nipple secretions: the "foam cell" and the "passive lining" duct cell. Normally only foam cells may be seen in nipple smears, especially during pregnancy, lactation, or in some women using oral contraceptives.

FOAM CELL

The normal columnar cell in nipple secretions is the foam cell, which is morphologically indistinguishable from the histocytic foam cell of nipple secretions. They usually arise from mammary acini and represent the bulk of the secretory elements of the epithelium. They occur singly and are round in shape with round to oval central or eccentric nuclei. The cytoplasm is abundant and foamy, being filled with multiple small vacuoles which do not coalesce into single vacuole (Figures 2.123 and 2.124). These changes are more prominent during lactation. Foamy macrophages tend to become denser with less obvious vacuoles in ductal blockage, such as in fibrocystic changes (Figure 2.125).

THE PASSIVE LINING CELLS

The presence of these cells is most important. Normally shed singly, they are not usually identifiable. However, when shed as a tissue fragment, especially with an identifiable epithelial luminal border and occurrence in papillary or acinar formations, this cell type is recognizable and signifies papillary proliferation of duct epithelium. The nuclei of such cells crowd and frequently mold. The

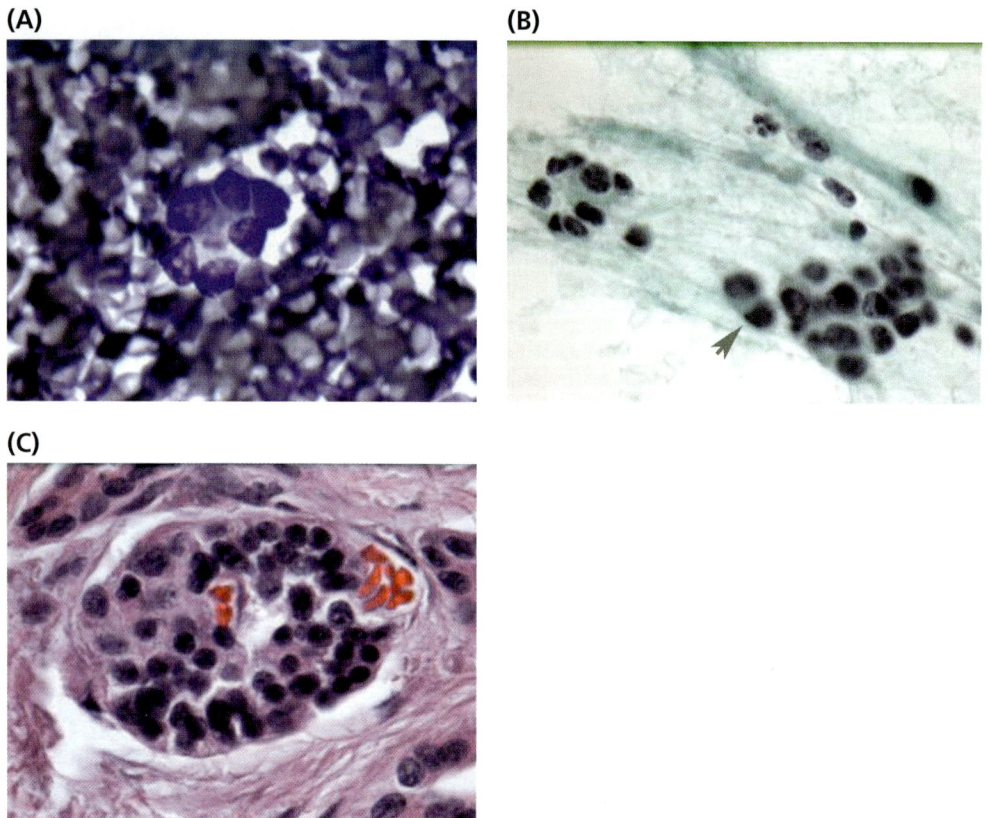

Figure 2.120 (A) Islet cells, plasmacytoid appearance. (B) Pleomorphic lymphoid forms, notice scant cytoplasm (arrow). (C) Tissue section showing similar features. Case of chronic pancreatitis. EUS specimen (A, B). (A) Diff-Quik, (B) Pap, (C) H/E tissue section.

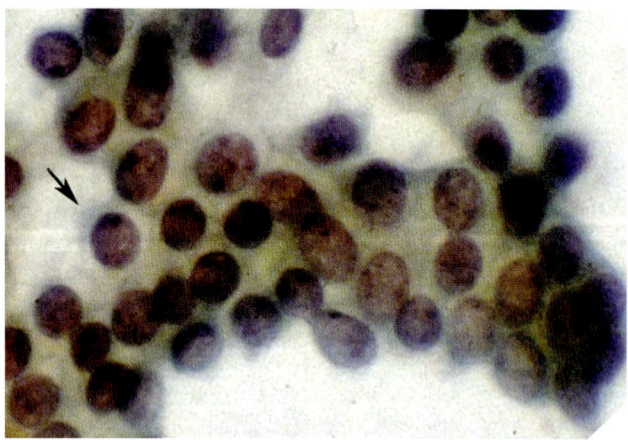

Figure 2.121 Pancreatic ductal cells. Notice the polygonal shapes (arrow) of the cells. EUS, LBP, Pap stain.

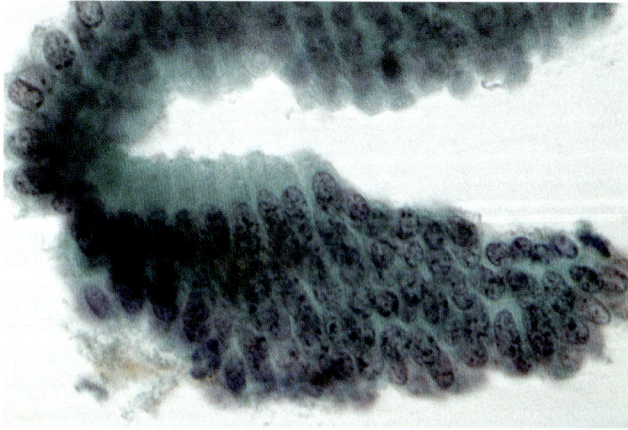

Figure 2.122 Bile duct cell. Notice the tall columnar appearance and pseudostratification of the cells. EUS, LBP, Pap stain.

cytoplasm is scanty, clear, and may be singly vacuolated – often pouched out in hyperdistention (Figure 2.126). Myoepithelial cells occur as elongated, dark and generally cigar-shaped with scant cytoplasm. They are intermixed with ductal cells and almost always denote the benign nature of the lesion (Figure 2.127).

Transitional (urothelial)

Transitional cells within the urinary bladder orient either parallel or perpendicular to the basement membrane. They may appear as thin flat squames or thick, cuboidal, and dense. These alterations are dependent upon the distention of the urinary bladder and stretching of the wall. Vaginal

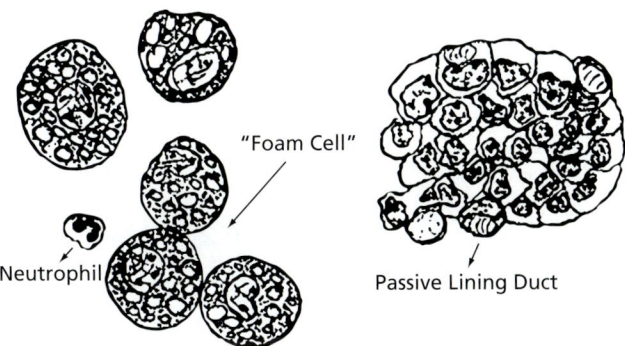

Figure 2.123 Line drawings depicting the development of "foam cell" of ductal origin.

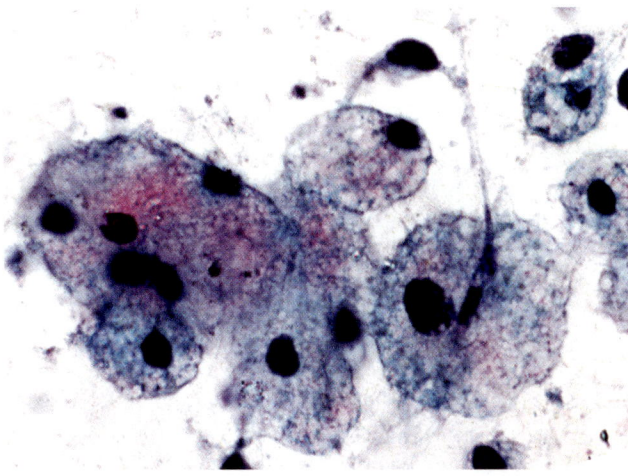

Figure 2.124 "Foam cells" of ductal origin. Notice the numerous fine intracytoplasmic secretory vacuoles. Nipple discharge, pregnancy. Conventional smear, Pap stain.

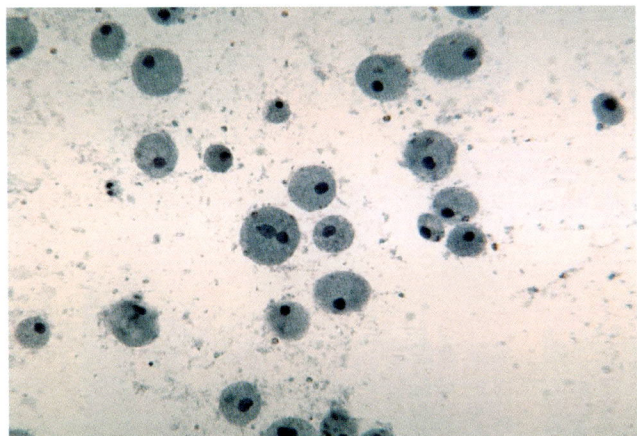

Figure 2.125 Foam cells. Notice the relatively dense cytoplasm and less obvious secretory vacuoles. Fibrocystic change. Conventional smear, Pap stain.

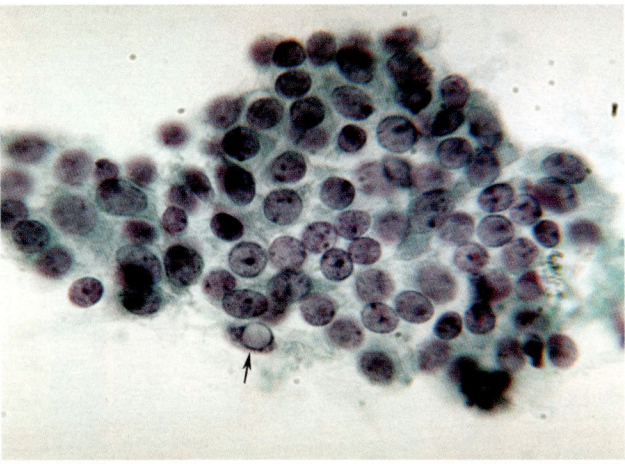

Figure 2.126 Group of lining ductal cells. Notice the intracytoplasmic vacuole (arrow). Fine needle aspiration, breast, and conventional smear, Pap stain.

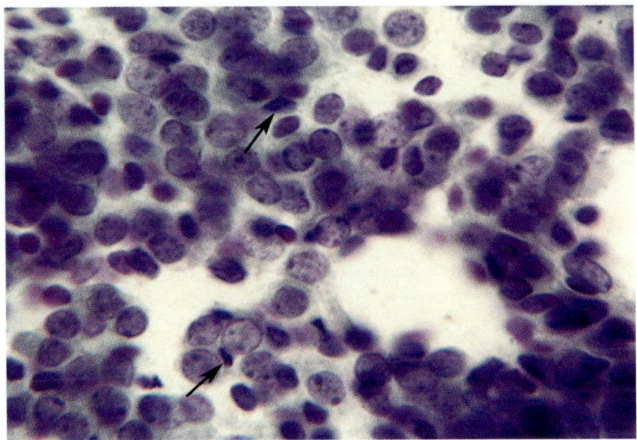

Figure 2.127 Myoepithelial cells (arrows) intermixed with ductal cells. Breast fine needle aspiration. Conventional smear, Pap stain.

contamination is common in voided urine specimens, and squamous metaplasia resulting from chronic inflammation, irritation and obstruction may render the identification of urothelial cells difficult. These changes are, however, less pronounced in specimens obtained from the ureters and upper urinary tract.

When exfoliated, these cells vary from uni-caudate ("columnar") cells with moderately thick cytoplasm, through rounded cells of parabasal appearance, to flat squamous cells not unlike the intermediate cells of squamous epithelium. The nuclei of this whole series of cells tend to be larger than those of the squamous series, without a proportionate increase of cytoplasm (Figure 2.128). Normal transitional cells in voided urine specimens are shed singly or in small clumps, unless "reamed-out" by a catheter, instrumentation, or irritation. When such a tissue fragment occurs, its margin lacks the dependent "community border" of a papillary frond, appearing to be made up

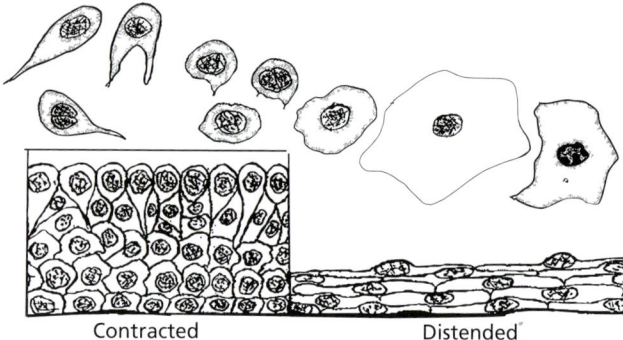

Figure 2.128 Line drawings depicting the appearances of urothelial cells in a voided urine specimen. These cells have nuclei that are larger than the intermediate squamous cells and they vary in size and shape according to the distention of the bladder.

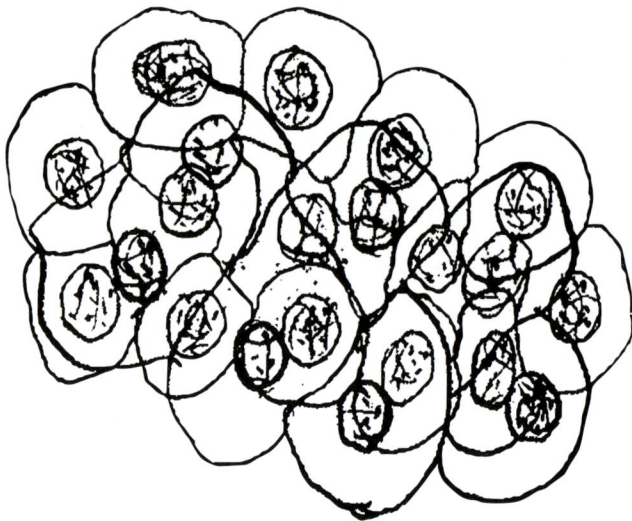

Figure 2.129 Line drawing showing the shedding of single urothelial cells. They tend to produce clumps of overlapping epithelial cells.

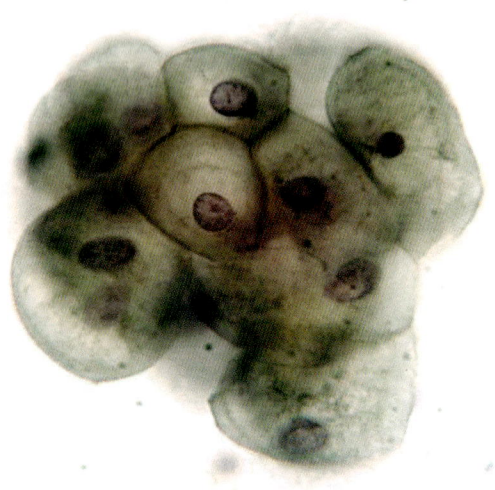

Figure 2.130 Group of normal urothelial cells, voided urine specimen. Notice lack of intercellular molding. Voided urine, Millipore filter, Pap stain.

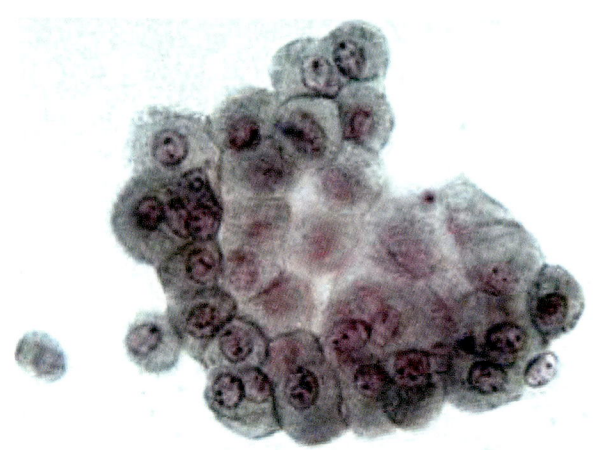

Figure 2.131 Tissue fragment of urothelial cells showing community border and surface maturation. Bladder wash specimen, Millipore filter, Pap stain.

of independent cell borders of individual cells in a "haphazard" fashion (Figures 2.129 and 2.130). Multinucleation and hyperchromasia are very frequent in umbrella cells, especially in irritation due to infection, calculi, and instrumentation (Figure 2.131). Urothelial cells can also appear columnar as well as spindle-shaped (Figure 2.134).

Presence of true urothelial tissue fragments is voided urine specimens is uncommon; often associated with an irritative (stone, catheterization), inflammatory, invasive procedure, or neoplastic processes. Urothelial cells can occur in pseudo-papillary formation. These structures may appear to contain immature abnormal-appearing cells (Figures 2.129–2.132) but almost always reveal surface maturation (Figure 2.130). At times, proper identification of urothelial cell tissue fragments can be problematic; renal tubular cells and cells from prostatic urethra and ducts are

a common cause of misrecognition. Multinucleation among urothelial cells occurs commonly in irritative processes such as stone, infections, and undulating catheter (Figure 2.133) is frequent. Vaginal contamination in voided urine specimens.

Renal tubular

These occur rarely and may be seen in urine specimens from persons over 60 years of age. They are generally cuboidal with prominent nucleoli and pale, soft, and finely vacuolated cytoplasm (Figure 2.135). Renal parenchymal disease (diabetes, hypertension, nephrosclerosis, renal infarction) often result in the exfoliation of renal tubular cells. Some of the most bizarre forms of renal tubular cells are observed following immunosuppression and renal

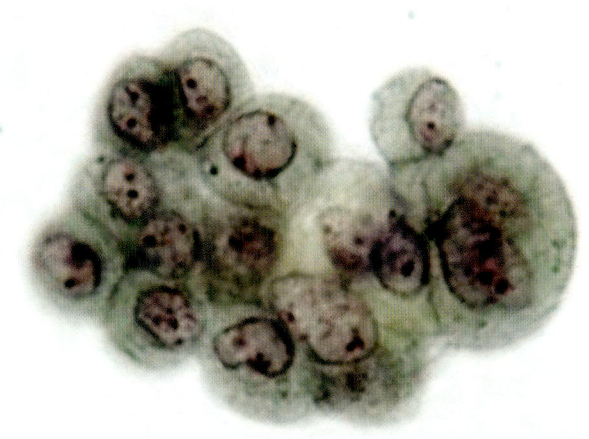

Figure 2.136 Fragment of extremely atypical renal tubular cells, kidney transplant rejection. Compare to Figure 2.135C. Voided urine specimen, Millipore filter, Pap stain.

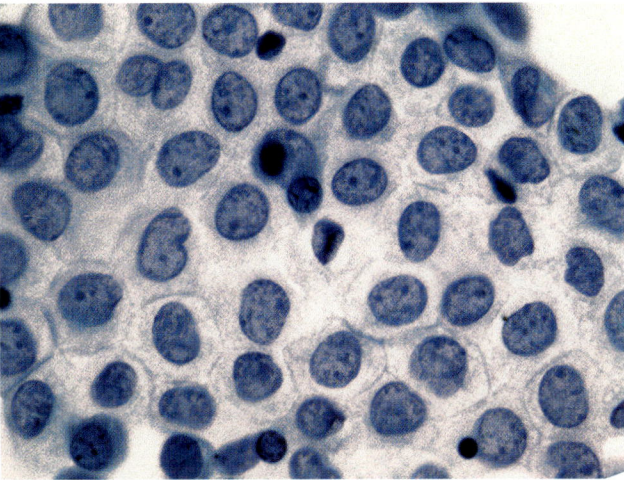

Figure 2.137 Group of mesothelial cells in an abdominal wash specimen. Notice the pavement-like pattern of cells with polygonal-shaped cells. Abdominal wash, Millipore filter, Pap stain.

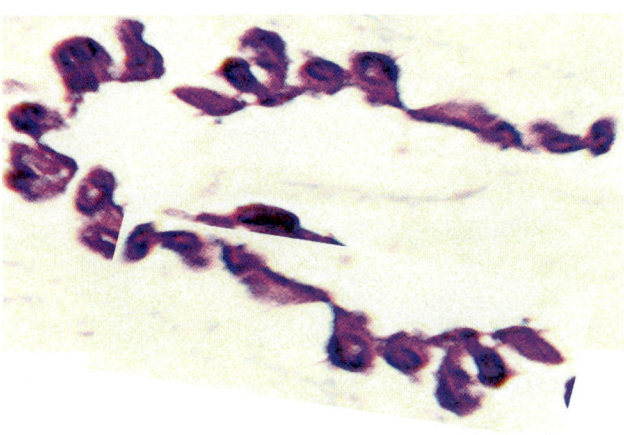

Figure 2.138 Cell block, mesothelial cells. Notice the cuboidal to columnar to flat squamoid appearance, H/E stain.

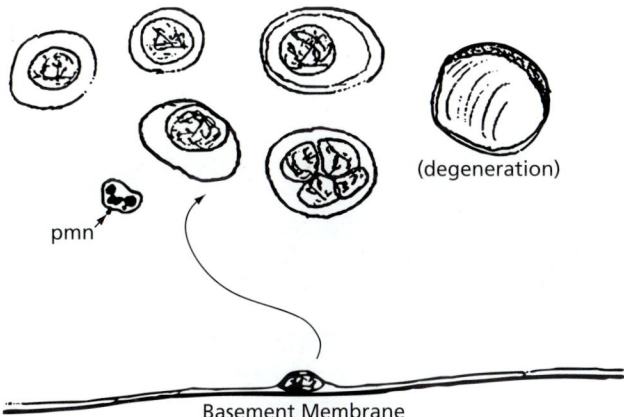

Figure 2.139 Line drawings depicting the exfoliation of mesothelial cells. When shed, cells become rounded; multinucleation, signet cell changes may occur. PMN, polymorphonuclear leucocytes.

transplant (Figures 2.135 and 2.136). They can occur with hyperchromasia and extremely prominent nucleoli and can be mistaken for renal cell carcinoma cells. Prostatic and seminal vesicle cells can sometimes mimic renal tubular cells. Renal tubular cells can have intracytoplasmic secretions and inclusions. Most often, intracytoplasmic orangophilic inclusions represent inspissated proteinous material (Figure 2.135D), but they may be viral in origin. Similarly, intracytoplasmic material may occur in certain metabolic diseases.

Mesothelial

"Normal" mesothelial cells should not be observed in body cavity specimens. Some cells may be recovered from rectovaginal space specimens. Mesothelial cells may, however, be forcibly removed or scraped during surgery or instrumentation. A monolayer of such cells with polygonal shapes, well-defined edges and centrally located nuclei may be observed in body cavity specimens (Figure 2.137). Cells occur as cuboidal to flat squames lining the various cavities (Figure 2.138).

The simple mesothelial cell usually sheds singly, and rounds up in the fluid with a round to oval nucleus and uniform chromatin pattern. These cells may appear in small clumps and are separated evenly spaced by intercellular partitions often termed as "windows." Depending upon the composition of the body cavity fluid, mesothelial cells may become multinucleate, or signet ring in shape (Figures 2.139–2.141).

When very "active," however, as in a pleural reaction over a pulmonary infarction, the chromatin pattern in

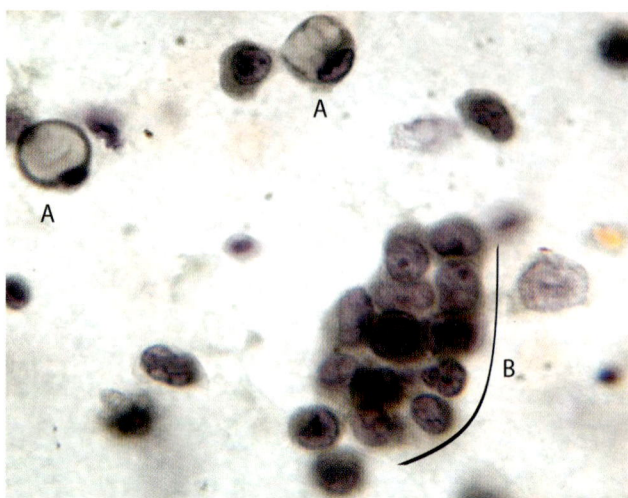

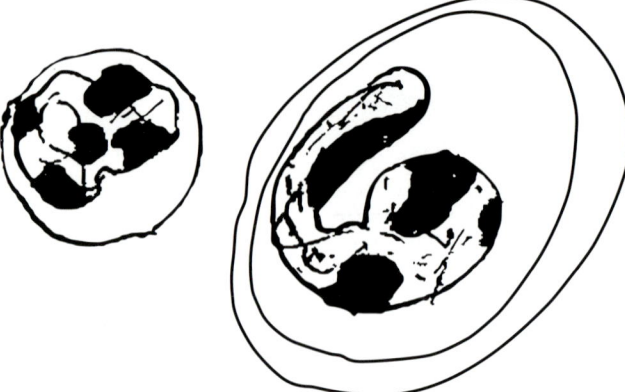

Figure 2.141 Line drawings depicting the nuclear changes in reactive mesothelial cells.

Figure 2.140 Mesothelial cell with degeneration. Notice the signet cell (A), and a group of high N:C ratio cells with dense hyperchromatic nuclei and scant cytoplasm (B). Such changes can be misinterpreted as malignant. Pleural fluid, congestive cardiac failure, Millipore filter, Pap stain.

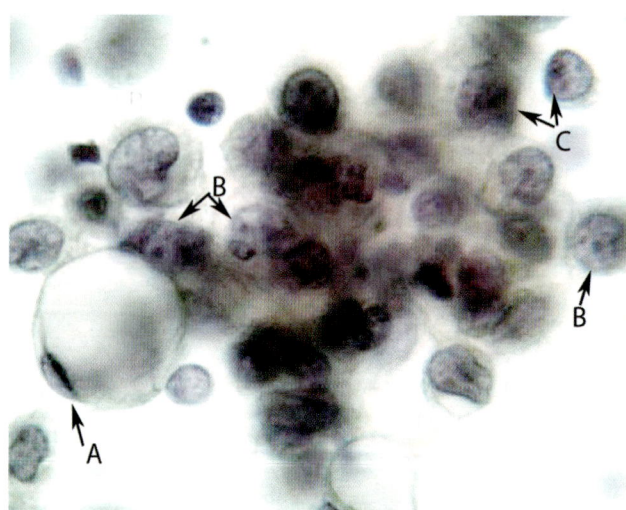

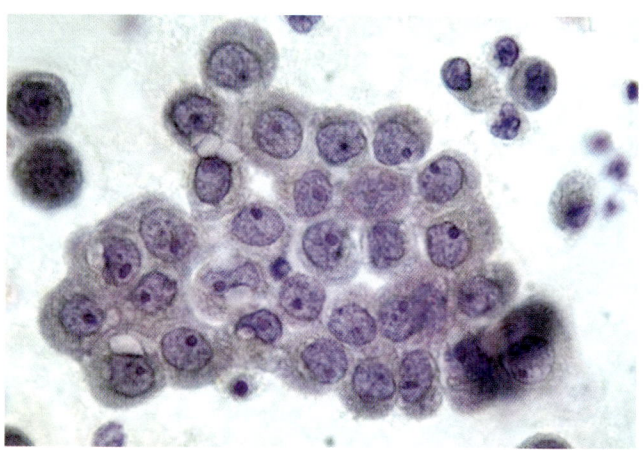

Figure 2.143 Reactive mesothelial cells. Notice the prominent nucleoli. Liver transplant, abdominal fluid, ThinPrep Pap stain.

Figure 2.142 Reactive and degenerating mesothelial cells. Signet cell (A), prominent nucleoli (B), and abnormal chromatin clumps (C). Pleural fluid. ThinPrep, Pap stain.

mesothelial cells may be markedly clumped and irregular with prominent nucleoli. Both chromatin clumps and nucleoli, even though massive in size, tend not to be sharply pointed, but are rounded and somewhat fuzzy (Figures 2.139–2.143). These mesothelial cells may proliferate and occur in papillary and tissue fragment formations that are often a hallmark of malignancy in the body cavity fluid specimens (Figure 2.144).

Such proplastic mesothelial cells may have many malignant criteria, so that the relationships of cells in a group take on great importance with this material. When

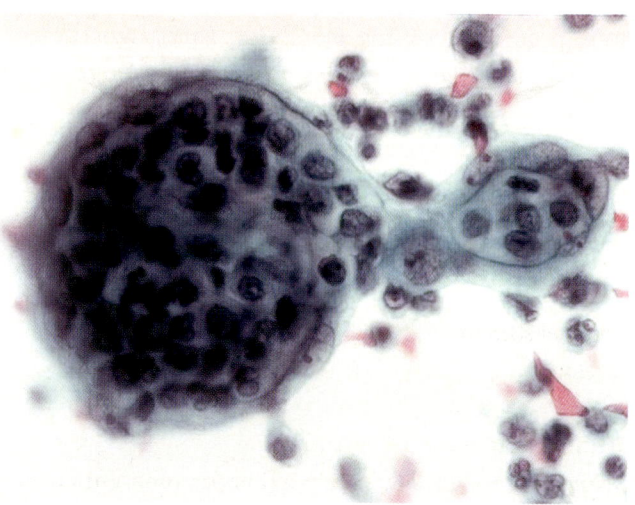

Figure 2.144 Tissue fragment and papillary formation in reactive mesothelial cells. Abdominal fluid. Post liver transplant specimen. Direct smear, Pap stain.

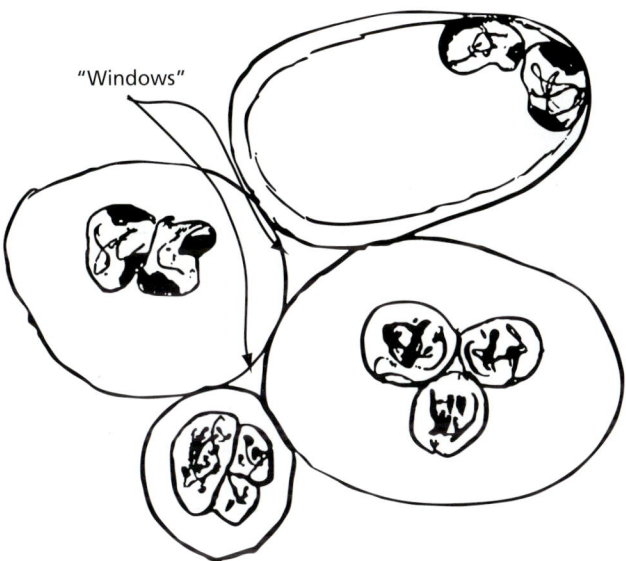

"Windows"

Figure 2.145 Line drawing showing the reactive mesothelial cells with "windows," multinucleation, degeneration, and chromatin changes.

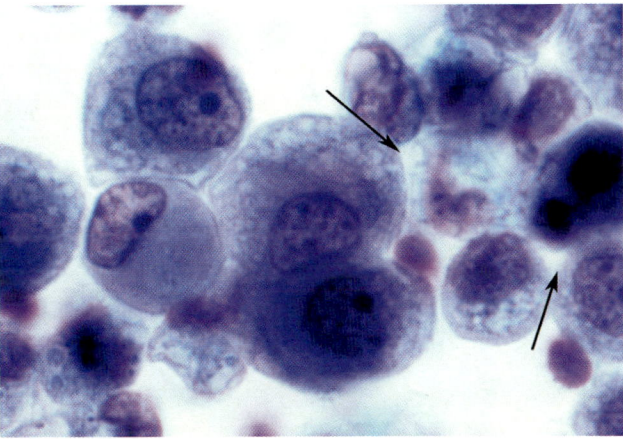

Figure 2.146 Group of reactive mesothelial cells with "windows" (arrows). Notice the prominent nucleoli and chromatin changes. Viral pleuritis. Pleural fluid, Millipore filter, Pap stain.

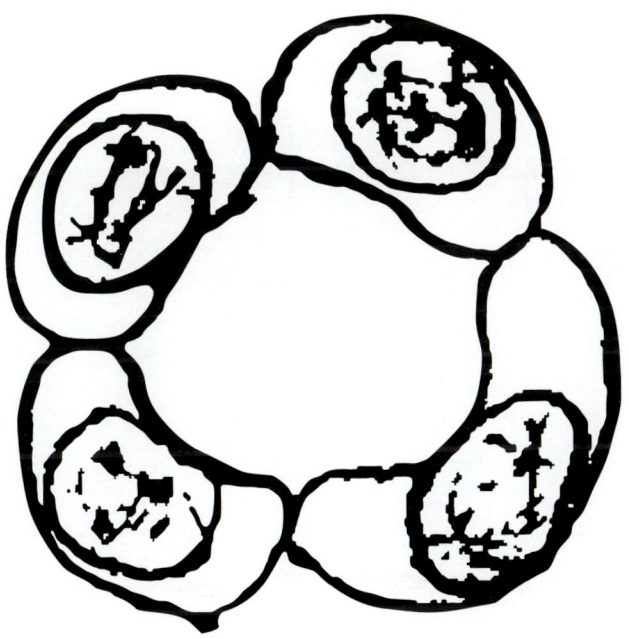

Figure 2.147 Line drawing showing the loop-to-loop arrangement of mesothelial cells that most commonly represents reactive changes.

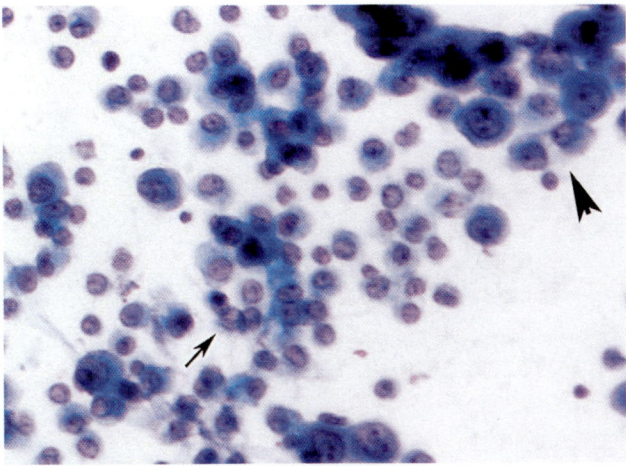

Figure 2.148 Glandular (arrow) and loop-to-loop (arrowhead) arrangement of reactive mesothelial cells. Pleural effusion patient with congestive cardiac failure. Millipore filter, Pap stain.

mesothelial cells clump, they appear as though they "came together secondarily," rather than "grew together primarily" as a true tissue fragment. (i) They associate loosely with each other; (ii) they have occasional intercellular spaces, or "windows;" and (iii) the outer margin of their clump lacks the "community border" appearance of an epithelial surface, appearing to be made up of the cellular membranes of individual cells in a "loop-the-loop," haphazard fashion rather than a true tissue fragment (Figures 2.145–2.148).

Multinucleation is a common occurrence in reactive mesothelial cells. Specifically, they may be observed in cases with intracavitary intervention such as medication or surgery, and may be seen following trauma and pneumothorax. Multinucleation can sometimes be seen in granulomatous infections such as tuberculosis and syphilis (Figures 2.149 and 2.150). Mesothelial cells can wrap around collagen tissue and produce multinucleate collagen balls (Figure 2.150B).

Mesothelial cells can acquire phagocytic activities and are commonly seen with ingested red blood cells in cases with hemorrhagic effusions. They can also ingest bile material and, rarely, amyloidal proteins (Figures 2.151–2.154).

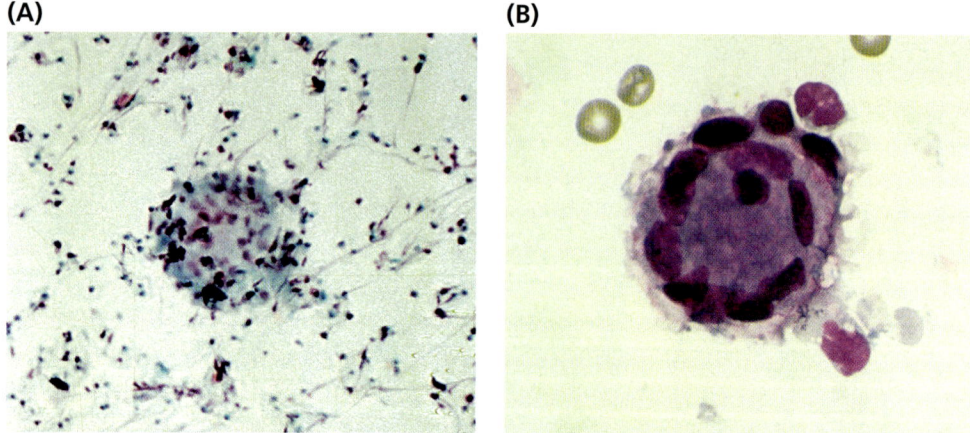

Figure 2.149 Multinucleation in cerebrospinal fluid. (A) Patient with cerebral tuberculoma (case courtesy of Dr. Sandra Bigner MD, Duke University). (B) Patient with secondary syphilis. (A) Millipore filter. (B) Diff-Quik.

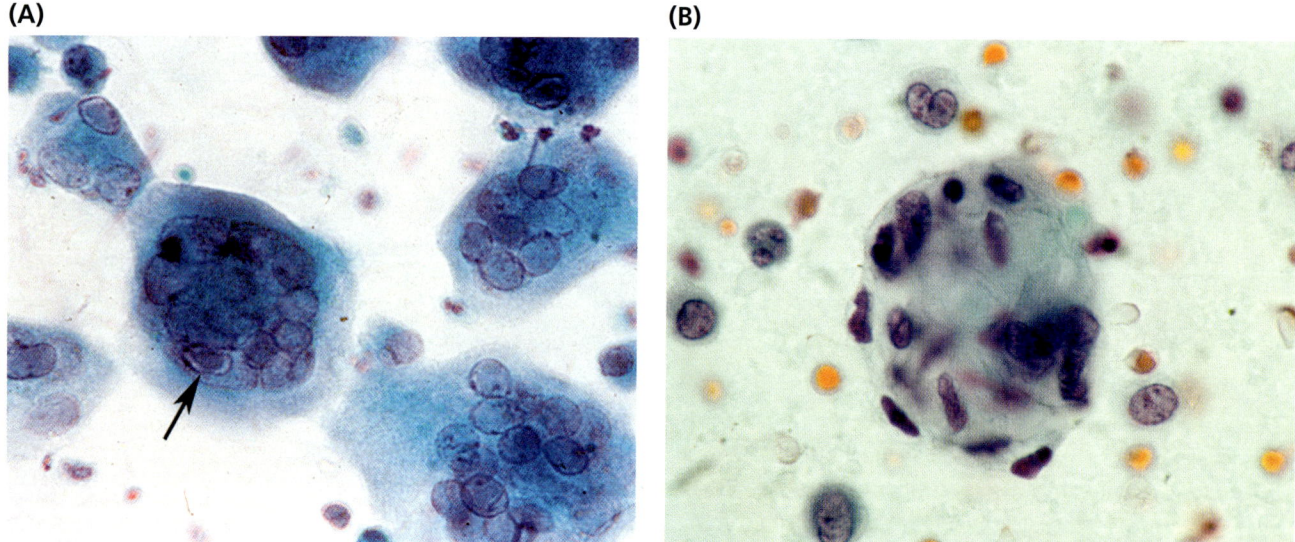

Figure 2.150 (A) Multinucleated mesothelial giant cells viral pleuritis, notice the intranuclear inclusion (arrow) (case courtesy of Dr. Ruth Katz MD, MD Anderson Houston). (B) Collagen ball abdominal fluid, notice the multinucleation of mesothelial cells surrounding collagen material, abdominal fluid, uterine fibroids. (A) Direct smear, (B) Millipore filter, Pap stain.

Groups of mesothelial cells may come together around an air bubble, mucus, mucopolysaccharides, foreign substances and other similar material. This is often seen in the inflammatory response and following intracavitory intervention. Mesothelial cells can appear to form an acinus; careful scrutiny, however, fails to reveal the identifying layers of an acinus (p. 31), and the cells appear to be loosely arranged, as if they "came together secondarily." This pseudoacinus is, of course, not a true epithelial tissue fragment and has limited diagnostic value (Figure 2.155). Sometimes mesothelial cells can occur as "pseudoacinic" structures enclosing amorphous mucopolysaccharide material

secreted by the cells. Such formations can be mistaken for intraluminal mucin secretion, such as in tumor.

Squamous metaplasia may be observed in mesothelial proliferation, most commonly representing a reactive process. Similar findings can be seen in cases of mesothelioma, metastatic squamous cell carcinoma, and occasional metaplastic tumors including breast and urothelium (Figure 2.156).

Histocytic

These cells are derived from the mesenchymal and bone marrow elements. At times many epithelial cells (mesothelium, squamous, alveolar lining, glandular

(A)

(B)

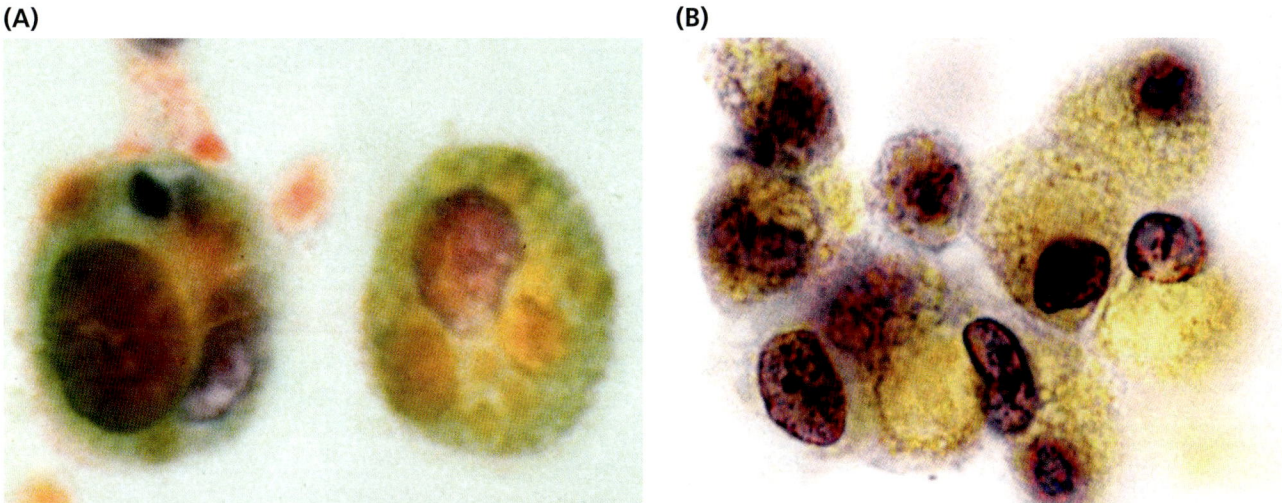

Figure 2.151 Ingested red blood cells (A) and bile (B) by mesothelial cells in case of hemorrhagic pleural effusion (A) and bile peritonitis. Cells in frame (B) stained for cytokeratin and were negative for macrophage markers. Cytospin slides, Pap stain.

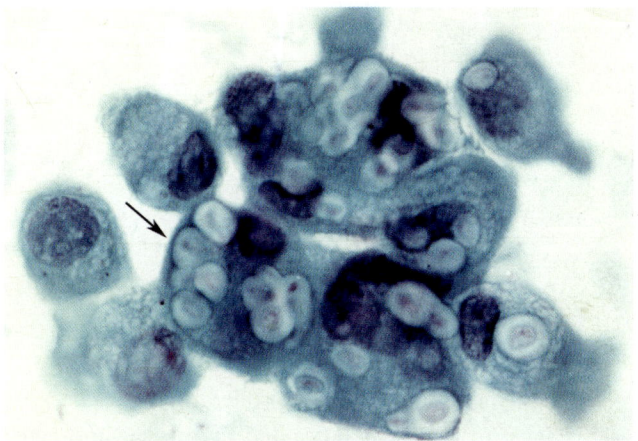

Figure 2.152 Mesothelial cells containing intracytoplasmic cryptococcus (arrow). Pleural fluid. Cytospin slide, Pap stain.

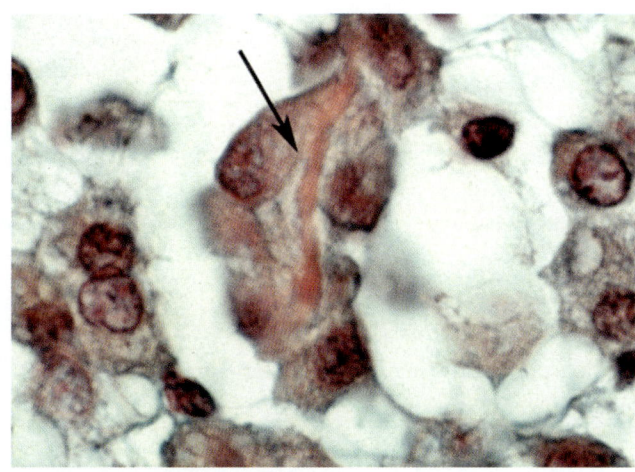

Figure 2.153 Amyloidal material surrounded by mesothelial cells (arrow). Pleural fluid, cell block, Congo red stain.

epithelial, as well as the tumor cells) may develop histiocytic functions resulting in macrophage-like activities and morphologic alterations that may mimic dyplastic and neoplastic changes. Histiocytes usually exfoliate singly. When they do group together, rounded clumped cells "come together secondarily" with intercytoplasmic "windows" and with a haphazard, non-epithelial border to the clump, rather than that of a true tissue fragment of cells derived from the same clone and which "grew together;" epithelial cells often associated with granulation tissue and reparative processes represent an extreme example of histiocytic look-alike cells (Figures 2.157–2.158).

They may exfoliate as single or multinucleated histiocytes (Figure 2.151). The cytoplasm of these cells

characteristically is foamy or vacuolated, with or without debris. The nucleus is round, oval or bean-shaped in the resting or euplastic state; with a uniform reticular and granular chromatin pattern it is eccentric, usually touching the nuclear membrane at one point, as if "bouncing off" of it (Figures 2.159 and 2.160).

Histiocytes present some of the most troublesome morphologic features. They may resemble both benign and neoplastic epithelial and mesenchymal cells (Figures 2.161–2.163). Often, immuno-markers are necessary for correct interpretation and diagnosis. Histiocytic cells in lymph node FNA specimens are particularly prone to misinterpretation, especially from cases with suspected metastatic epithelial tumors.

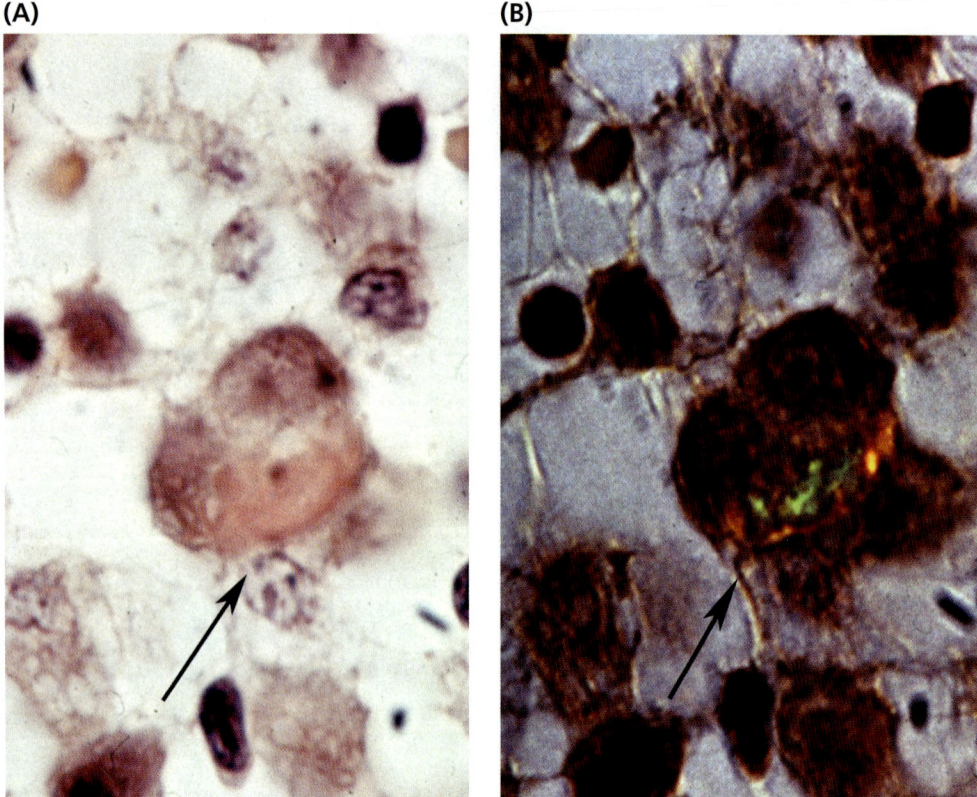

(A) **(B)**

Figure 2.154 (A) Amyloid deposit (arrow) within the mesothelial cells. (B) Congo red stain, bright field. Polarized light demonstrating apple-green birefringence. Notice the plasma cells in the background. Pleural fluid, direct smear.

At times, pulmonary alveolar macrophages can be morphologically indistinguishable from pneumocytes, and most often are not diagnosed in cytology specimens. They can, however, be more obvious when occurring as reactive cells, often causing a diagnostic dilemma. However, pneumocytes tend to be smaller, cuboidal with dense cytoplasm and prominent nucleolus (Figures 2.164 and 2.165).

Mostly, histiocytes perform phagocytic functions with minimal discernible morphologic features; they essentially remain "normal" or euplastic in appearance. They are able to ingest and digest mostly biological material without obvious alterations (Figure 2.166). These activities appear more commonly in chronic reactive processes and infections.

Cells may become enlarged and stick together as an epitheloid formation (Figures 2.167 and 2.168). They may phagocytose the foreign material, but more often metabolic and degenerative microbial and tissue products are present within the cytoplasm of epitheloid cells. Chronic granulomatous processes including sarcoid and mycobacterium often result in the formation of epitheloid cells. These are different from multinucleated giant cells (discussed below).

HISTIOCYTIC CELLS REFLEX RESPONSE

When challenged by an acute episode, histiocytes become "active," i.e. reactive. They respond by nuclear and cytoplasmic changes. Cells generally enlarge, with bi- and multinucleation bizarre forms and giant cell formations, and reveal alarming nuclear changes. Mitoses, generally normal and rarely abnormal in appearance, may occur. The nuclear distortions occur in five ways, each of which can be extremely odd, atypical, and prone to misinterpretation. Immunohistochemical staining (CD68 and keratin biomarkers) can often help in the accurate identification of macrophages and help diagnostically (Figure 2.169).

Nuclear changes

Shape. The cell may become extremely bizarre, and enlarged, resembling an epithelial cell occurring singly or as syncytial formations. Cytoplasmic borders can be sharp and distinct or pale and fuzzy (Figure 2.170). The nucleus becomes irregular, varying from round to oval to one side flattened (the side near the cell center) to indented

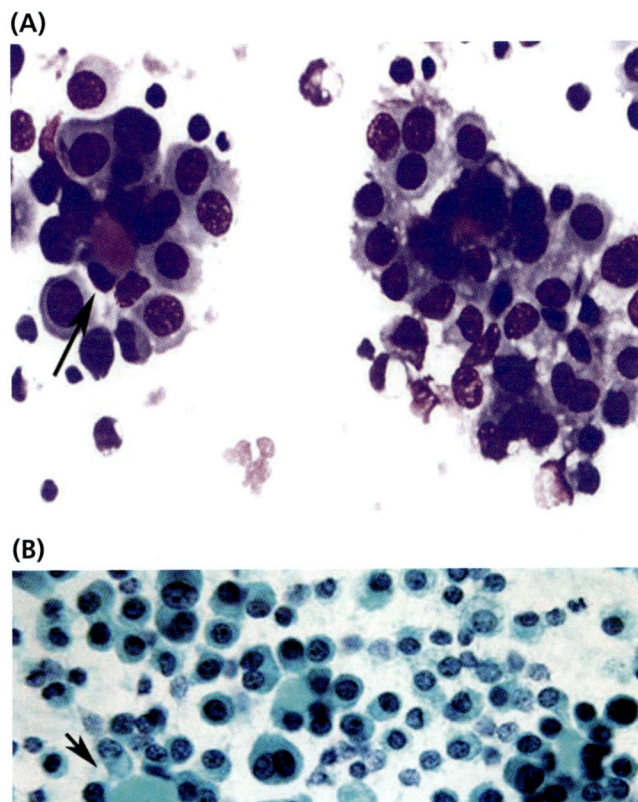

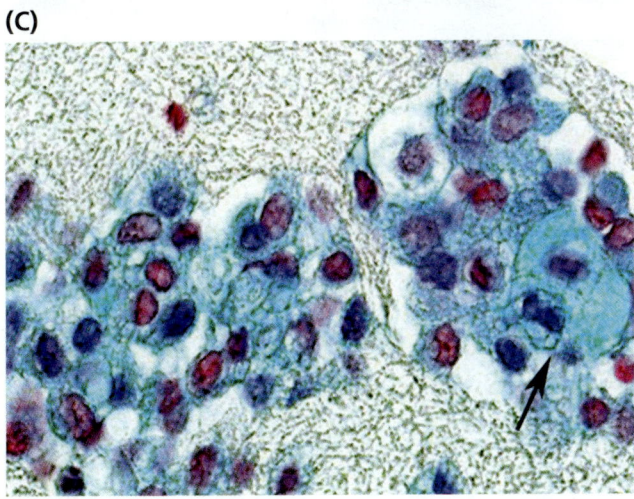

Figure 2.155 Mucopolysaccharide (arrows) material pleural fluid. Pseudoacinic formations surround the secretions. (A) Metachromasia seen by Diff-Quik. (B) Acellular material seen, Pap stain. (C) Staining by Alcian Blue reaction (case courtesy of Dr. Rana Hoda, Cornell Medical Center, New York).

(kidney-bean shape) or infolded, lobulation; nucleoli can be extremely prominent (Figures 2.171 and 2.172). These cells can pose diagnostic problems, especially when occurring in cases with epithelial malignancies and suspected lymph node metastasis.

Chromatin pattern. The chromatin may become dark and uneven or pale and homogenous with clumping, cleared areas (conspicuous parachromatin), prominent nucleoli, and unevenly thickened nuclear membrane. These chromatin clumps and nucleoli, however, are *rounded* and frequently smudged (rather than having the distinct, sharp "cookie-cutter" borders of preservation and ragged, jagged angles of malignancy). Extreme examples may occur in pulmonary infarcts, thyroid nodules following FNA, and from reactive lymph nodes following therapy (Figures 2.172–2.174).

Mitoses

These are frequent in active histiocytic activity, and uncommon in epithelial (reactive) cells exfoliated into non-physiologic material as mucus and debris. Mitotic activity within both histiocytic and epithelial cells can be more pronounced in cells bathing in cystic spaces such as a body cavity, breast and thyroid cysts. A nutrient-rich environment is most conducive to the proliferation of these cells. Such awareness is helpful diagnostically (Figures 2.161 and 2.175).

Histiocytes are among the most deceptive cells; they can have extremely variable cytoplasmic and nuclear features. They may be easily mistaken for malignant cells, especially when stimulated and irritated as by invasive procedure, infection, or therapy. Careful attention to morphologic details and clinical correlation is essential while examining histiocytic cells.

Phagocytosis

This occurs commonly and may be helpful diagnostically. Ingestion of nuclear debris occurs frequently in inflammatory reactions (Figures 2.176 and 2.177). A tangible macrophage is a typical example of such ingestion. Intracytoplasmic hemosiderin pigment is commonly seen within the pulmonary macrophages in cases of intra-alveolar hemorrhage. The pigment may be associated with inhalation of fumes and environmental elements. While melanin pigment may be seen in dermatopathic lymph node specimens, its presence in other localities may be

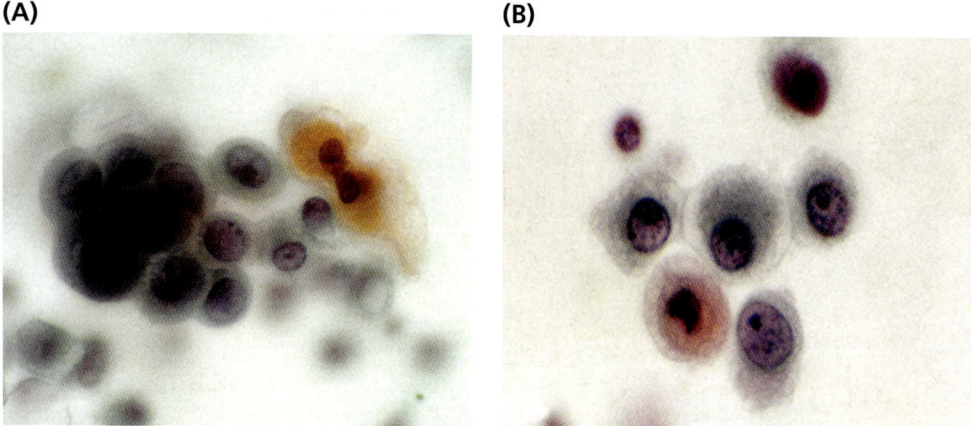

(A)   (B)

Figure 2.156 (A) Metaplastic mesothelial cells. (B) Adenocarcinoma breast pleural effusion. Tuberculosis under treatment, abdominal fluid. Millipore filter, Pap stain.

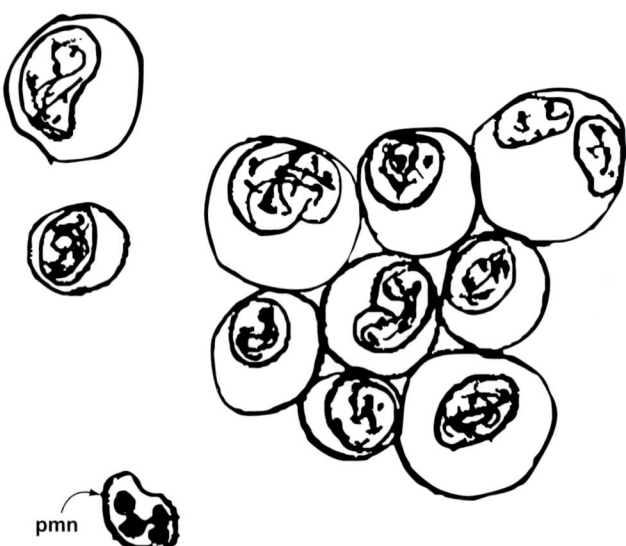

pmn

Figure 2.157 Line drawings depicting the morphology of macrophages. They are larger than a neutrophil, generally occur singly and are pleomorphic.

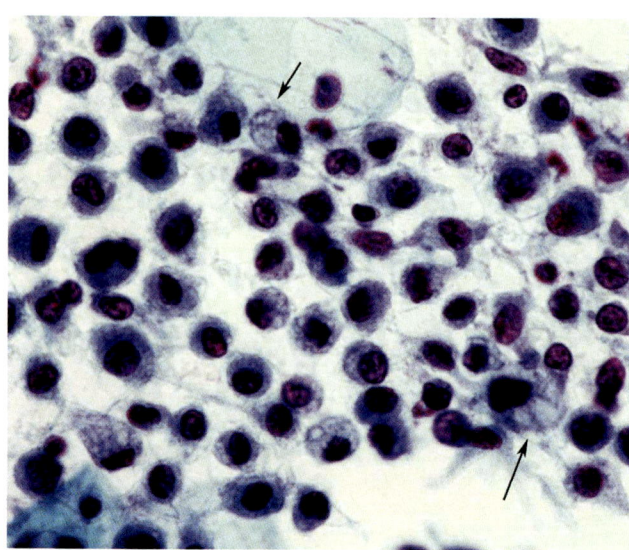

Figure 2.158 Group of histiocytes, notice the pleomorphism, N:C ratio, hyperchromasia, and cytoplasmic vacuolation (arrows). Vaginocervical smear, Pap stain.

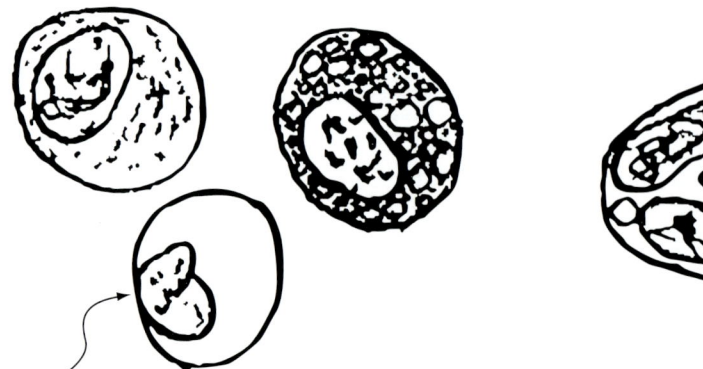

"Bouncing Off"

Figure 2.159 Line drawings showing the nuclear cytoplasmic relationship of the histocytic cells. Intracytoplasmic reticular appearance and ingestion are also depicted in these pictures.

(A)

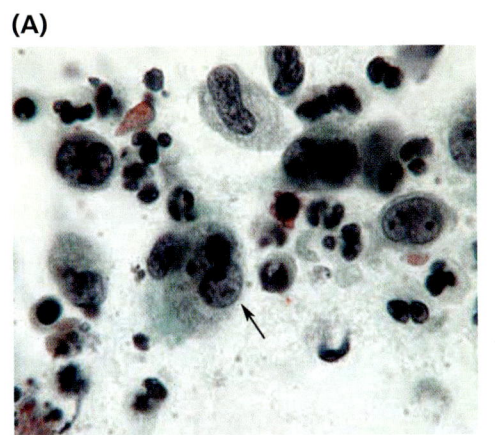

(B)

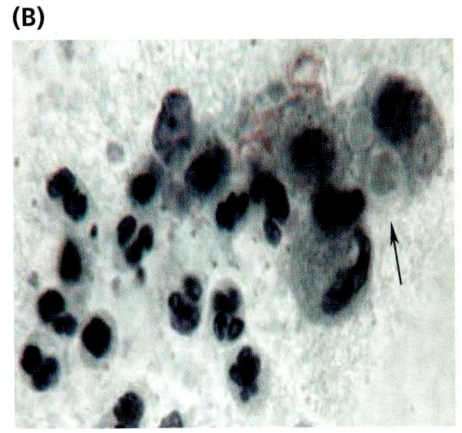

Figure 2.160 Macrophage (A) "bouncing off" the nuclear membrane (arrow), intracytoplasmic extraneous material (B) (arrow), bronchial wash specimen. Direct smear, Pap stain.

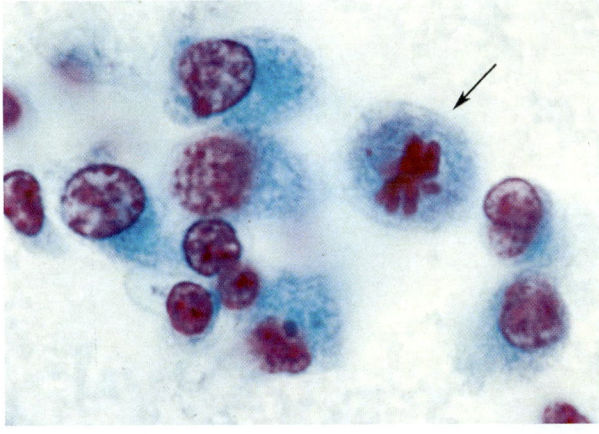

Figure 2.161 Histiocytes with epithelial cell appearance, note the mitosis (arrow), hyperchromasia, coarse chromatin, and prominent nucleoli; features commonly associated with neoplasia.

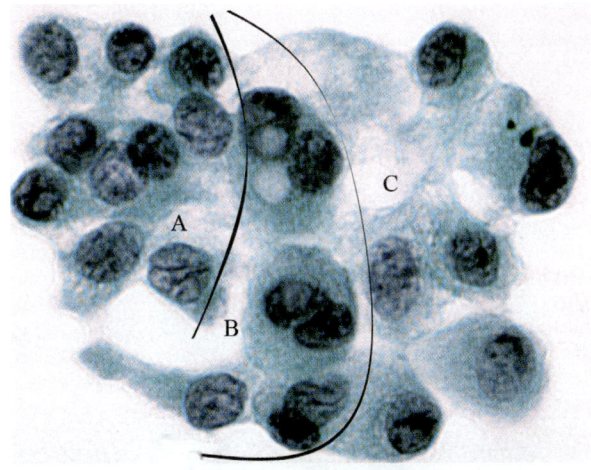

Figure 2.162 Morphologic similarity between neoplastic and histolytic cells. (A) represents a group of neoplastic epithelial cells, (B) shows cells that may pose diagnostic problems, and (C) represents histiocytic cells. Antibody studies are often helpful in such cases. Lung aspiration, direct smear, Pap stain.

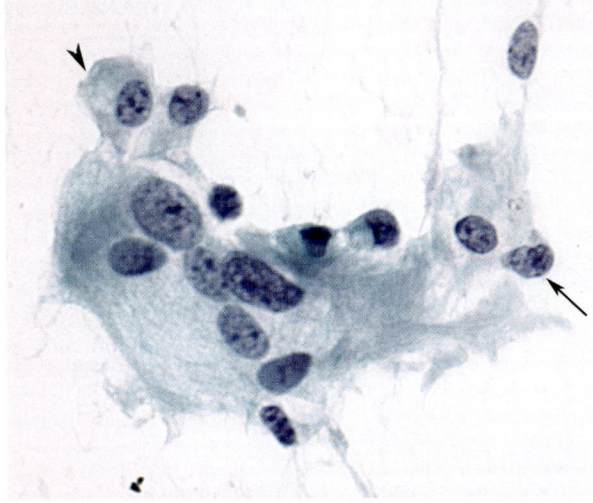

Figure 2.163 Histiocytic cells resembling mesenchymal cells. While the morphology is helpful (arrowhead), the nucleus is touching the cell membrane (arrow), and immunocytochemical stains are often helpful. Lung aspiration, direct smear, Pap smear.

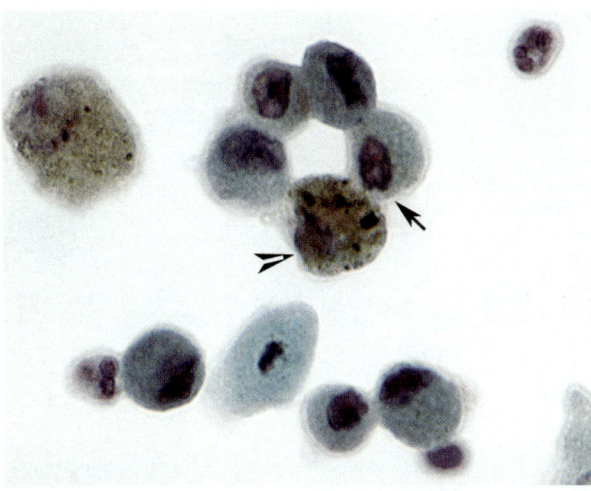

Figure 2.164 Type II pneumocytes (arrow), notice the cuboidal appearance with dense cytoplasm. Macrophages appear with pale nuclei and rarified cytoplasm (arrowhead). BAL specimen, ThinPrep slide.

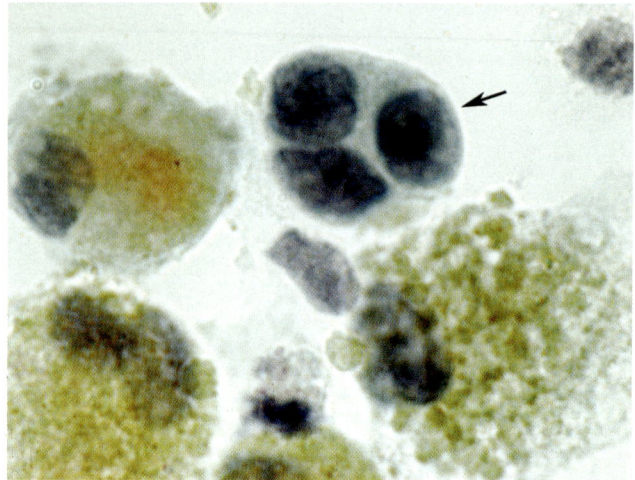

Figure 2.165 Pulmonary macrophages and a group of pneumocytes (arrow). BAL specimen, lung transplant, ThinPrep, Pap stain.

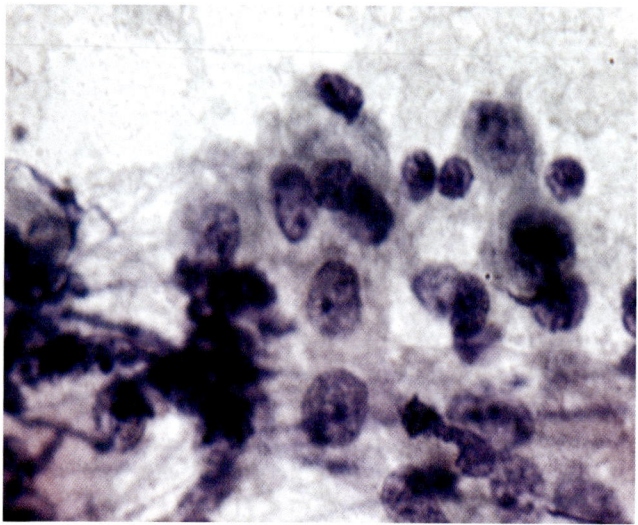

Figure 2.167 Epitheloid cells occurring as syncytial formation, lymph node aspiration, patient with sarcoidosis, Pap stain.

(A)

(B)

(C)

(D)

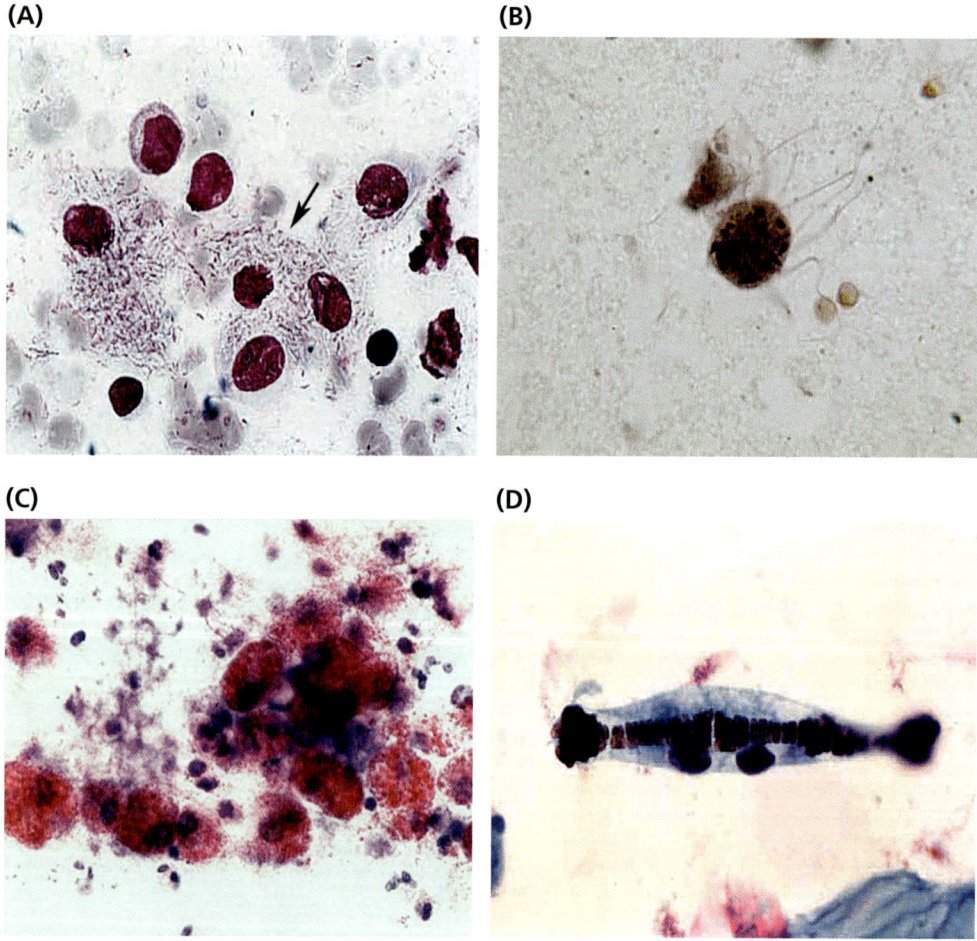

Figure 2.166 Macrophage functional activity. Notice the rather bland nuclei in these cells. Ingested atypical mycobacteria, lymph node fine needle aspiration (A), ingested spermatozoa, voided urine specimen, post prostectomy (B), ingested lipids, bronchial wash, lipid pneumonia lipid stain (C), ingested ferruginous body by two pulmonary macrophages (D). Pap stain.

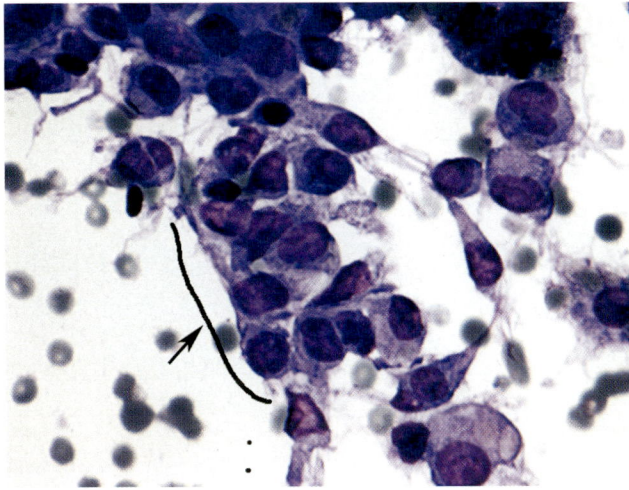

Figure 2.168 Thyroid aspiration specimen with a group of epitheloid cells (arrow). Diff-Quik stain.

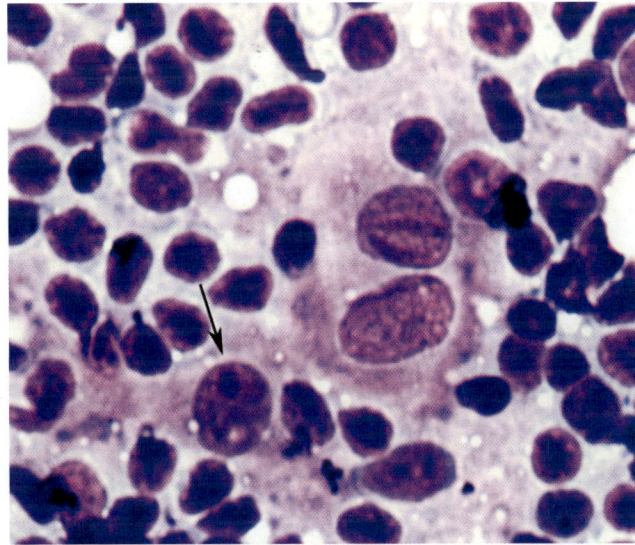

Figure 2.170 Atypical and bizarre histiocytic cells with prominent nucleolus (arrow). Neck node aspiration, patient with past history of squamous cell carcinoma of the tonsil.

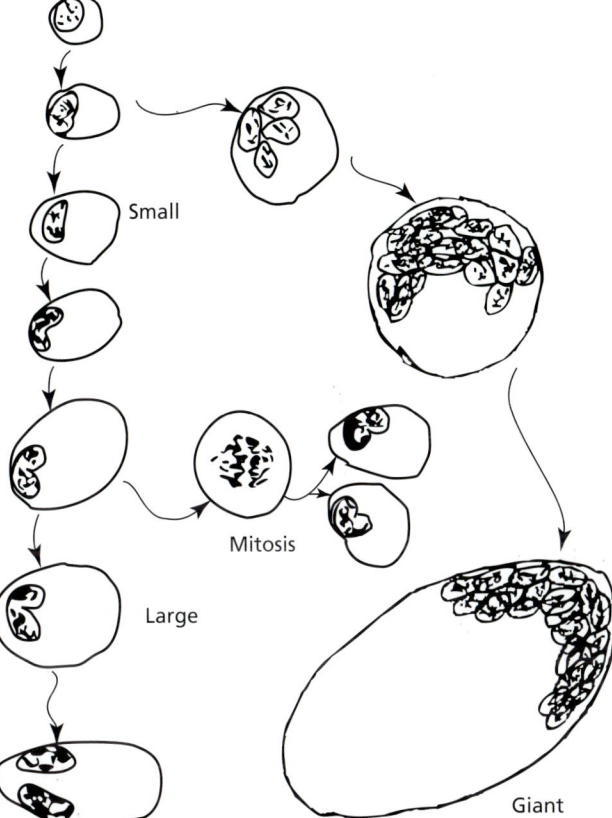

Figure 2.169 Line drawings depicting the reactive changes in macrophages.

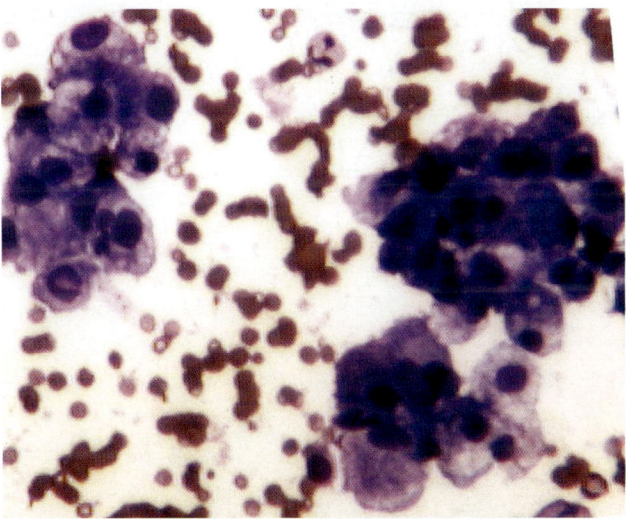

Figure 2.171 Foamy and atypical macrophages, neck lymph node aspiration, patient with history of papillary thyroid carcinoma. Direct smear, Diff-Quik stain.

MULTINUCLEATION

This is a common finding in histiocytes especially when certain types of debris and foreign bodies are encountered.

clinically important. Intracytoplasmic organisms including acid-fast bacilli, *Histoplasma*, and *Toxoplasma* are diagnostically important. It is important to recognize a histiocytic pseudo-syncytium as not a true single cell. Cytoplasmic inclusions bespeak the type of debris ingested. Carbon-bearing histiocytes ("dust" cells) are good evidence for a deeply raised sputum; hemosiderin-bearing histiocytes ("heart failure" cells) suggest old hemorrhage; when other cells have been phagocytosed, they are broken down in partial digestion: fat droplets ingested indicate tissue break down, or extrinsic fat (as in lipid pneumonia) (Figures 2.178, 2.179). Syncytial formation, asteroid, Schawman body, and various crystals may be helpful clinically (Figure 2.180).

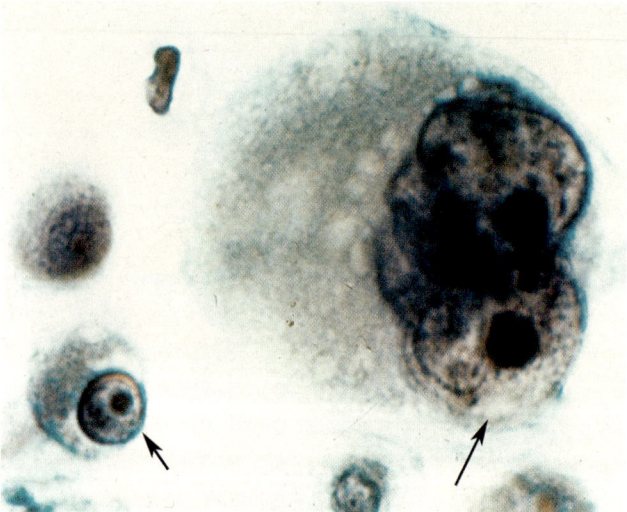

Figure 2.172 Pulmonary macrophage, notice the prominent nucleoli (arrows) and nuclear membrane changes. Case of pulmonary infarct. Sputum, direct smear, Pap stain.

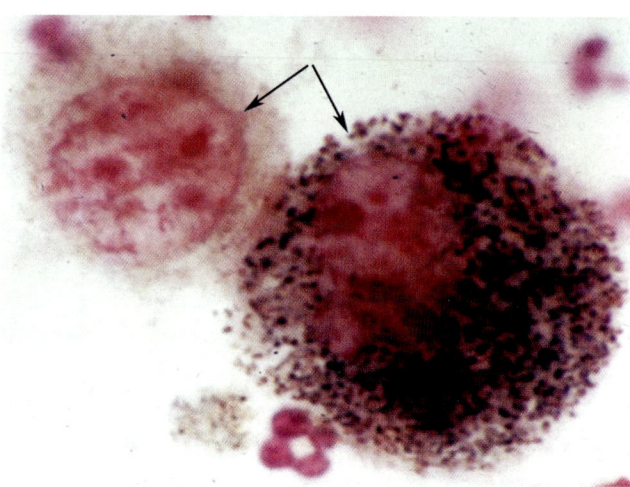

Figure 2.173 Pulmonary macrophage, notice the prominent nucleoli (arrows) and pale homogeneous chromatin. Same case as Figure 2.172, another sputum specimen, Pap stain.

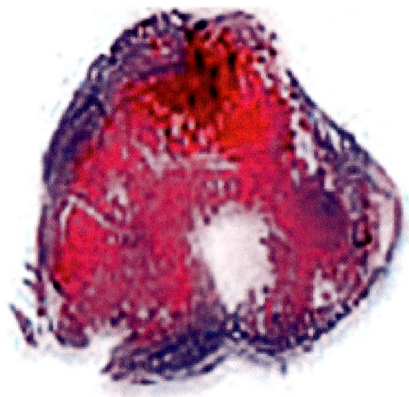

Figure 2.174 Full mount infracted lymph node following chemotherapy for squamous cell carcinoma of the tongue. H/E stain.

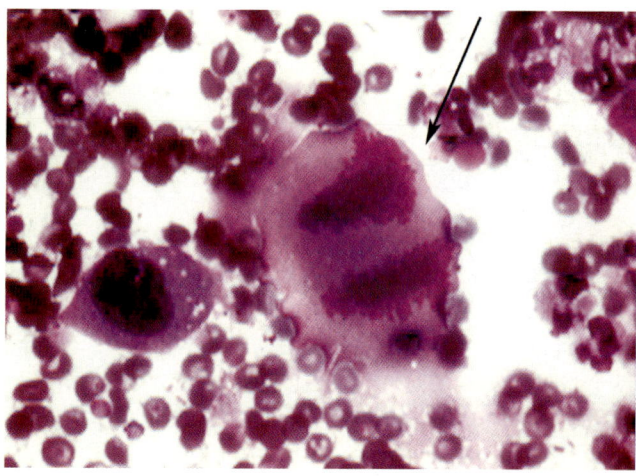

Figure 2.175 Mitosis (arrow) in a macrophage, reactive lymph node, neck fine needle aspiration. Diff-Quik stain.

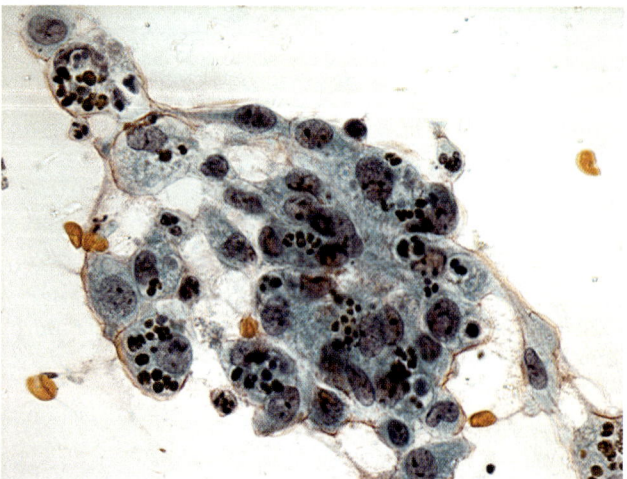

Figure 2.176 Macrophages with ingested nuclear debris in a case of chronic cervicitis. Vaginocervical smear, Pap stain.

It results in karyomegaly, binucleation or the multinucleation with foreign body giant cell formation. In addition, nuclear changes, essentially reactive in nature, are present. This results in creation of the small, large and multinucleated giant cell histiocytes that may resemble tumor giant cells, trophoblasts and other similar formations that may occur by processing and fixation techniques (Figures 2.180 and 2.182).

When histiocytes degenerate, their cytoplasmic borders become sticky and adhere to neighboring cells, lose their cellular borders, and form syncytia. As the cells making up this pseudo-syncytium were *firstly* individual cells (arising

(A)

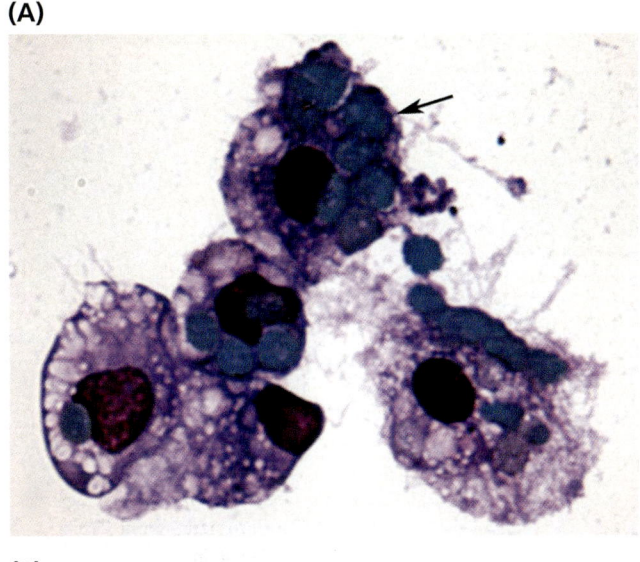

(B)

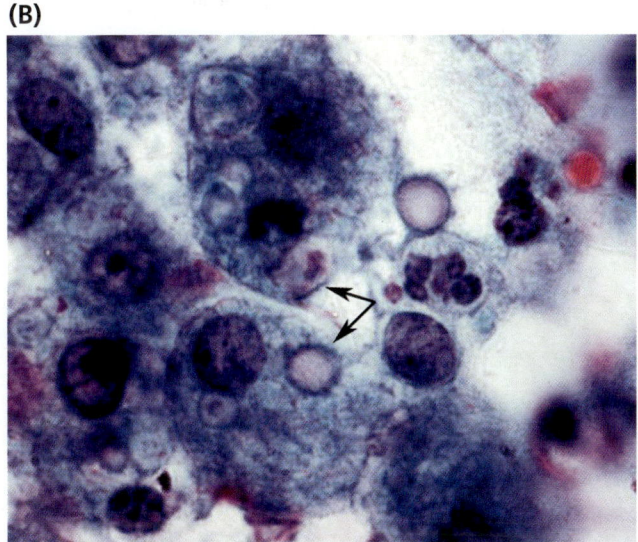

Figure 2.177 (A, B) Thyroid fine needle aspiration. (A) Macrophages containing thyroglobin droplets (arrow). Diff-Quik stain. (B) Macrophages containing Michaelis Gutmann bodies (arrows). Gastric brush specimen, Pap stain.

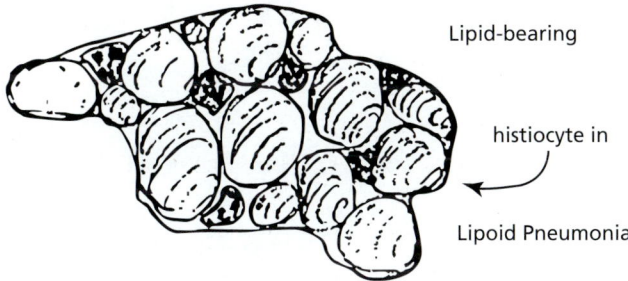

Lipid-bearing

histiocyte in

Lipoid Pneumonia

Figure 2.178 Line drawings showing the lipid-laden histiocytes in lipid pneumonia.

differently and reacting to different stimuli in different ways) and came together *secondly*, they may contain nuclei very different in development and appearance from each other (Figure 2.183).

(A)

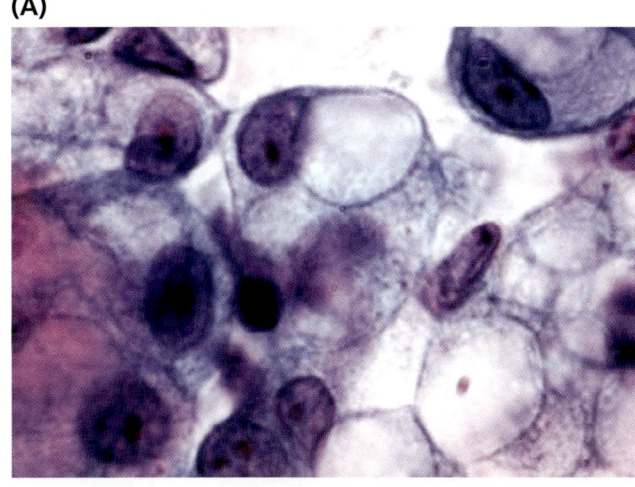

(B)

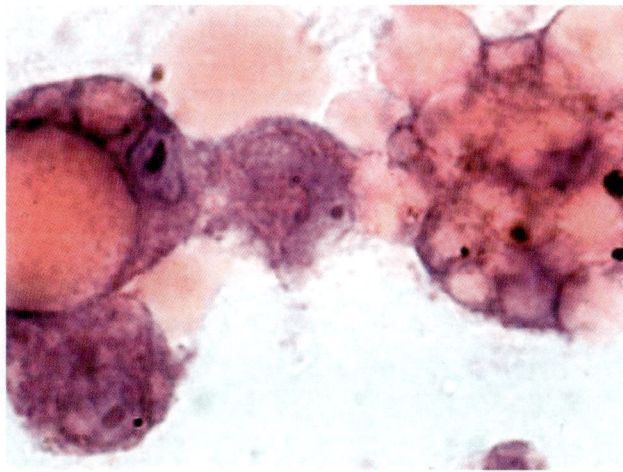

Figure 2.179 Pulmonary macrophages filled with lipid. (A) Pap stain, (B) lipid stain. Bronchial wash specimen.

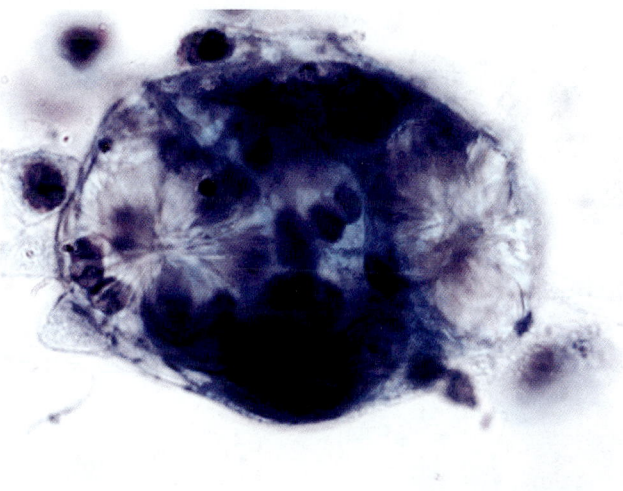

Figure 2.180 Intracytoplasmic oxalate crystals in a pulmonary specimen, patient with *Aspergillus* infection. Bronchial brush, direct smear, Pap stain.

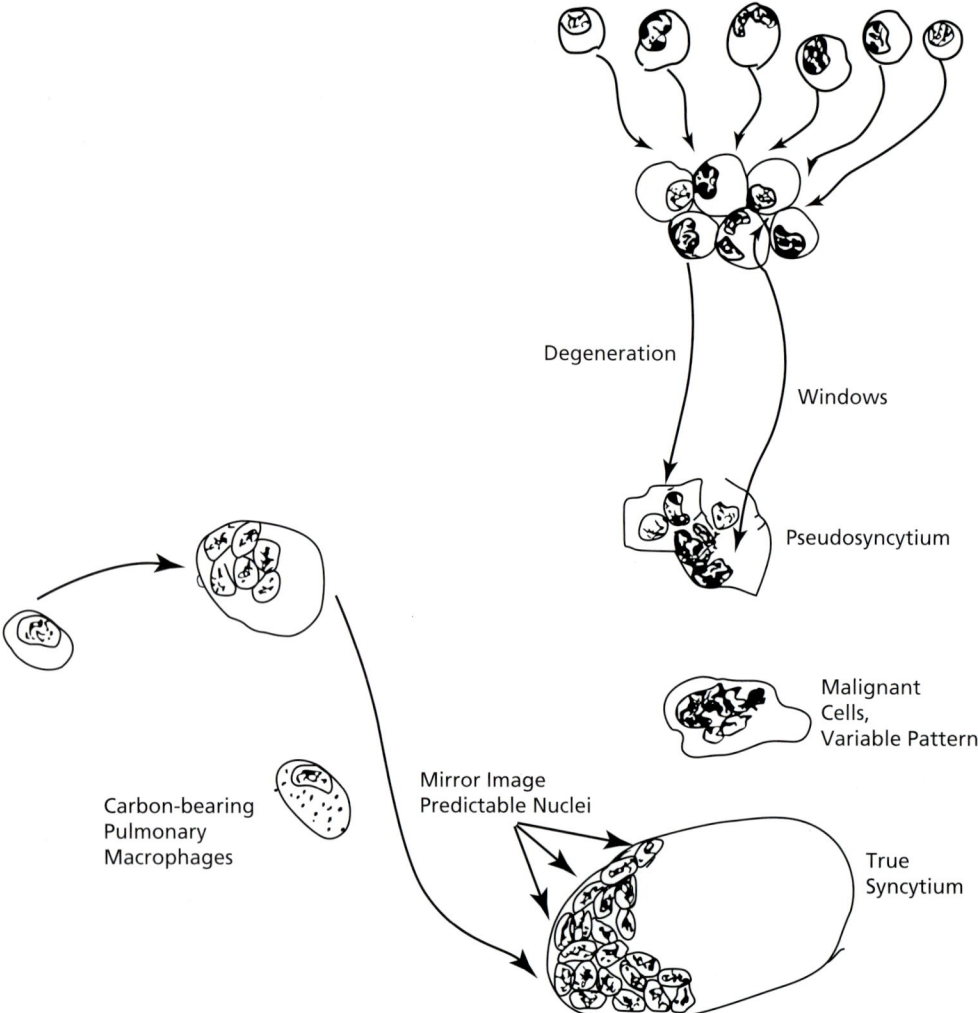

Degeneration

Windows

Pseudosyncytium

Malignant
Cells,
Variable Pattern

Carbon-bearing
Pulmonary
Macrophages

Mirror Image
Predictable Nuclei

True
Syncytium

Figure 2.181 Line drawings showing the development of giant cells. Degeneration and pseudosyncytium formation and degenerative changes that may result in similar appearances.

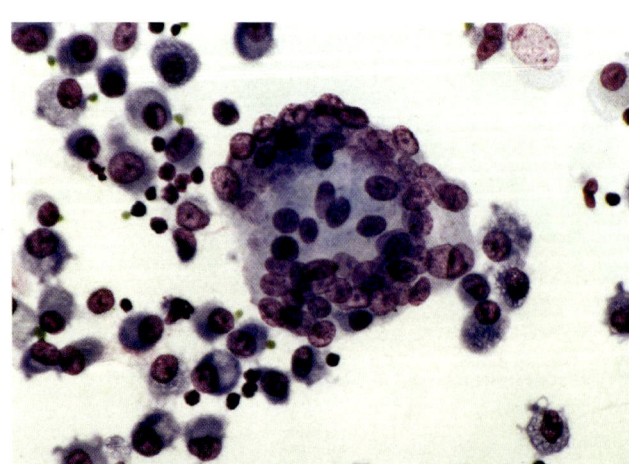

Figure 2.182 Multinucleated giant cell with nuclear syncytial formation case of pulmonary sarcoidosis. Bronchial brush specimen, Diff-Quik stain.

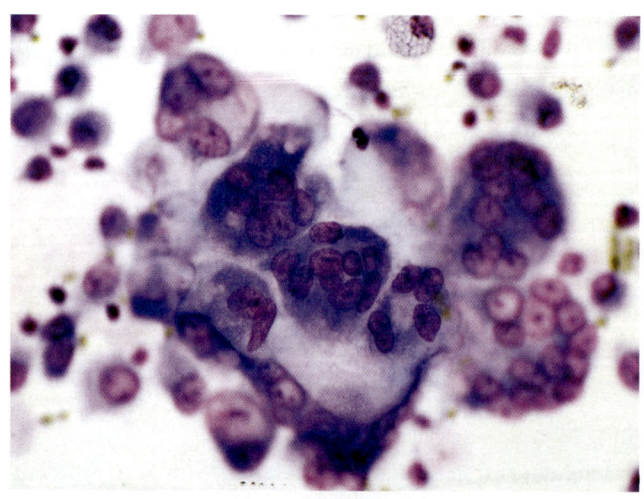

Figure 2.183 Multinucleated giant cells with degenerative cytoplasmic changes. Patient with Berylliosis. Bronchial lavage specimen, Pap stain.

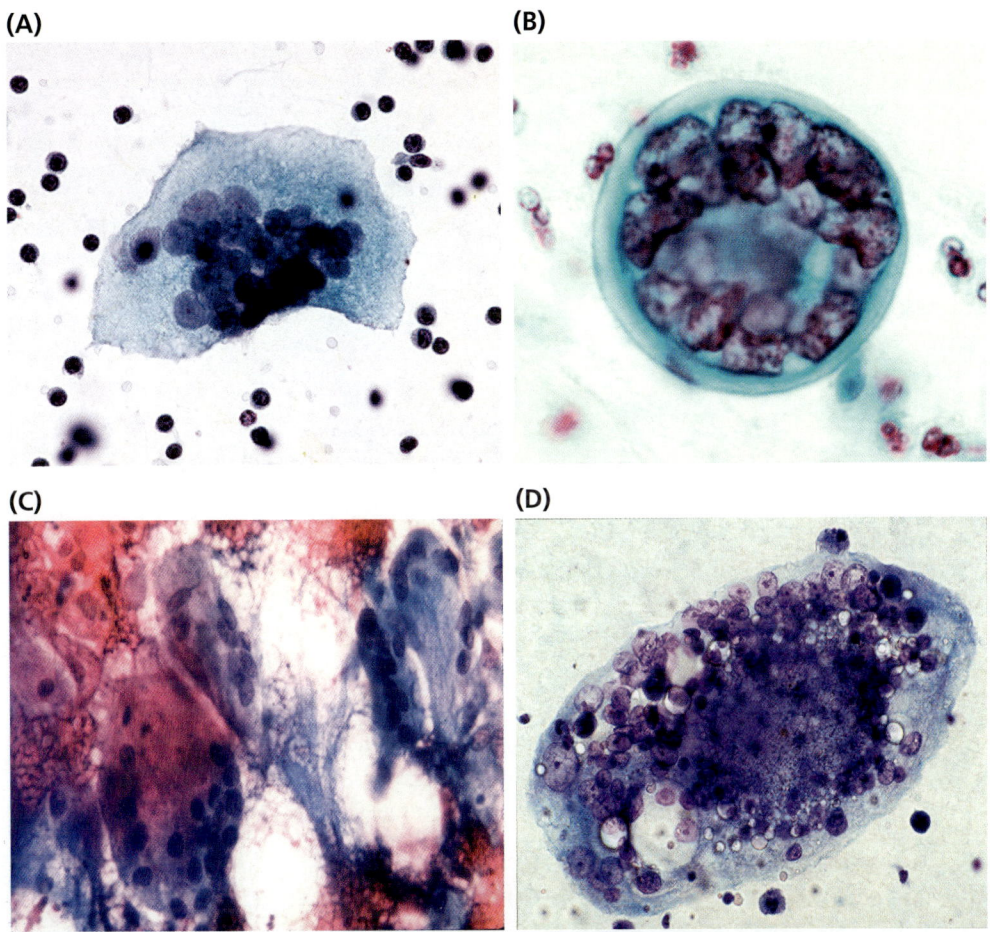

Figure 2.184 Composite of various types of multinucleated giant cells. (A) cells associated with viral pleural effusion, (B) single multinucleated cell of endometrial origin in a woman with prolonged IUD usage, (C) foreign body type multinucleated giant cell after IUD 3 weeks after IUD insertion, endometrial specimen, (D) foreign body type multinucleated giant cell, cerebrospinal fluid specimen 48 h after spinal interventional study.

It is important to recognize degenerated individual cells coming together secondarily; while a truly multinucleated giant histiocyte has "mirror-image" nuclei (chromatin pattern, size, shape), a good malignant criterion for a single malignant cell is to find multiple nuclei having greatly different patterns within the single cell (Figure 2.184).

FURTHER READING

Ahmed, M. N. (1987). *Urinary Tract Cytology.* New York, NY, Thieme Medical Publishers.

Ajit, D., S. B. Dighe, *et al.* (2006). "Cytology of ileal conduit urine in bladder cancer patients: diagnostic utility and pitfalls". *Acta Cytol* **50**(1): 70–3.

Akinwale, O. P., G. C. Oliveira, *et al.* (2008). "Squamous cell abnormalities in exfoliated cells from the urine of *Schistosoma haematobium*-infected adults in a rural fishing community in Nigeria". *World Health Popul* **10**(1): 18–22.

Al-Badri, A. and A. Pridmore. (2007). "An endocervical polyp with an unusual cytology finding". *Cytopathology* **18**(5): 316–8.

Alsharif, M., R. S. Andrade, *et al.* (2008). "Endobronchial ultrasound-guided transbronchial fine-needle aspiration: the University of Minnesota experience, with emphasis on usefulness, adequacy assessment, and diagnostic difficulties". *Am J Clin Pathol* **130**(3): 434–43.

Anagnostopoulou, I., R. Rammou-Kinia, *et al.* (1995). "Urine cytology evaluation in cases of uretero-ileal cutaneous diversion". *Cytopathology* **6**(4): 268–72.

Bhadani, P. P., M. C. Sharma, *et al.* (2004). "Paget's disease of the nipple diagnosed on cytology: a case report". *Indian J Pathol Microbiol* **47**(2): 246–8.

Bhagavan, B. S. and P. K. Gupta. (1978). "Genital actinomycosis and intrauterine contraceptive devices. Cytopathologic diagnosis and clinical significance". *Hum Pathol* **9**(5): 567–78.

Boldorini, R., M. Brustia, *et al.* (2005). "Periodic assessment of urine and serum by cytology and molecular biology as a diagnostic tool for BK virus nephropathy in renal transplant patients". *Acta Cytol* **49**(3): 235–43.

Boon, M. E., F. M. van Dunne, *et al.* (1995). "Recognition of atypical reserve cell hyperplasia in cervical smears and its diagnostic significance". *Mod Pathol* **8**(7): 786–94.

Bourne, G. H., International Society for Cell Biology, *et al.* (1952). *International Review of Cytology.* New York, NY, Academic Press.

Bulten, J., P. C. de Wilde, *et al.* (2000). "Proliferation in 'atypical' atrophic pap smears". *Gynecol Oncol* **79**(2): 225–9.

Burja, I. T., S. K. Thompson, *et al.* (1999). "Atypical glandular cells of undetermined significance on cervical smears. A study with cytohistologic correlation". *Acta Cytol* **43**(3): 351–6.

Chen, K. T. (1995). "Cytodiagnostic pitfalls in pulmonary coccidioidomycosis". *Diagn Cytopathol* **12**(2): 177–80.

Chien, C. R., L. L. Ting, *et al.* (2005). "Post-radiation Pap smear for Chinese patients with cervical cancer: a ten-year follow-up". *Eur J Gynaecol Oncol* **26**(6): 619–22.

Cibas, E. S. and B. S. Ducatman. (2009). *Cytology: Diagnostic Principles and Clinical Correlates.* Philadelphia, PA, Saunders Elsevier.

Connolly, T. P. and A. C. Evans. (2005). "Atypical Papanicolaou smear in pregnancy". *Clin Med Res* **3**(1): 13–8.

Davidson, B., B. Risberg, *et al.* (2003). "Effusion cytology in ovarian cancer: new molecular methods as aids to diagnosis and prognosis". *Clin Lab Med* **23**(3): 729–54, viii.

Demay, R. M. (2000). "Hyperchromatic crowded groups: pitfalls in pap smear diagnosis". *Am J Clin Pathol* **114**(Suppl): S36–43.

Ducatman, B. S., H. H. Wang, *et al.* (1993). "Tubal metaplasia: a cytologic study with comparison to other neoplastic and non-neoplastic conditions of the endocervix". *Diagn Cytopathol* **9**(1): 98–103; discussion 103–05.

Ehya, H. (1991). "Effusion cytology". *Clin Lab Med* **11**(2): 443–67.

Elsheikh, T. M., J. L. Kirkpatrick, *et al.* (2006). "Comparison of Thin-Prep and cytospin preparations in the evaluation of exfoliative cytology specimens." *Cancer* **108**(3): 144–9.

Emerson, R. E., M. L. Randolph, *et al.* (2006). "Endoscopic ultrasound-guided fine-needle aspiration cytology diagnosis of intraductal papillary mucinous neoplasm of the pancreas is highly predictive of pancreatic neoplasia". *Diagn Cytopathol* **34**(7): 457–62.

Filotico, M. and S. Grasso. (1981). "Atypical reserve cell hyperplasia of cervical glands, simulating adenocarcinoma. An undescribed reversible lesion in a woman taking oral contraceptives". *Tumori* **67**(5): 491–6.

Gupta, R. K., D. Gaskell, *et al.* (2004). "The role of nipple discharge cytology in the diagnosis of breast disease: a study of 1948 nipple discharge smears from 1530 patients". *Cytopathology* **15**(6): 326–30.

Harshan, M., J. P. Crapanzano, *et al.* (2009). "Papillary thyroid carcinoma with atypical histiocytoid cells on fine-needle aspiration". *Diagn Cytopathol* **37**(4): 244–50.

Hata, S., Y. Mikami, *et al.* (2002). "Diagnostic significance of endocervical glandular cells with 'golden-yellow' mucin on pap smear". *Diagn Cytopathol* **27**(2): 80–4.

Hayhoe, F. G. J., R. J. Flemans, *et al.* (1982). *Color Atlas of Hematological Cytology.* New York, NY, Wiley.

Herzberg, A. J., D. S. Raso, *et al.* (1999). *Color Atlas of Normal Cytology.* New York, NY, Churchill Livingstone.

Hoda, R. S. and S. A. Hoda. (2007). *Fundamentals of Pap Test Cytology.* Totowa, NJ, Humana Press.

Hwang, E. C., S. H. Park, *et al.* (2007). "Usefulness of liquid-based preparation in urine cytology". *Int J Urol* **14**(7): 626–9.

Kanbour, A. and N. Doshi. (1980). "Psammoma bodies and detached ciliary tufts in a cervicovaginal smear associated with benign ovarian cystadenofibroma". *Acta Cytol* **24**(6): 549–52.

Kazerooni, T. and A. Mosalaee. (2002). "Does contraceptive method change the Pap smear finding?" *Contraception* **66**(4): 243–6.

Kelten, C., M. Akbulut, *et al.* (2009). "Signet ring cells in fine needle aspiration cytology of breast carcinomas: review of the

cytological findings in ten cases identified by histology". *Cytopathology* **20**(5): 321–7.

Kline, T. S. (1981). *Handbook of Fine Needle Aspiration Biopsy Cytology.* St. Louis, MO, C.V. Mosby.

Kobayashi, T. K., M. Ueda, *et al.* (1997). "Scrape cytology of pemphigus vulgaris of the nipple, a mimicker of Paget's disease". *Diagn Cytopathol* **16**(2): 156–9.

Kobayashi, T. K., M. Ueda, *et al.* (1998). "Brush cytology of herpes simplex virus infection in oral mucosa: use of the ThinPrep processor". *Diagn Cytopathol* **18**(1): 71–5.

Koss, L. G., M. R. Melamed, *et al.* (2006). *Koss' Diagnostic Cytology and its Histopathologic Bases.* Philadelphia, PA, Lippincott Williams & Wilkins.

Koukoulaki, M., M. O'Donovan, *et al.* (2008). "Prospective study of urine cytology screening for BK polyoma virus replication in renal transplant recipients". *Cytopathology* **19**(6): 385–8.

Laucirica, R. and M. L. Ostrowski. (2007). "Cytology of nonneoplastic occupational and environmental diseases of the lung and pleura". *Arch Pathol Lab Med* **131**(11): 1700–08.

Lee, A., Z. W. Baloch, *et al.* (2000). "Mesothelial hyperplasia with reactive atypia: diagnostic pitfalls and role of immunohistochemical studies – a case report". *Diagn Cytopathol* **22**(2): 113–6.

Leung, K. M., W. Y. Chan, *et al.* (1994). "Invasive squamous cell carcinoma and cervical intraepithelial neoplasia III of uterine cervix. Morphologic differences other than stromal invasion". *Am J Clin Pathol* **101**(4): 508–13.

Macfarlane, E. W., G. H. Ceelen, *et al.* (1964). "Urine cytology after treatment of bladder tumors". *Acta Cytol* **8**: 288–92.

Malik, S. N., E. J. Wilkinson, *et al.* (2001). "Benign cellular changes in Pap smears. Causes and significance". *Acta Cytol* **45**(1): 5–8.

McKee, G. T. (2004). *Atlas of Gynecologic Cytology.* London, Taylor & Francis.

Montz, F. J. (2001). "Significance of 'normal' endometrial cells in cervical cytology from asymptomatic postmenopausal women receiving hormone replacement therapy". *Gynecol Oncol* **81**(1): 33–9.

Mori, M., Y. Imamura, *et al.* (2003). "Cytology of pleural effusion associated with disseminated infection caused by varicella-zoster virus in an immunocompromised patient. A case report". *Acta Cytol* **47**(3): 480–4.

Murugan, P., N. Siddaraju, *et al.* (2008). "Significance of intercellular spaces (windows) in effusion fluid cytology: a study of 46 samples". *Diagn Cytopathol* **36**(9): 628–32.

Nassar, A., P. Gupta, *et al.* (2003). "Histiocytic aggregates in benign nodular goiters mimicking cytologic features of papillary thyroid carcinoma (PTC)". *Diagn Cytopathol* **29**(5): 243–5.

Owens, C. L. and S. Z. Ali. (2005). "Atypical squamous cells in exfoliative urinary cytology: clinicopathologic correlates". *Diagn Cytopathol* **33**(6): 394–8.

Papanicolaou, G. N. (1954). *Atlas of Exfoliative Cytology.* Cambridge, MA, Published for the Commonwealth Fund by Harvard University Press.

Papanicolaou, G. N., E. L. Bridges, *et al.* (1961). "Degeneration of the ciliated cells of the bronchial epithelium (ciliocytophthoria) in its relation to pulmonary disease". *Am Rev Respir Dis* **83**: 641–59.

Patton, A. L., L. Duncan, *et al.* (2008). "Atypical squamous cells cannot exclude a high-grade intraepithelial lesion and its clinical significance in postmenopausal, pregnant, postpartum, and contraceptive-use patients". *Cancer* **114**(6): 481–8.

Pitman, M. B. and V. Deshpande. (2007). "Endoscopic ultrasound-guided fine needle aspiration cytology of the pancreas: a morphological and multimodal approach to the diagnosis of solid and cystic mass lesions". *Cytopathology* **18**(6): 331–47.

Renshaw, A. A. (2005). *Aspiration Cytology*. Philadelphia, PA, Elsevier Saunders.

Saad, R. S., A. Kanbour-Shakir, *et al.* (2006). "Cytomorphologic analysis and histological correlation of high-grade squamous intraepithelial lesions in postmenopausal women". *Diagn Cytopathol* **34**(7): 467–71.

Shih, S. R., H. Y. Li, *et al.* (2006). "Prognostic significance of cytologic features in fine-needle aspiration cytology samples of papillary thyroid carcinoma: preliminary report". *Thyroid* **16**(8): 775–80.

Sidawy, M. K. and S. Z. Ali. (2007). *Fine Needle Aspiration Cytology*. Philadelphia, PA, Churchill Livingstone Elsevier.

Touijer, A. K. and G. Dalbagni. (2004). "Role of voided urine cytology in diagnosing primary urethral carcinoma". *Urology* **63**(1): 33–5.

Tweeddale, D. N. (1977). *Urinary Cytology*. Boston, MA, Little, Brown.

Wang, N., S. N. Emancipator, *et al.* (2002). "Histologic follow-up of atypical endocervical cells. Liquid-based, thin-layer preparation vs. conventional Pap smear". *Acta Cytol* **46**(3): 453–7.

Zajicek, J. (1974). *Aspiration Biopsy Cytology, Part 1: Cytology of Supradiaphragmatic Organs*. Basel, S. Karger.

3 MALIGNANT CELL MORPHOLOGY

GENERAL PERSPECTIVE

The morphologic findings referred to in this chapter as "malignant criteria" are those changes which, when found together in a recognized pattern, have been most useful for identifying malignant cells in cytological material. It must be recognized that there is a constellation of morphologic changes that help in diagnosis. Most commonly, this interpretation is critically influenced by clinical and relevant information. There is no single cytologic feature which, by itself, unequivocally indicates malignancy; nor is there a cytologic change which, when absent, bespeaks benignancy.

One must be careful not to include a cellular finding as a malignant criterion only because it happens to be present in a cell known to be malignant. As far as possible, the criteria should exclusively be observed using malignant cells with minimal overlap with benign conditioning. It is necessary to employ an extremely conservative approach in malignancy diagnosis; specifically, is more important than specificity. To quote the late Dr. Frost,

> It being my philosophy that we should strive for a cytologic unequivocal diagnosis of malignancy having the reliability of a tissue diagnosis. Only this unequivocally cancer group, do I call "Positive" in my own practice (0.8% of Gyn-Ob patients). To the normal or bizarre benign group, I refer as "Negative" (95.4%). Then there is the group containing the "shaded" lesions, (3.8%).

A malignant diagnosis is based upon the evaluation of multiple parameters. These include clinical history, relevant investigational studies, precise location of the lesion, manner of specimen collection, and processing. While a population is "screened," a cytoslide/preparation is examined, evaluated, and interpreted in view of the above enumerated features. We detect and diagnose an underlying pathological lesion based upon the cytomorphology and integration of the numerous factors mentioned before. All necessary resources must be utilized to develop a meaningful interpretation valuable to the patient and health care providers. A number of important clinical and life and death management decisions are made upon cyto diagnosis. This is especially applicable to non-gynecologic specimens, tumor recurrences, effect of therapy, and follow-up studies. The value of ancillary investigation and or cyto-histo correlation in this regard cannot be overemphasized. While evaluating and diagnosing single cell abnormalities, microbiopsies and tissue groups, cell accompaniments, specimen gross appearance, slide background, and all relevant resources should be utilized to provide an accurate and correct diagnosis, always cognizant of the fact that there is a person dependent upon this report.

Regardless of the reporting system, it is communication with other health care providers that is pivotal in cytodiagnosis; however, this should not become a wastebasket for indecision. The pathologist must always strive to place his report in either the "cancer" or "no cancer" category within his experience and the quality of the specimen. In other words, we do *not* have a mandate to say "cancer" or "no cancer" on every case, in either cellular or tissue pathology, but should reserve the right to say "we do not know" or "it may be becoming cancer." Only those morphologic features which discriminate well will be referred to herein as malignant criteria.

The quality of cellular preparations is the single most important factor in the evaluation, interpretation, and diagnosis of cancer. First and foremost, malignant criteria found in *well preserved* cells are most diagnostic. Disregard for this one feature is the greatest cause for false cancer diagnoses.

Cytohistology: Essential and Basic Concepts, Prabodh Gupta and Zubair Baloch. Published by Cambridge University Press. © Cambridge University Press 2011.

MALIGNANT CELL CHANGES

Malignancy is a growth disorder and nuclear changes form the linchpin of cancer diagnosis. Rarely, cytoplasmic features may help in such cancer diagnoses. Three major "trends" run through the most valuable malignant criteria. For normally regularly occurring structures, these are to be found in a pattern of *irregularity* (nuclear shapes, chromatin patterns, etc.), *sharp angularity* (chromatin clumps, nucleoli, etc.) and *extremes* (N:C ratio, thickness of nuclear membrane, etc.).

Nucleus (classic)

The nucleus is the conductor of the cell orchestra. It controls, determines and displays its growth activity. Cytoplasm, on the other hand, provides the functional differentiation of the cell. The nucleus showcases the diagnostic features of malignancy, whereas cytoplasm determines the differentiation or the type of malignancy, e.g. squamous, glandular, neuroglial, mesenchymal, and others.

As students of cytopathology, we have been primed to consider the following features as hallmarks of malignancy.

High N:C ratio

High N:C ratio in cytopathology does not have the same diagnostic connotation as in paraffin-processed tissue slides fixed by aldelydes (formalin). A high N:C ratio in small cells (<4 lymphocytes) generally should not be used as a feature of malignancy (Figures 3.1 and 3.2a,b). It is important to appreciate that this feature may not be used as the single criterion for the diagnosis of malignancy.

Although often seen in malignant nuclei, a high N:C ratio may occur in benign lesions. Intranuclear inclusion of BK virus-infected urothelial cells is a classic example. In

Malignant Features: N/C Ratio

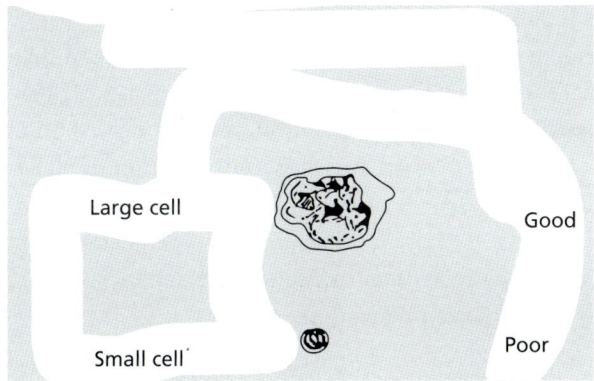

Figure 3.1 This line drawing depicts the value of high nucleocytoplasmic ratio; it is important as a diagnostic feature only among large cells.

(A)

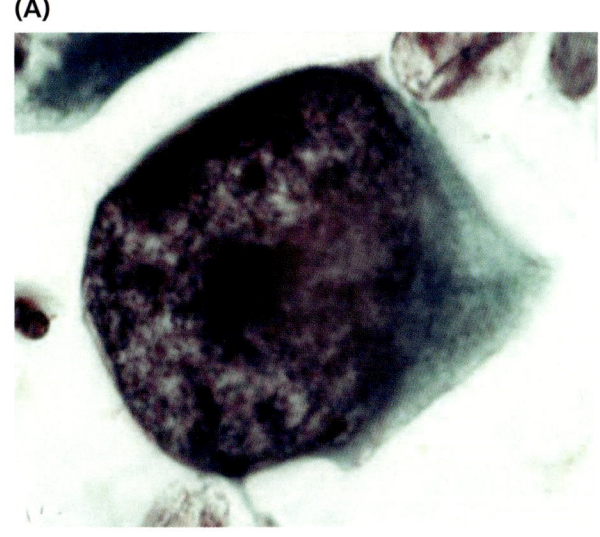

(B)

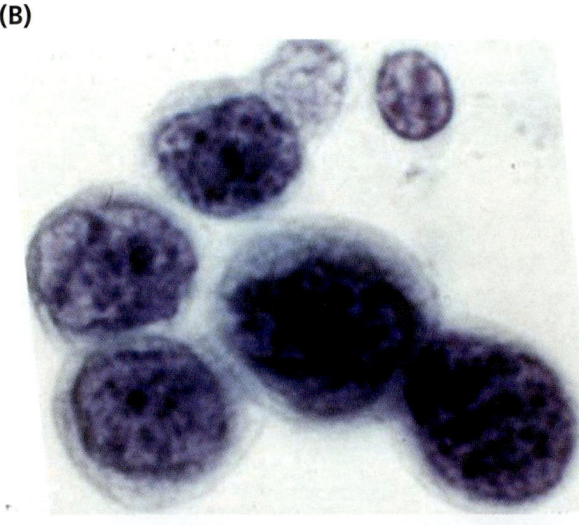

(C)

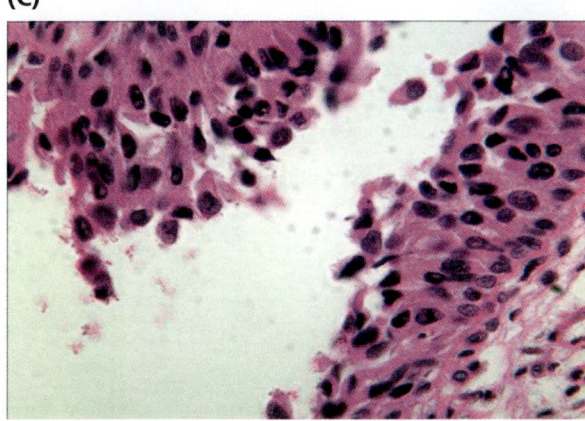

Figure 3.2 (A–C) These two pictures in composite reveal high N:C ratio malignant cells. The single cell in (A) has scant cytoplasm, hyperchromasia, and some malignant nuclear changes. (B) shows a group of well-preserved high N:C ratio cells. Notice the associated nuclear membrane and chromatin changes. Lung FNA (A), direct smear, bladder wash (B), Millipore filter. Pap stain. (C) Represents the corresponding urinary bladder biopsy, H/E stain.

(A)

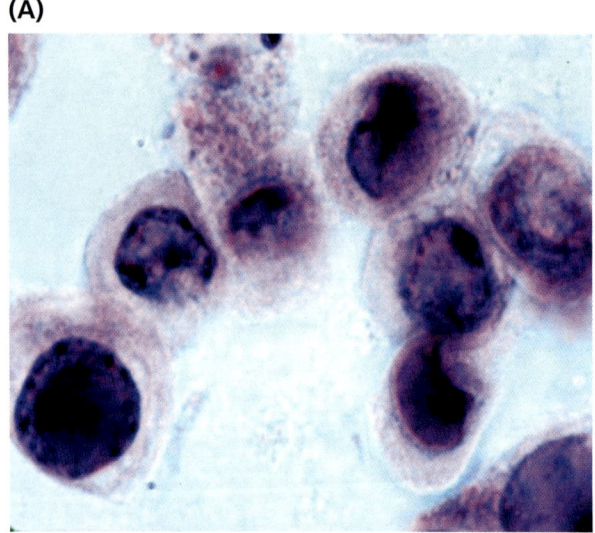

(B)

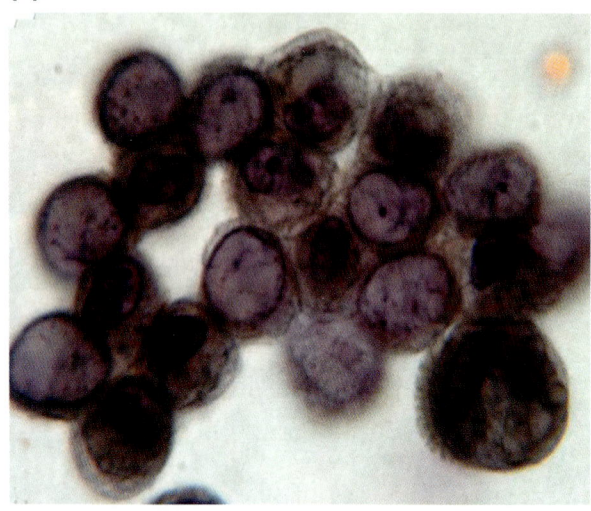

(C)

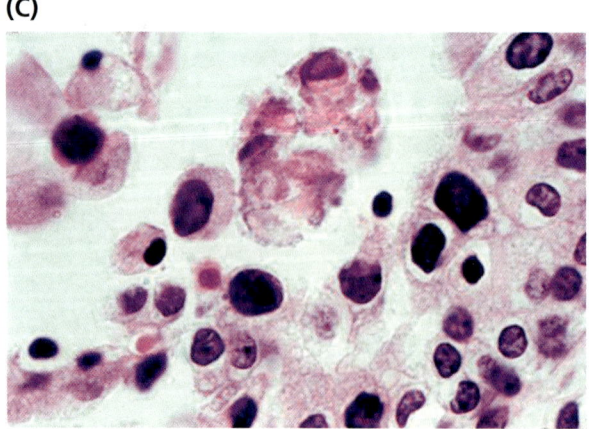

Figure 3.3 (A–C) (A) depicts a group of urothelial cells infected with BK virus. Notice the high N:C ratios and hyperchromasia. (B) shows a group of epithelial cells infected with BK virus showing high N:C ratios. Renal transplant cases, voided urine, Millipore filter, Pap stain. (C) represents the corresponding urinary bladder biopsy, H/E stain.

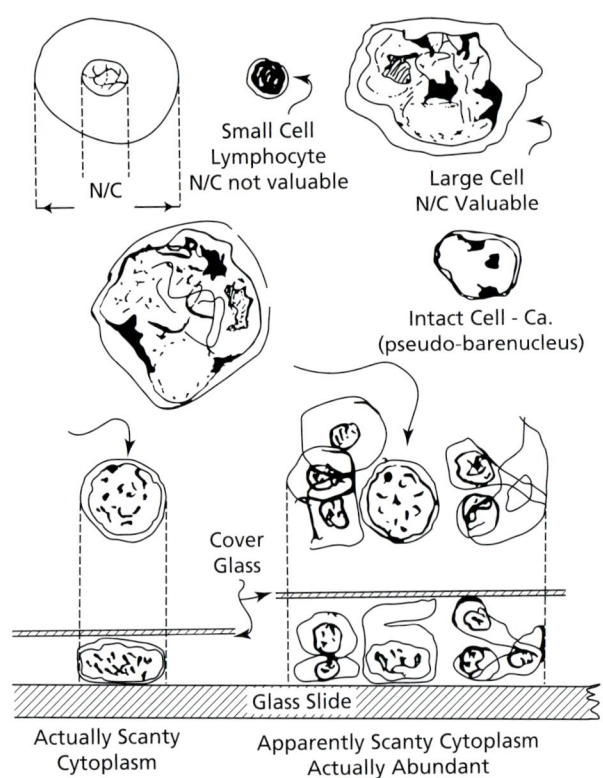

Figure 3.4 Line drawings depicting the vertical disposition of cytoplasm and the value of high N:C ratio.

fact, these cells infected with the polyoma virus were dubbed as "decoy cells," as they are morphologically similar to the urothelial carcinoma in-situ cells (Figure 3.2a,b, 3.3). Similar nucleocytoplasmic changes can be observed with adenovirus infection affecting epithelial cells.

When occurring on-end or within a mass of cells or debris, cells can appear to have high N:C ratios. Adequate cytoplasm may lie above or below such a nucleus, while the cytoplasmic profile about the nuclear rim may appear to be scanty. It is important to focus up and down, to establish a true feeling for this third dimension. Cells fixed before spreading appear falsely to have a scantier cytoplasm than fresh cells spread and then fixed (Figures 3.4–3.6). Bare nuclei represent poor preparation and cell degeneration and should not be used as a diagnostic criterion of malignancy (Figure 3.7). It is true that certain neoplastic processes, such as those of hepatobiliary, alimentary, and respiratory systems, may reveal a large number of bare nuclei in cytologic preparations.

Nuclear chromasia

Although hyperchromasia is often seen among malignant nuclei, a number of aggressive and high-grade epithelial

(A)

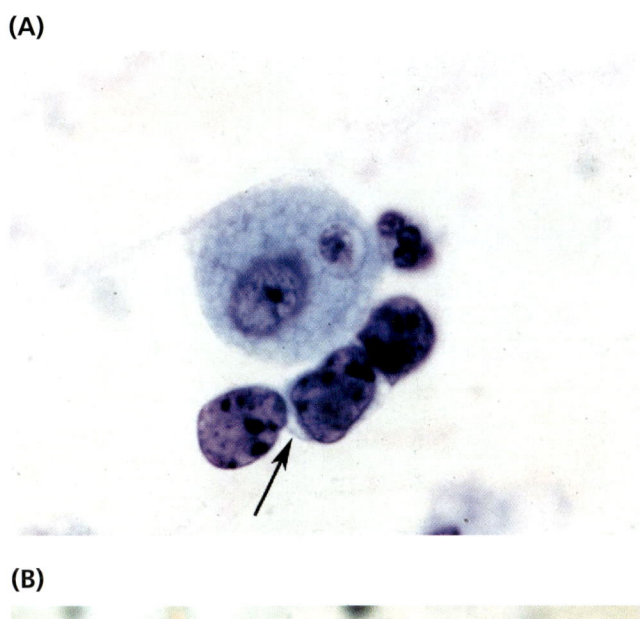

(B)

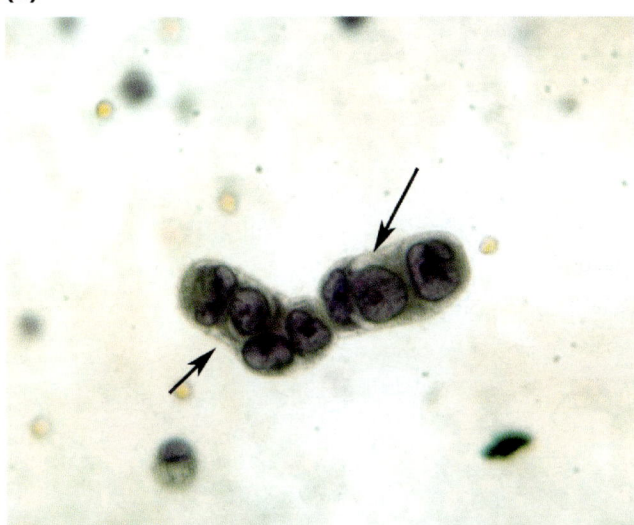

Figure 3.5 Small-cell carcinoma lung, note the scant cytoplasm (A, arrows), sputum specimen, direct smear, neuroendocrine carcinoma (B), notice the scant cytoplasm(arrows). FNA pancreas, Millipore filter, pap stain. Such morphologic details may not be always recognizable in prefixed specimens.

malignant cells often present with pale, normochromic or hypochromic nuclei (Figure 3.8). Adenocarcinomas of the hepatobiliary, genitourinary, and pulmonary tracts often appear pale and hypochromatic. Similarly, thyroid papillary tumors may reveal comparable nuclear features.

Mitosis

Mitosis is often used as an indicator of malignancy. "Normal" mitoses occur more commonly in non-neoplastic, reactive and reparative processes and have no diagnostic value in cytological specimens. "Abnormal" mitosis, however, offers a good criterion of malignancy. In the body cavity fluids abnormal mitosis can be occasionally

Cytoplasmic Features

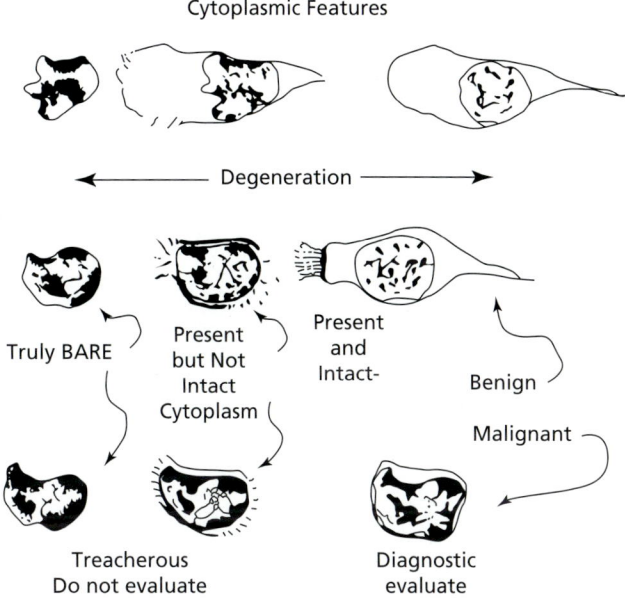

Figure 3.6 The pitfalls of evaluation of cells with varying degrees of cytoplasmic degeneration and bare nuclei. It is critical that only well-preserved cells be examined for cytodiagnoses. Varying degrees of these changes are often seen in poor quality specimens and may be over-interpreted.

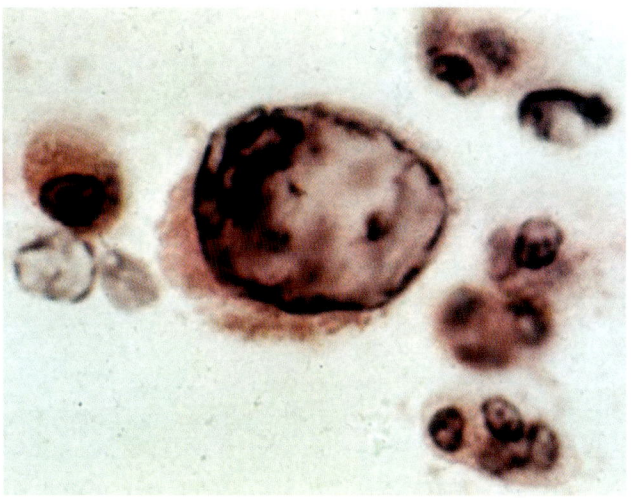

Figure 3.7 Degenerated bronchial cell with a shroud of cytoplasm. High N:C ratio and nuclear changes closely mimic malignant transformation. Sputum specimen, direct smear, Pap stain.

observed in reactive and non-neoplastic processes (Figures 3.9–3.12). Cells stored in preservative sometimes continue to go through the replication cycle and exhibit increased mitotic activity; these are of limited diagnostic value.

Nuclear characteristics

In a well-preserved (discussed below) and representative cell, a number of nuclear characteristics must be carefully

(A)

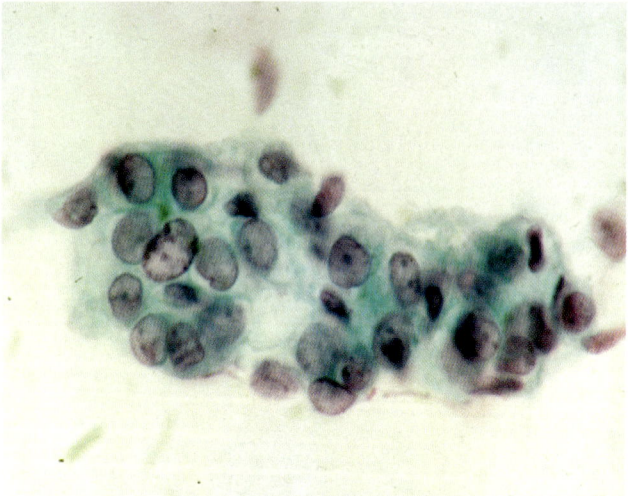

(B)

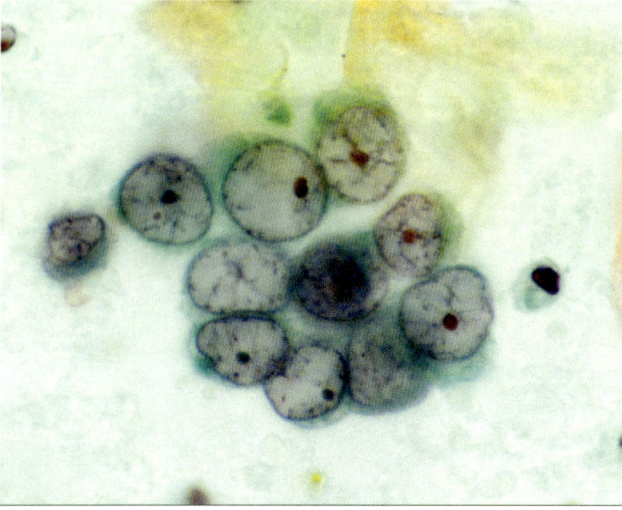

Figure 3.8 Malignant epithelial tumors with hypochromatic nuclei. Adenocarcinoma, (A) pancreas, (B) prostate. (A) FNA, direct smear, (B) voided urine, Millipore filter, Pap stain.

Mitosis and N:C Ratio Features

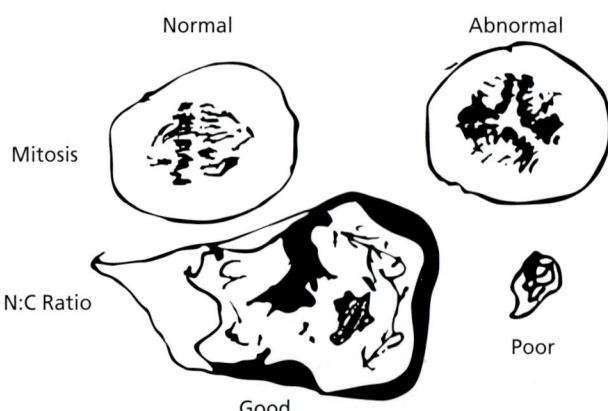

Figure 3.9 These line diagrams depict the value of abnormal mitosis and high N:C ratio in malignant diagnosis.

(A)

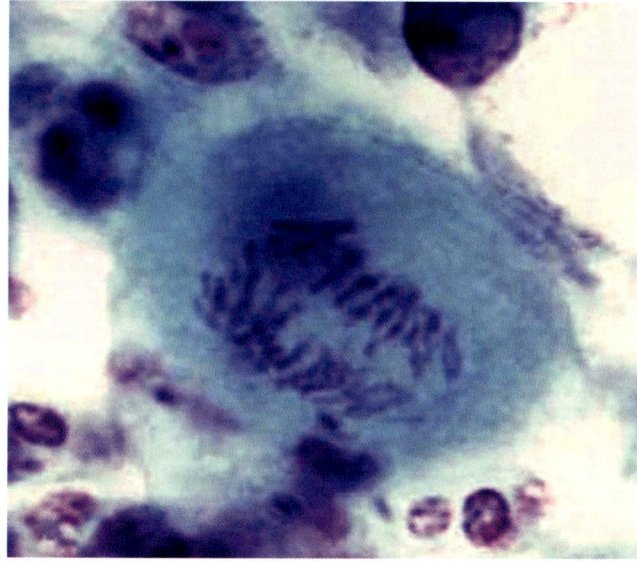

(B)

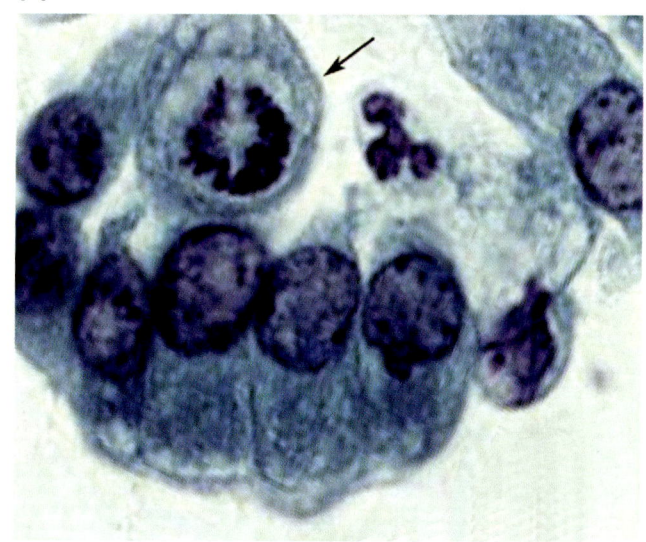

Figure 3.10 (A) depicts a normal mitosis in a pulmonary specimen; (B) depicts an endocervical cell with unevenly distributed chromatin material and mitosis (arrow). Such nuclear changes do not reflect a neoplastic process. Vaginocervical smear, Pap stain.

evaluated when assessing the malignancy or biological behavior of cells in cytologic preparations. Not all the alterations may occur or be discernible in a single cell, preparation or specimen. The following nuclear features should be examined:

1. chromatin,
2. parachromatin (nuclear sap),
3. nuclear membrane (envelope),
4. nucleoli,
5. intranuclear inclusions, and
6. intranuclear grooves.

(A)

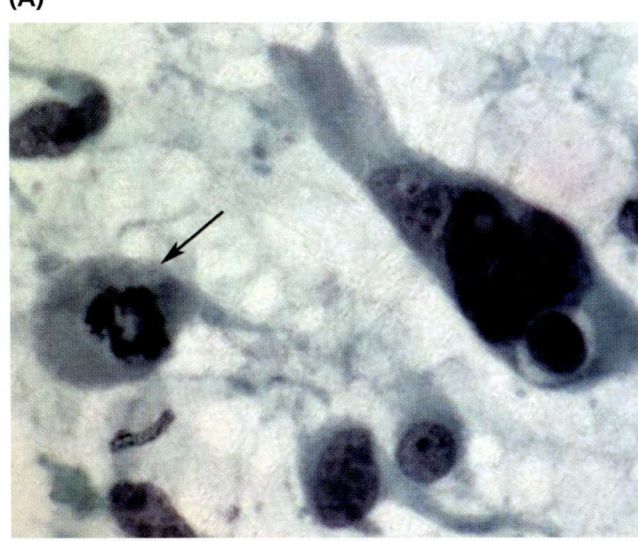

(B)

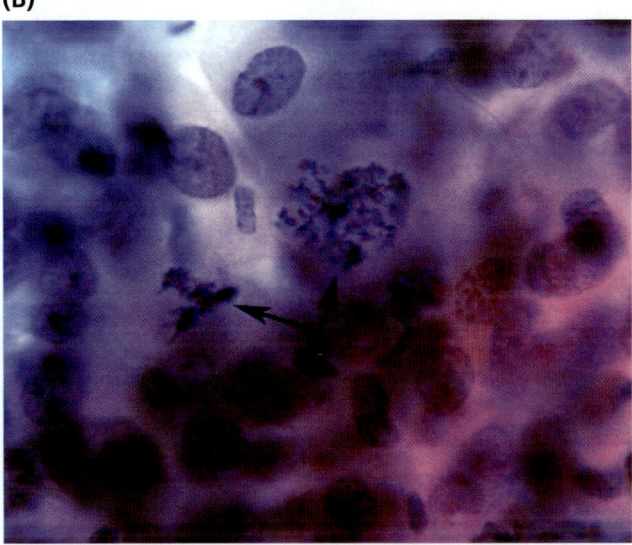

Figure 3.11 Photomicrographs (A) and (B) depict abnormal mitoses (arrow) in malignant cells. Vaginal melanoma (A), endocervical adenocarcinoma (B). Vaginocervical smears, Pap stain.

CHROMATIN (HEMATOXYLINOPHILIC)

Chromatin is mostly made up of the nuclear DNA. When stained with Papanicolaou recipe, chromatin exhibits variable tinctorial characteristics. It may appear almost black to reddish brown, most commonly staining as a shade of purple or lavender. Chromatin features of diagnostic importance are depicted (Figure 3.13).

(a) **Alterations in pattern with irregularity**.

(b) **Massive chromatin clumps:** with

    (a) Sharp "cookie-cutter" borders. Good preservation is important in this regard.

(A)

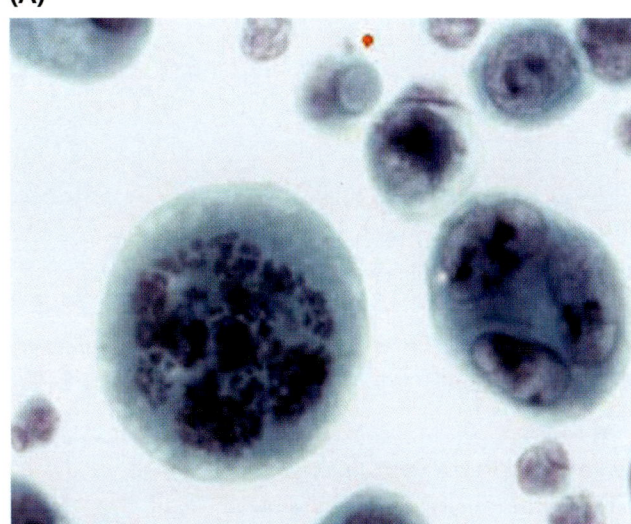

(B)

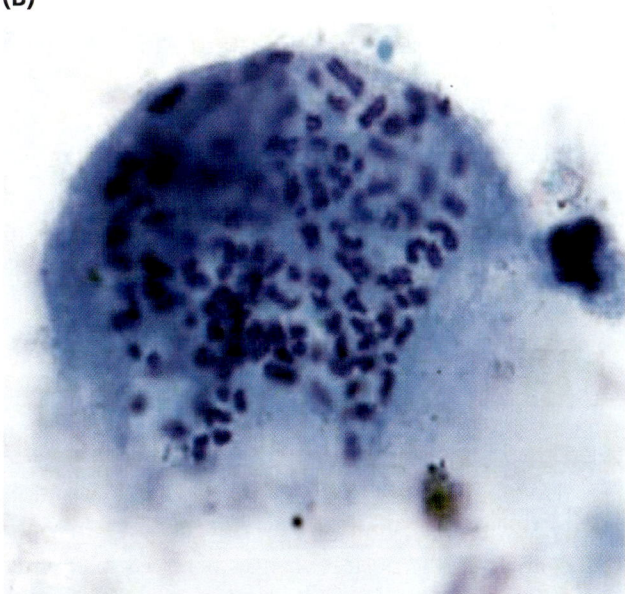

Figure 3.12 (A) represents abnormal mitosis in a pleural effusion from a case of metastatic adenocarcinoma. Cells can continue to go through the division cycle when suspended in protein-rich fluids. (B) represents an abnormal mitosis in a sputum specimen collected and preserved in Saccomanno's preservatives. (A, B) Pap stain.

    (b) Pointed projections and indentations. This is an excellent malignant criterion.

    (c) Hyperchromasia with good preservation. This feature should not be exclusively utilized for cancer diagnosis.

(c) **Coarse granularity**. This is a good measure, if cytoplasm is scant.

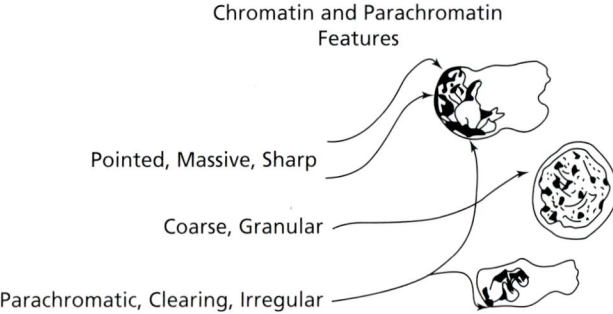

Chromatin and Parachromatin
Features

Pointed, Massive, Sharp

Coarse, Granular

Parachromatic, Clearing, Irregular

Figure 3.13 Chromatin and parachromatin alterations associated with malignant transformation. These include pointed, sharp, irregular aggregates, and abnormal clearing of the nuclear sap.

PARACHROMATIN (NUCLEAR SAP)

This is the nuclear matrix visible by light microscope that contains chromatin and nucleoli. In the literature various terms such as nuclear sap, nucleoplasm, chromatin, interchromatin, and euchromatin have been used to identify the parachromatin. In relation to malignancy, the following parachromatin features are important diagnostically.

(a) **Abnormally "cleared" areas.** Unpredictable and uneven extremes of parachromatin clearing occur in malignant cells. At times the clearing is so pronounced that the background of the slide is visible through the nucleus (Figure 3.14a,b). Although such parachromatin alterations may be observed in reactive and degenerated cells (discussed below), they are good criteria for malignancy.

(b) **Large, unevenly distributed areas.** This clearing is random through the same nucleus; and alteration of symmetry. This unpredictable distribution is in sharp contrast to the nuclear changes observed in reactive (proplastic) and carcinoma in situ cells.

(c) **"Cookie-cutter" borders.** As mentioned earlier, the chromatin aggregates in well-preserved malignant cells have sharp borders. Parachromatin adjacent to these areas of abnormal chromatin distribution tends to have valuable diagnostic significance.

NUCLEAR MEMBRANE (ENVELOPE)

(a) The nuclear membrane (nuclear envelope) or rim is the single most important nuclear organelle for malignant diagnosis. Instead of being uniformly thin, the nuclear rim develops irregular clumps and thickens up often alternating with extreme and almost imperceptible thinness. When observed on alternate areas within

(A)

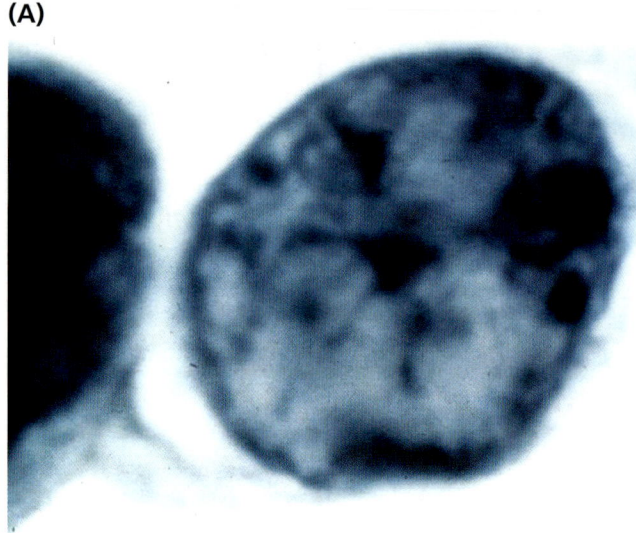

(B)

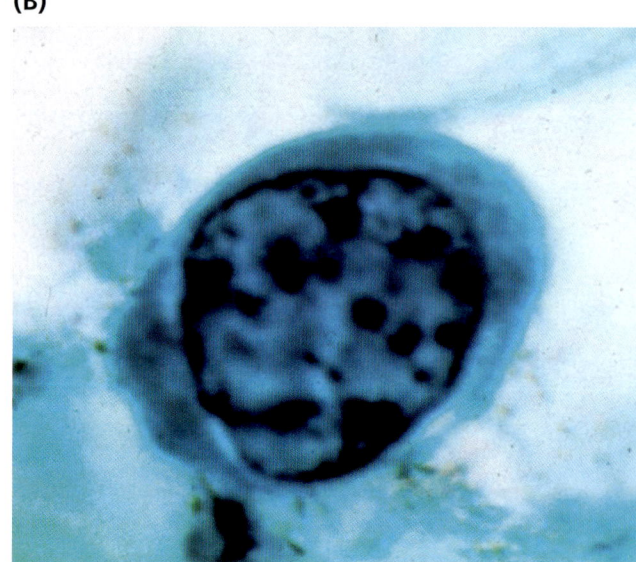

Figure 3.14 (A, B). (A) represents a malignant nucleus. Notice the nuclear membrane and chromatin changes. Abnormal chromatin clearing is less pronounced in (B). Vaginocervical smear, Pap stain.

the same nucleus, this is a good feature of a malignant nucleus (Figure 3.15a,b).

(b) The nuclear membrane shape in a well-preserved nucleus offers good evidence of malignancy. The membrane, instead of being smooth and uniformly taught, maintaining a parallelism with the outer border of the cell, may show out-pouching into the cytoplasm as "blebs" or projections. Similar membrane extensions can develop inwards within the nucleus as sharp bits or spicules.

(A)

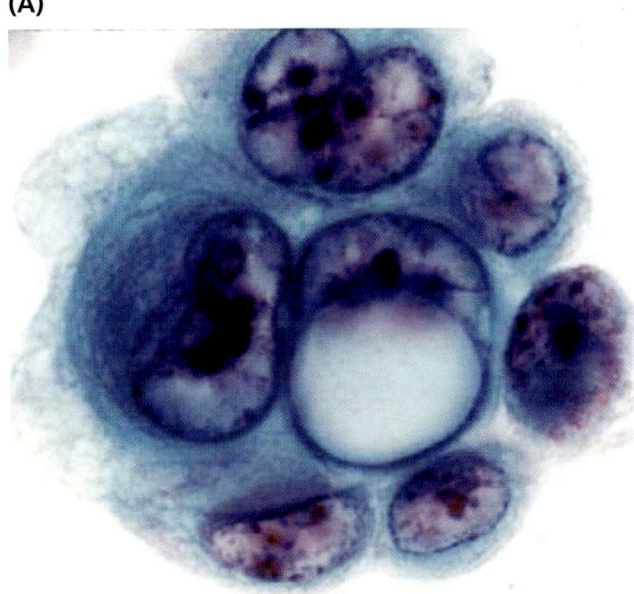

Nuclear Membrane

Thickness variation

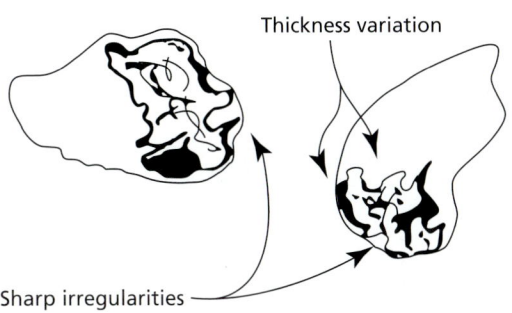

Sharp irregularities

Figure 3.16 The salient features of nuclear membrane changes that are most valuable in malignant diagnosis. These include extreme, alternate thinning and thickening, irregular sharp projections into and away from the nucleus and nuclear membrane irregularities towards the outside or away from the cytocentrum of the cell.

(B)

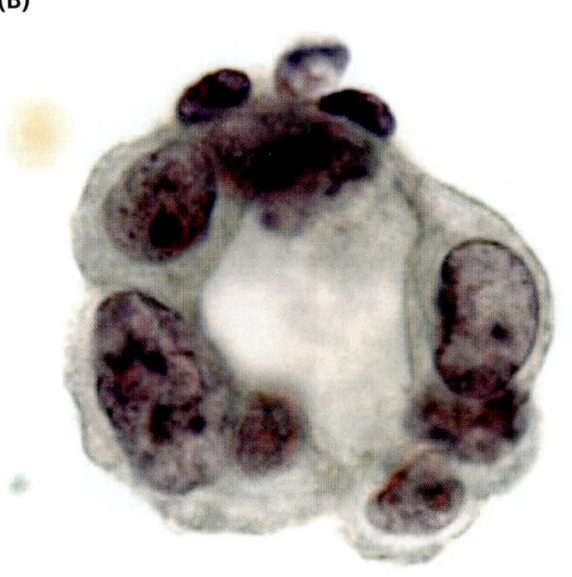

Figure 3.15 (A, B) Malignant nuclei. Notice the relative uniformity of the nuclear membranes. Parachromatin, however, is variable in distribution and clearing. FNA lung specimens, direct smears, Pap stain.

(c) Nuclear membrane irregularities away from the cytocentrum: physiologically active cells have a predictable nuclear orientation within them; it reflects the biological behavior. There is a convexity of the nuclear membrane away from the cytocentrum or nuclear "hilum." The nuclear shape conforms to the cell profile, remaining equi-spaced and smooth. In malignant cells, one may get extremely sharp irregularities of the nuclear membrane towards the anti hoff or away

from the cytocentrum location. These irregularities may occur in degenerative cells, but extremes in well-preserved cells evidence malignancy (Figures 3.16–3.18).

NUCLEOLI

These represent rapid cell proliferation and production of nucleoproteins by the cell. Depending upon the preparation, nucleoli may be identifiable to varying degrees. Many times nucleolar-associated chromatin may obliterate its acidophilia, making correct recognition difficult. Similarly, the three-dimensional nature of the cell and Papanicolaou stain with its transparency may be compromised by the quality of the cytopreparation.

(a) **Irregular shape** and sharp pointed projections and indentations. These characteristics of nucleoli almost mirror similar changes observed in the chromatin structure in malignant cells. Sharp, outward-pointed nuclear extensions may be associated with inward indentations and are an excellent criterion of malignancy (Figures 3.19–3.22a).

(b) **Large size**. Massive acidophilic nucleoli per se are poor criteria of malignancy. Similar changes may occur in extremely reactive (proplastic) nuclei. In the latter situation, however, the nucleoli tend to be round and prominent (Figure 3.20b).

(c) **Large irregular shapes**. This is a good criterion of malignancy (Fig. 3.21a–c).

(d) **Variation in the number of nucleoli**. Nucleoli multiply in cellular proliferations and nucleoprotein production. The number of nucleoli is dependent upon

(A)

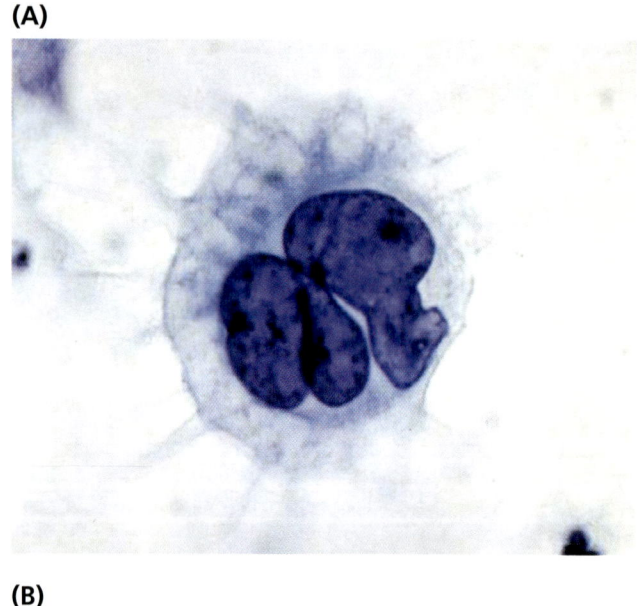

(B)

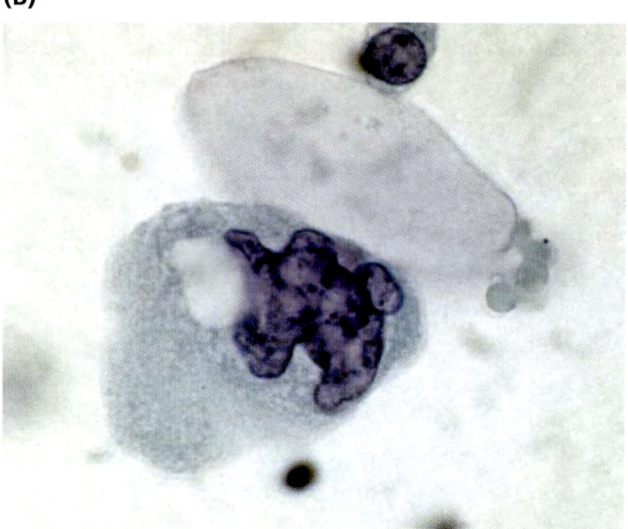

Figure 3.17 (A, B) Demonstration of the extremes of nuclear membrane irregularities seen among malignant nuclei. These changes need to be distinguished from the membrane wrinkling often associated with degeneration (see Figure 5.28, 5.29 and 5.33). FNA pancreas. Direct smear (A), voided urine, Millipore filter (B), Pap stain.

(A)

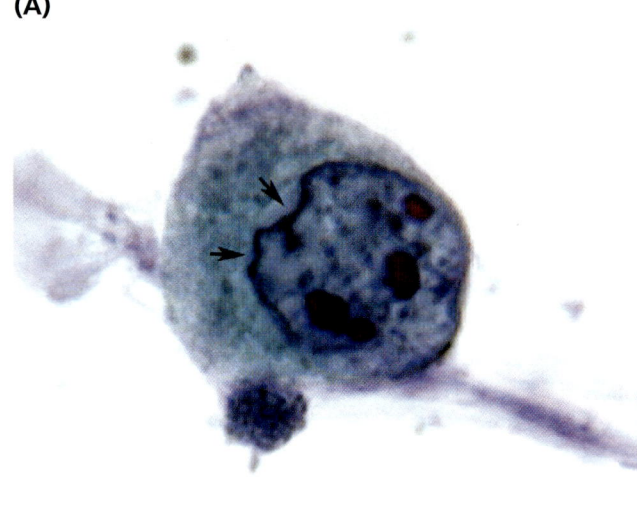

(B)

Figure 3.18 (A, B) Nuclear membrane changes, malignant cells. Notice the fine membrane irregularities (A) and marked variation in membrane thickness (B). Bronchial washings, Pap stain.

the type of stimulation and activity. The mere number of nucleoli has little relevance to the neoplastic process and should not be used as a malignant criterion.

In most proliferative activities, within the same clone or a group of cells the number of nuclei either remains the same or may vary but not more than $2n+1$. In malignant transformation the number of nucleoli may depart by more than $2n+1$. If there is a dramatically different nucleoli number variation, that is a good feature of malignancy (Figure 3.22).

INTRANUCLEAR INCLUSIONS

These are also known as intranuclear invaginations, and are produced by protrusion of the underlying cytoplasm through the nuclear chromatin. Typical intranuclear inclusions have a peripheral chromatin condensation surrounding a well-defined area of intranuclear clearing. In papillary thyroid carcinoma cells these are typically round and single (Figure 3.23a–d). Occasionally, these inclusions can be multiple and variable in size, showing a "soap-bubble"-like appearance.

Nucleolar Features

Shape

Size, Number

Figure 3.19 This line drawing depicts the salient features of nucleoli seen among malignant cells. The shapes of nucleoli are irregular, pointed, sharp, and enlarged. The number of the nucleoli varies by more than $2n+1$. While these are some of the most valuable malignant features, nulceolar size per se is a weak malignant criterion.

(A)

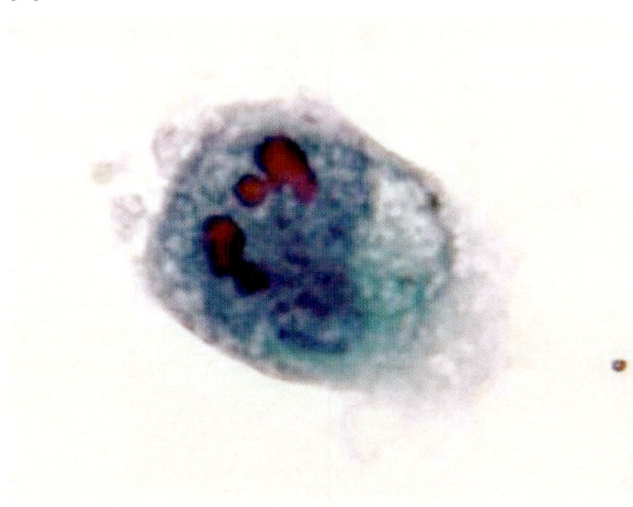

(B)

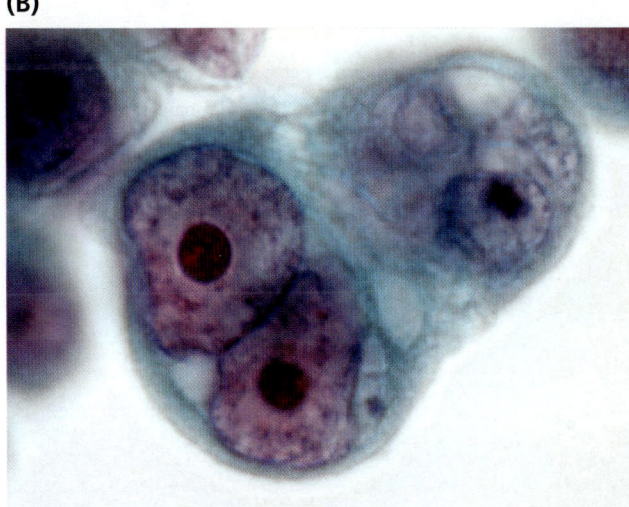

Figure 3.20 (A, B) These show the irregular shapes (A), and large, massive nucleoli (B) among malignant cells. (A) lung FNA, (B) bronchial brush, direct smears, Pap stain.

(A)

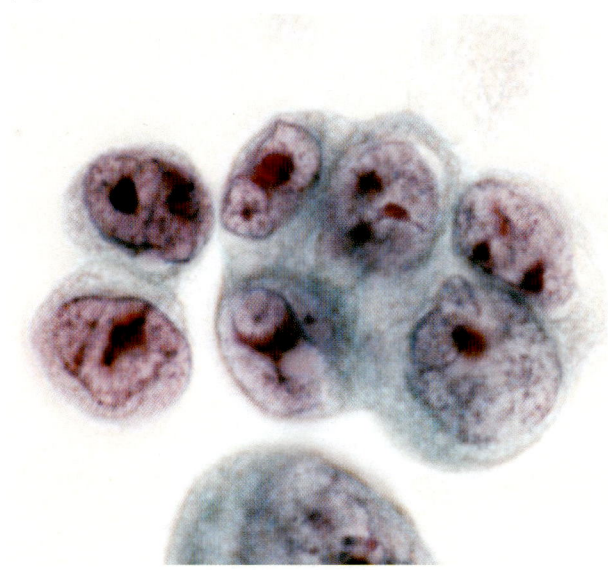

(B)

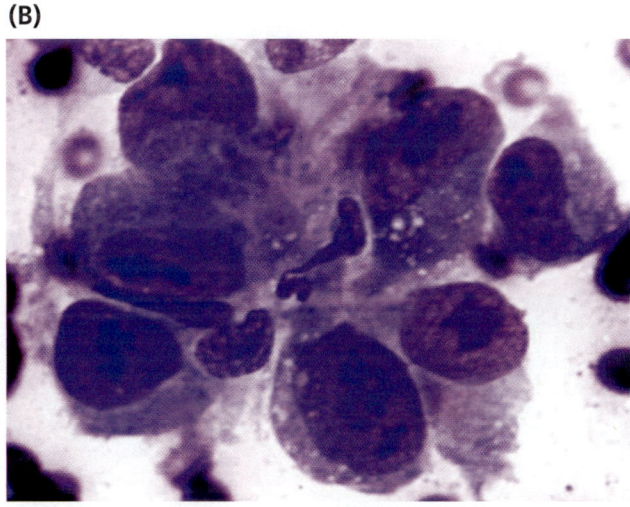

(C)

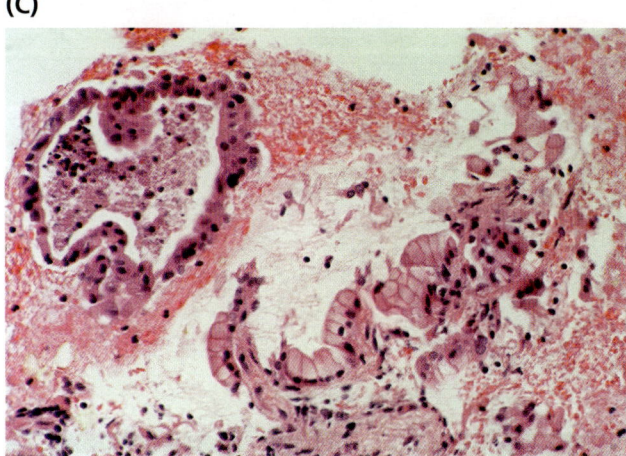

Figure 3.21 (A–C) Demonstration of the nucleolar abnormalities observed among malignant cells seen in Papanicolaou (A) and Diff-Quik (B) stains. FNA lung, same specimen. (C) Represents the cell block specimen from the same case, H/E stain.

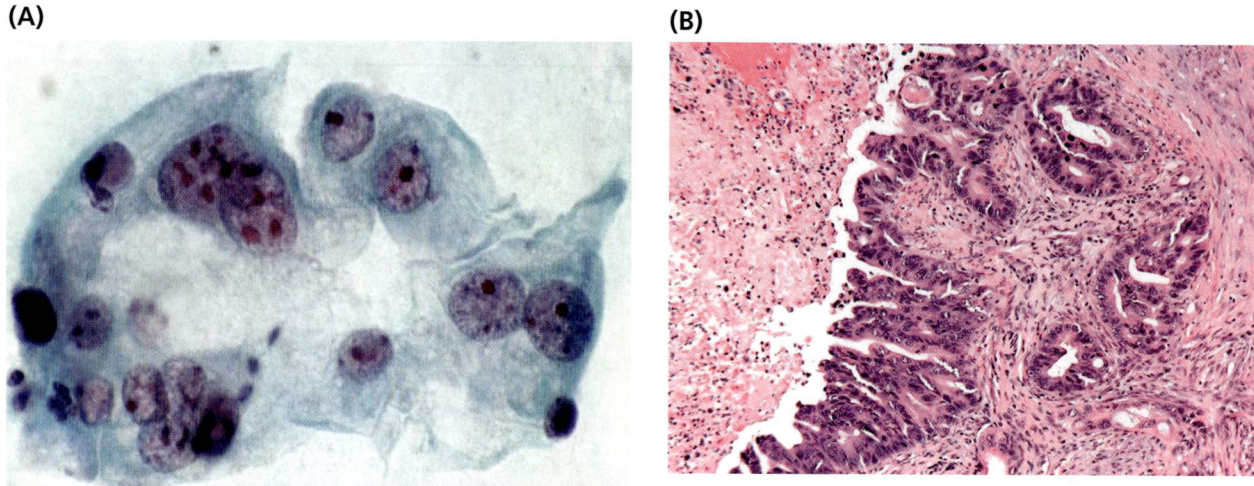

(A)

(B)

Figure 3.22 Tissue fragment of malignant cells showing nucleolar numbers variation (A). Pancreas FNA, direct smear, Pap stain. (B) represents cell block from the same case, H/E stain.

(A)

(B)

(C)

(D)

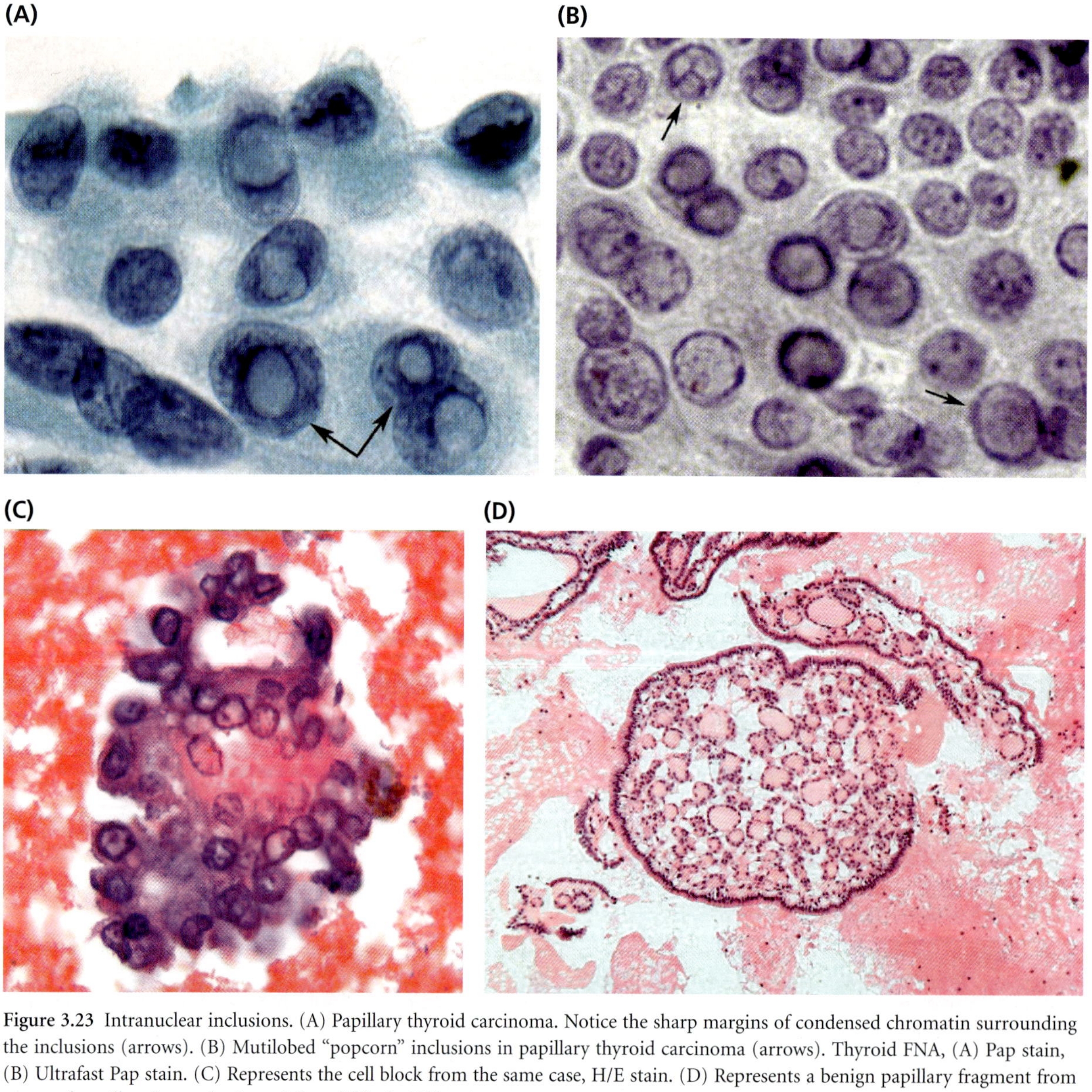

Figure 3.23 Intranuclear inclusions. (A) Papillary thyroid carcinoma. Notice the sharp margins of condensed chromatin surrounding the inclusions (arrows). (B) Mutilobed "popcorn" inclusions in papillary thyroid carcinoma (arrows). Thyroid FNA, (A) Pap stain, (B) Ultrafast Pap stain. (C) Represents the cell block from the same case, H/E stain. (D) Represents a benign papillary fragment from a case of papillary hyperplastic nodule, cell block, H/E stain.

(A)

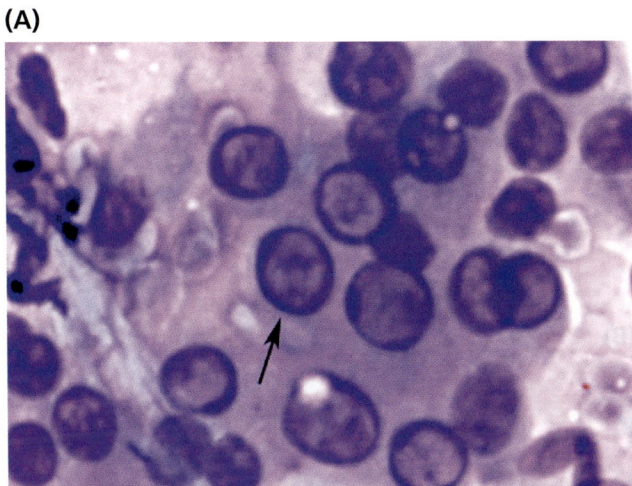

(B)

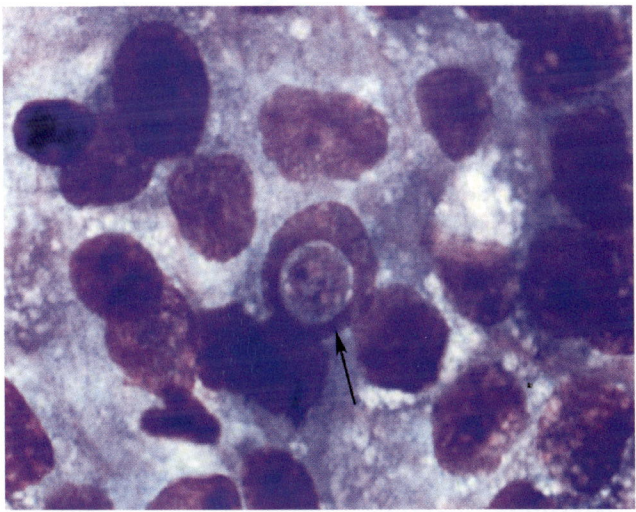

Figure 3.24 Intranuclear inclusions (arrow) adenocarcinoma lung (A) and hepatocellular carcinoma (arrow) (B). FNA specimens, Diff-Quik stain.

Intranuclear inclusions per se are insufficient for diagnosing malignancy. Similar inclusions may occur in bronchial cells and in bronchoalveolar carcinoma, and melanoma.

Intracytoplasmic inclusions may be observed in case of hepatoma with alpha fetoprotein occurrences (Figures 3.24 and 3.25). Similarly, intracytoplasmic deposits may occur in papillary thyroid carcinoma cells as well as in other neuroendocrine tumors.

INTRANUCLEAR GROOVES

These represent an intranuclear condensation of chromatinic material in a linear fashion. These most often are

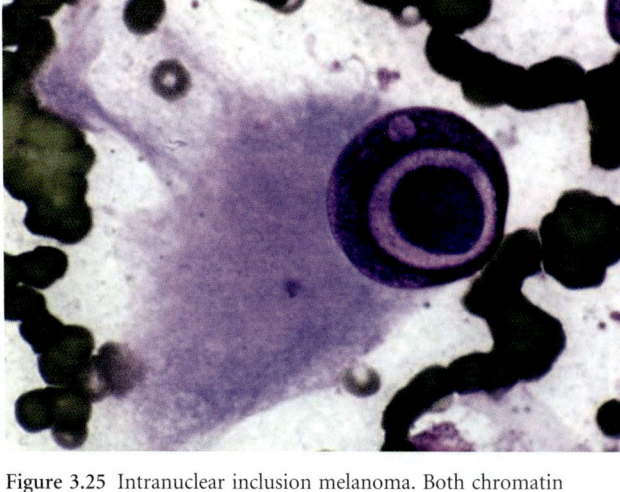

Figure 3.25 Intranuclear inclusion melanoma. Both chromatin and cytoplasmic invagination inclusions may be observed in these and other malignant cases. FNA, inguinal lymph node, Diff-Quik stain.

single and stretch the complete diameter of the affected nucleus (Figure 3.26). Sometimes more than one intranuclear groove may be observed. These may occur in papillary thyroid carcinomas, but may also be seen in benign oncocytic cells, intermittent squamous cells, and bronchial and a number of other epithelial cells (Figure 3.26a–c).

Nucleocytoplasmic relationship

Relationship of nuclear membrane to cytoplasmic membrane. Almost always in benign cells, an uncanny, uniform distance and parallelism is maintained between the borders of these two cellular membranes. This feature is predictable and independent of abundance of cytoplasm in the rest of the cell.

These changes acquire added importance when observed in small tissue fragments. In malignant cells, this relationship becomes unpredictable and bizarre. These include:

1. *molding:* nuclear molding to follow cell membrane or a small cytoplasmic vacuole. This appears as a pinching of the nuclear membrane of a vacuole by the cytoplasmic membrane (Figures 3.27–3.29);
2. *intrusion:* nucleus intrusion into the cell membrane for an appreciable distance. In this appearance, the two sides of the cell membrane appear to "mold" and push against the nuclear membrane for variable distance before flaring up and moving away from the nuclear membrane (Figures 3.27–3.33);

77

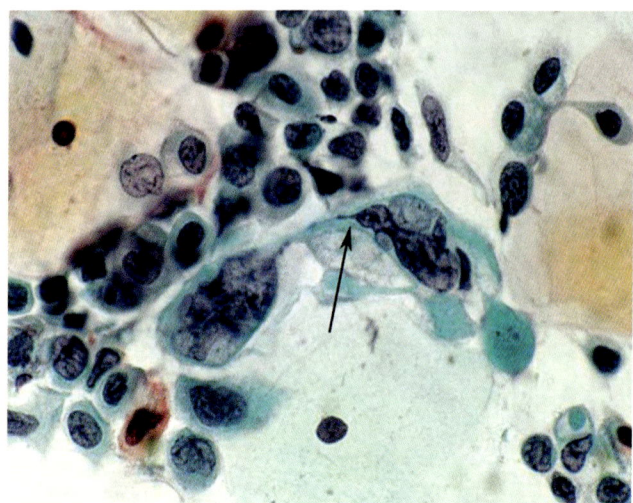

Figure 3.32 Malignant cell showing nuclear intrusion into the cytoplasm. LBP, Pap stain.

diagnostic significance cytologically, as it only reflects the growth of the cells together as a microbiopsy or tissue fragment.

3. Cytonuclear molding: as discussed, nucleus to nucleus, as well as cytoplasm to cytoplasm, kinship (molding) is of little diagnostic value; it only establishes the clonal nature of cells without any indication about their biological behavior. It is extremely important to recognize that cytoplasmic/nuclear molding, a cytoplasmic vacuole may indent the nucleus and create a concavity (Figures 3.35 and 3.36). Similarly, a cytoplasmic wedge may alter the shape of the two adjacent nuclei. These nuclei in non-neoplastic cells conform to each other and are not attached by the adjacent cytoplasm.

(A)

(B)

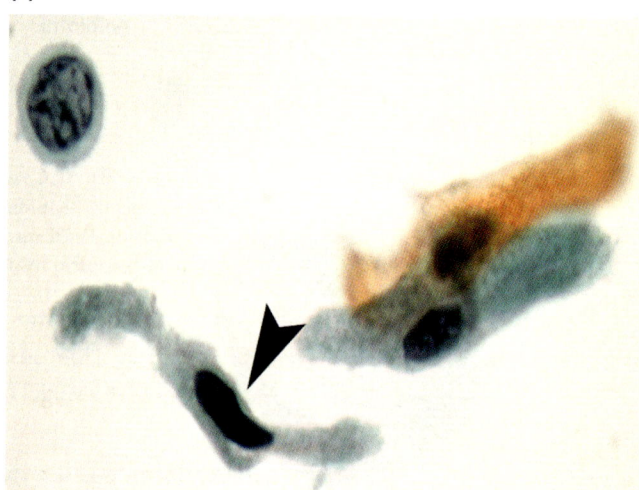

(C)

(D)

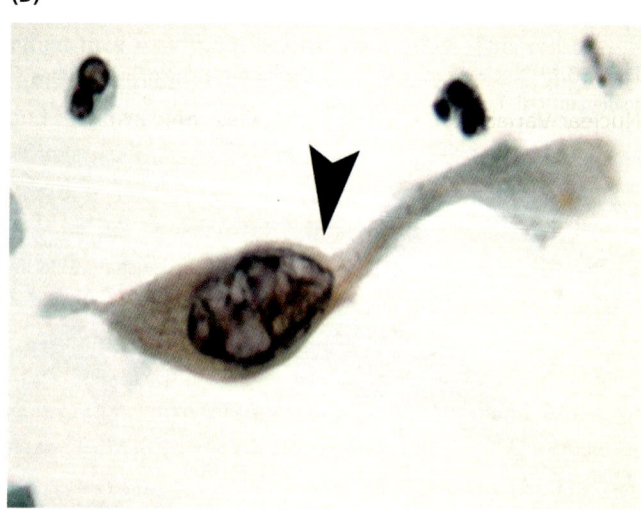

Figure 3.33 Nuclear intrusion into the cytoplasm in malignant cells (A) (arrows). These two cells, although hyperchromatic and elongated, are not diagnostic of malignancy; there is no cytoplasmic extension of the nuclei. (B–D) (arrowheads) These reveal varying degrees of cytoplasmic penetration by the nuclei and are malignant. (A, B) bronchial wash, (C, D) FNA lung, same patient, Pap stain.

(A)

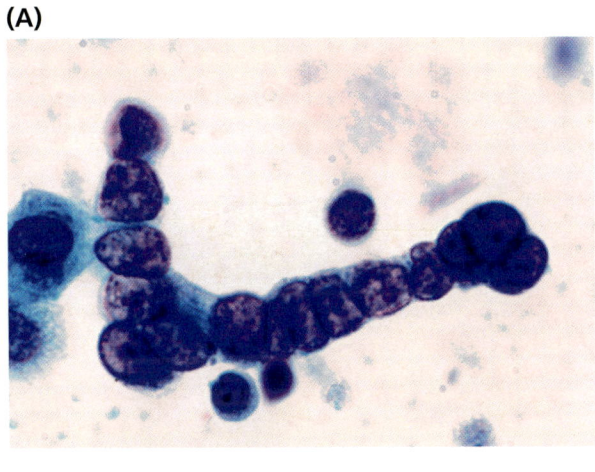

(B)

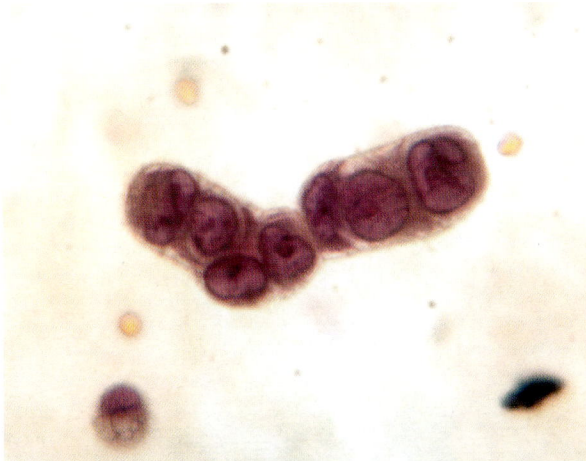

Figure 3.34 Internuclear molding-Indian file pattern, notice the malignant nuclear features. Breast adenocarcinoma, vaginocervical smear (A), small-cell carcinoma lung, pleural fluid (B), Pap stain.

Malignant Criteria: Intercellular Features

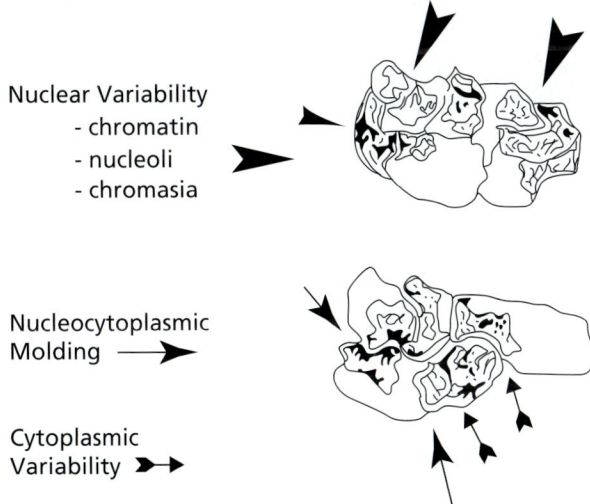

Nuclear Variability
- chromatin
- nucleoli
- chromasia

Nucleocytoplasmic Molding ⟶

Cytoplasmic Variability ➤➤

Figure 3.35 The salient features of intercellular relationship in malignant transformation.

(A)

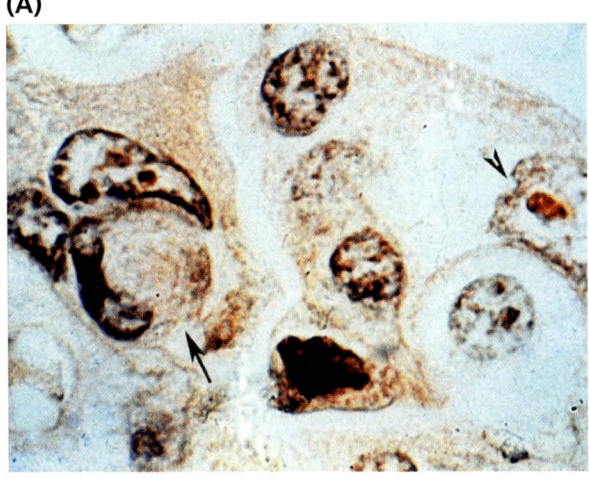

(B)

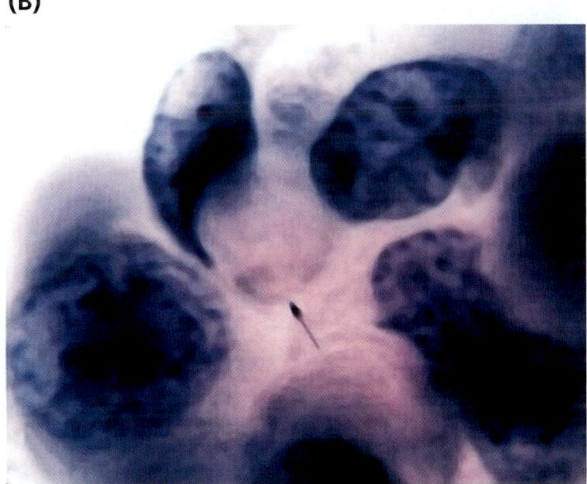

Figure 3.36 Cytoplasm to nuclear molding (arrow). Notice the molding of the nuclear shape by the cytoplasmic secretory vacuole. This is a good and reliable feature of malignant transformation. Nuclear membrane bite (arrowhead) at the antihof margin is another excellent malignant criterion. Sputum specimen (A), lung FNA specimen (B), Pap stain.

Tissue fragments

Most of these features have been discussed previously. In a tissue fragment of two or more cells, the following features are diagnostically important.

(a) While the size among nuclei within the same tissue fragment may vary up to 4 or 5 times, extreme variation in nuclear size is often associated with malignant change (Figure 3.37 and 3.38).

(b) Chromatin pattern and variability. Extreme variation in the chromatin "quantity." Pale/normochromatic and hyperchromasia is a good malignant criterion.

(c) Chromatin pattern. Extremely variable chromatin clumping among adjacent nuclei is a valuable malignant criterion (Figure 3.38).

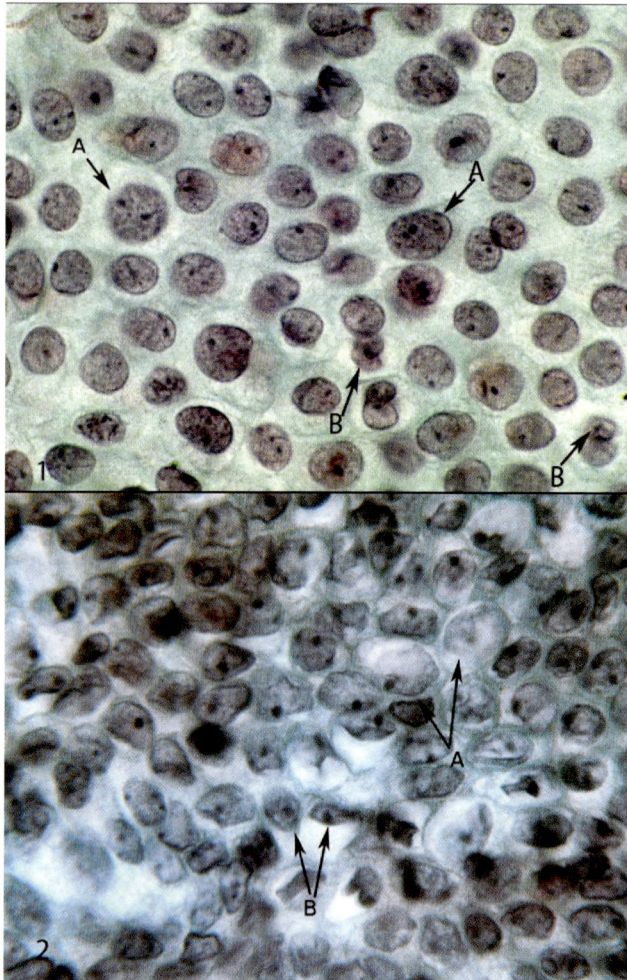

Figure 3.37 Nuclear size variation among malignant cells. (A) depicts minimum nuclear atypia, but size variation which is pronounced in (B) points to the chromatin pattern and other variabilities. Chromatin quantity and pattern, size, shape, and number of nucleoli EUS, pancreas (1), direct smear, ELBP (2), Pap stain.

(A)

(B)

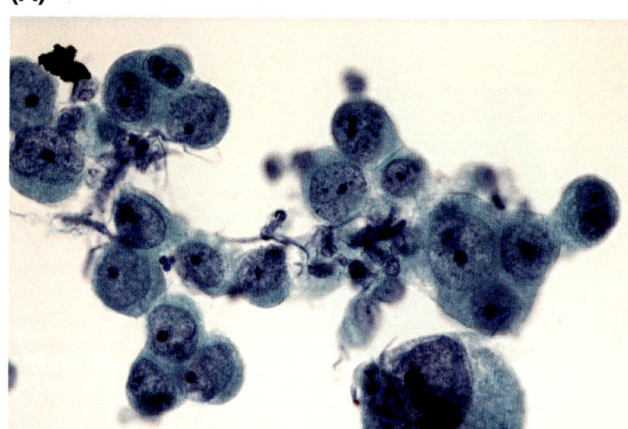

Figure 3.38 Malignant cells with nuclear size variation. (A) Cells resemble histiocytes. Lung FNA, cells resemble bronchial columnar cells. (B) Bronchial brush. Bronchi alveolar carcinoma, Pap stain.

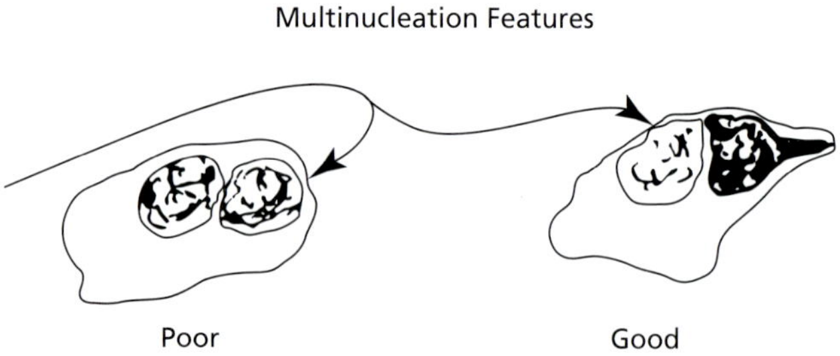

Multinucleation Features

Poor   Good

Figure 3.39 Chromatin variation among the nuclei in a multinucleated cell is a good criterion of malignancy.

(d) Nuclear variation. As already mentioned, number of nucleoli when fluctuating by more than $2n+1$ is a goal benchmark for malignant diagnosis (Figures 3.22 and 3.39).

MULTINUCLEATION

This, per se, is a poor criterion of malignancy. Multinucleation is more commonly observed in non-neoplastic processes such as infections, healing, and repair. It is valuable if the nuclei in a multinucleated cell reveal variations in intranuclear structures such as chromatin quantity, parachromatin clearing, and variations in the number of nucleoli (Figures 3.40 and 3.41).

ECTOPIC TISSUE OCCURRENCE

a. Acini, polyps, ducts and stalks extremely uncommonly occur in body cavity fluids in benign conditions. True papillary fragments of mesothelial cells can be observed in rectovaginal (cul-de-sac) pouch aspirations. Occasionally, calcified, psammoma bodies

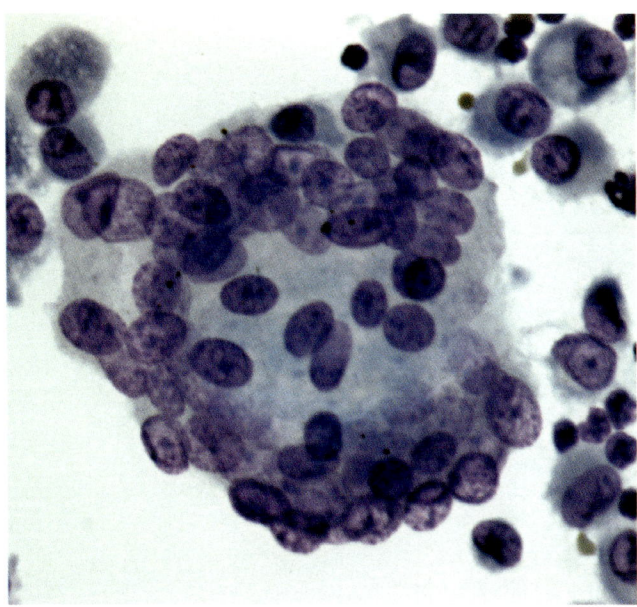

Figure 3.40 Benign multinucleated cell. Notice the uniformity of the chromatin pattern. BAL sarcoid, Pap stain.

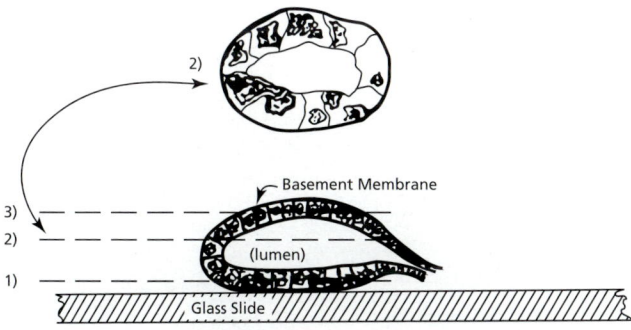

Figure 3.42 Line diagram depicting the three-dimensional nature of a true acinic structure. Such formations are uncommonly observed in LBP.

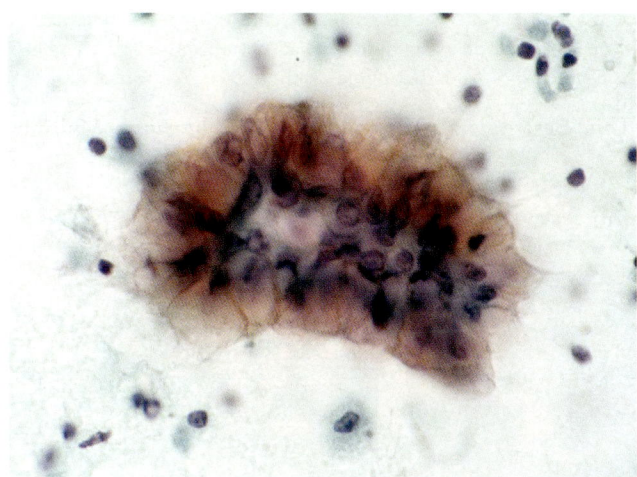

Figure 3.43 Mucinous carcinoma of the pancreas metastatic to pleural cavity. Although this lacks classic malignant criteria, its occurrence at an irrelevant location and clinical history are useful for diagnosis. Millipore filter, Pap stain.

(A)

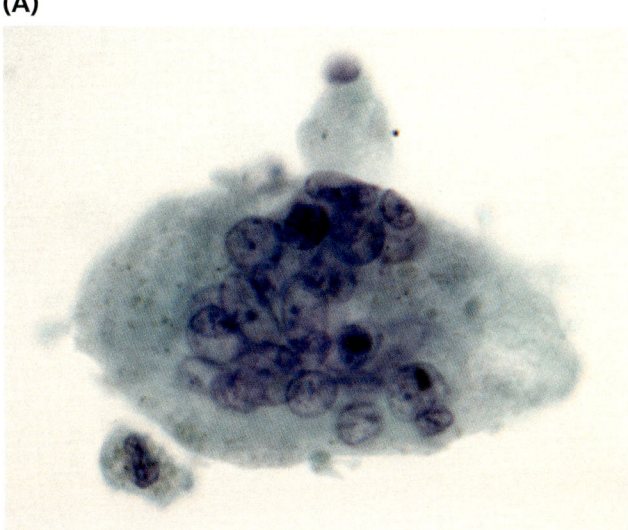

(B)

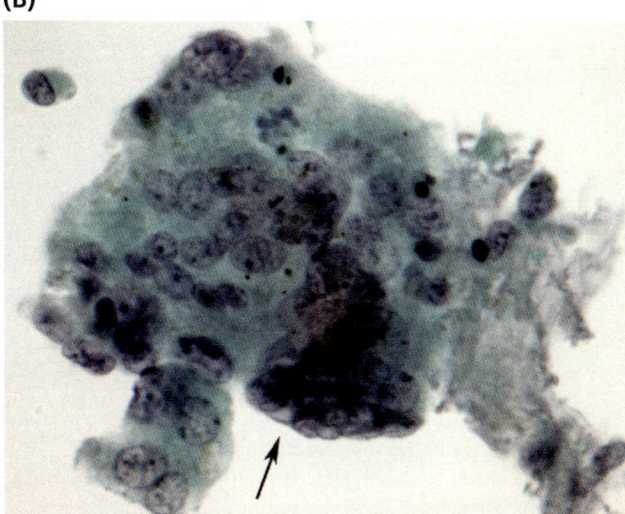

Figure 3.41 Benign and malignant multinucleated cell. Notice the nuclear uniformity in benign cell (A), and obvious variation in chromatin pattern (arrow) (B). Lung FNA, LBP, Pap stain.

may be seen. Occurrence of concentrically laminated calcified – psamomma – bodies is a well-known association with ovarian, endometrial, and papillary thyroid and rarely with bronchoalveolar, mesothelioma and other tumors. However, these should only be used for diagnosis once the malignancy has been established using nuclear features discussed earlier.

Polypoidal fragments of mesothelial cells may occur in body cavity fluids in collagen, vascular and autoimmune diseases, viral infections, following intracavitary medication, radiation, chemotherapy, and endometriosis. True tissue fragment of urothelial cells in voided urine may be seen after instrumentation or therapy; otherwise their

(A)

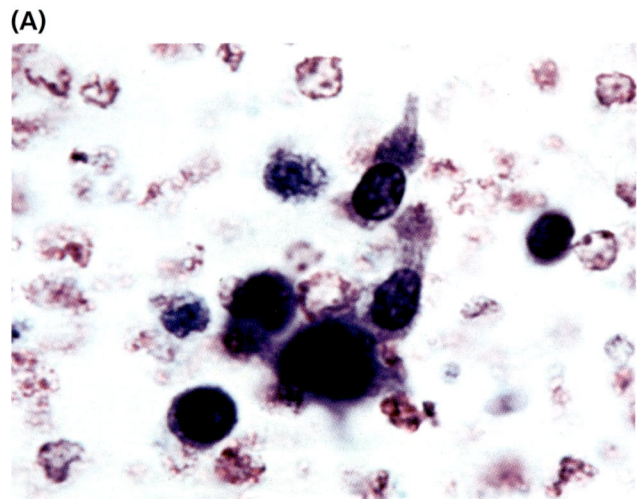

(B)

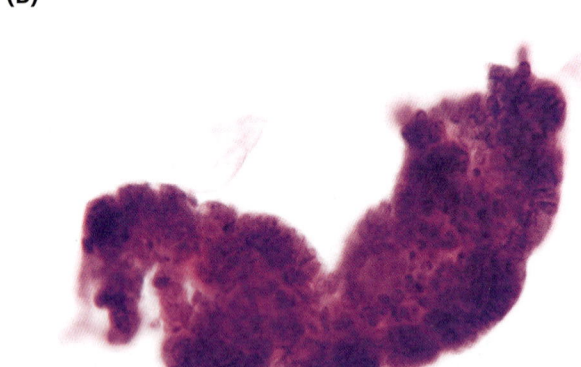

Figure 3.44 Right-sided pleural effusion in a young woman.
(A) Presence of columnar cells and macrophages with hemosiderin in this location is abnormal. This is a case of pleural endometriosis.
(B) Fragment of columnar cells with stroma, bladder wash, patient with urinary bladder endometriosis. Millipore filter, Pap stain.

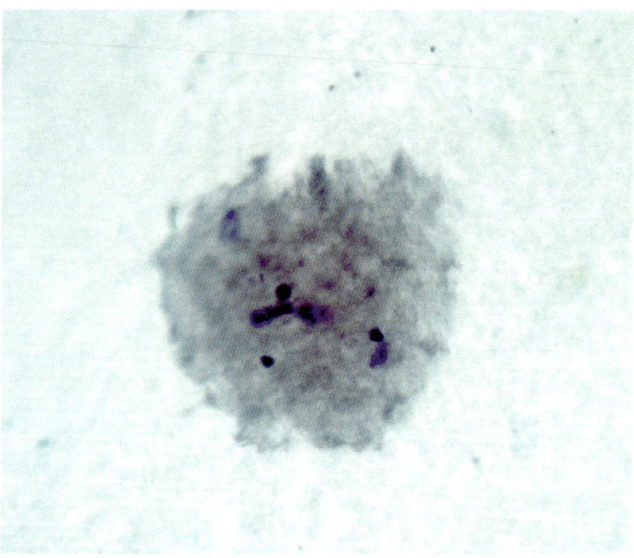

Figure 3.45 Fragment of cerebral cortical tissue in a spinal cerebrospinal fluid specimen. Patient had a ventricular shunt implanted for hydrocephalus. Millipore filter, Pap stain.

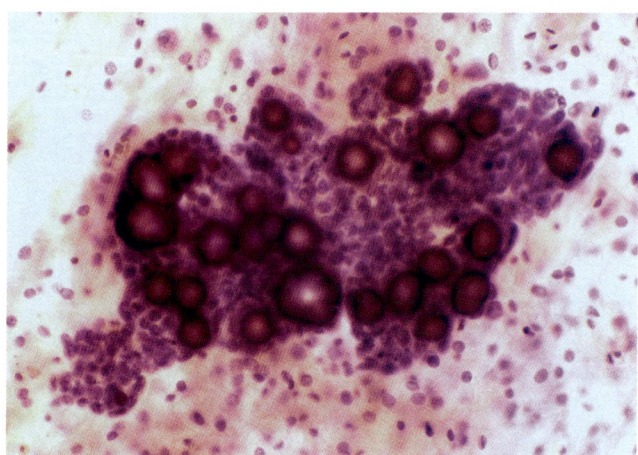

Figure 3.46 A number of laminated calcified psammoma bodies in a vaginal smear from a case of ovarian adenocarcinoma. These should be distinguished from dystrophic calcification and calcispherules that may occur in pulmonary specimens. Pap stain.

presence is a cause for concern and may indicate malignancy (Figures 3.42–3.46).

b. Papillary epithelial fragments in a nipple secretion generally indicate an underlying ductal lesion.

c. Cortical tissue in spinal fluid. Small fragments of cerebral cortical tissue may be seen in spinal or ventricular fluid specimens from patients with high-grade malignant tumors, after intracranial surgery, cerebral death, certain infectious processes, or neurovascular lesions.

Cytoplasmic features

Cytoplasmic features may occasionally reveal a malignant cytoplasmic differentiation, such as cross striations in elongated mesenchymal type or melanin, and bile pigment in cells at ectopic locations may suggest malignancy.

However, cytoplasmic changes must not be used as the only feature of malignancy diagnosis (Figures 3.47–3.54).

Background

These changes generally represent tell-tale evidence of an underlying or associated malignancy and may include background or not-so-classic cellular features.

Preparation background

This is a minor criterion that at times directs to the underlying malignancy. They are most helpful when evaluated in fresh smear slides. Background features are considerably

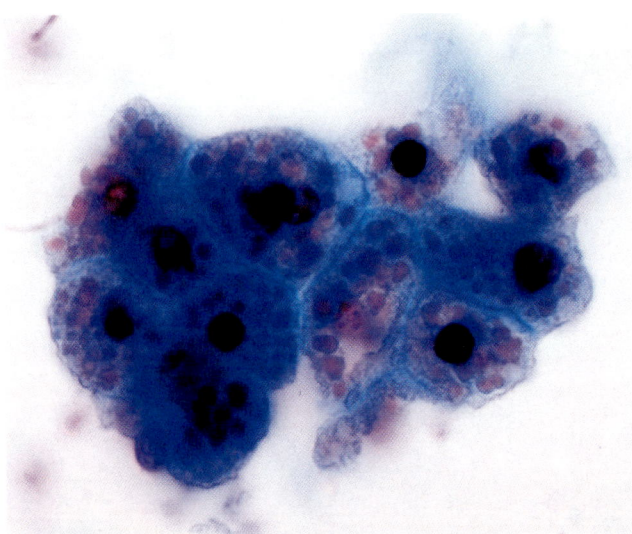

Figure 3.47 Hepatocytes with numerous alpha-1-antitrypsin intracytoplasmic globules. These vary in size, are diastase-resistant PAS-positive, and need to be distinguished from other intracytoplasmic organelles. FNA liver, Pap stain.

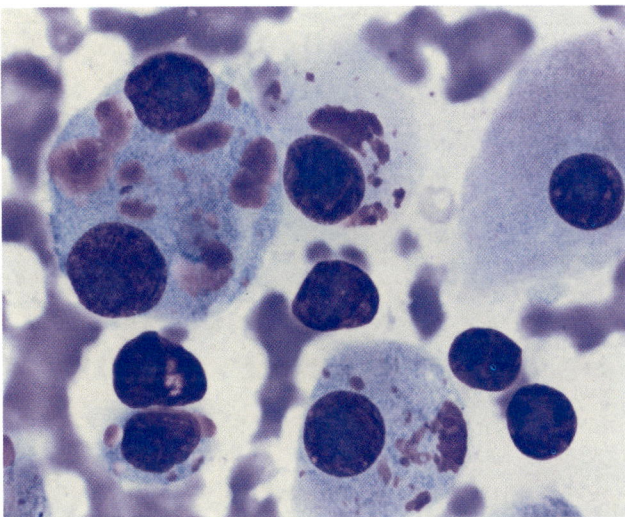

Figure 3.48 Liver fine needle aspiration showing numerous intracytoplasmic globules of alfa fetoproteins in hepatoma cells. These exhibit metachromasia by Diff-Quik stains.

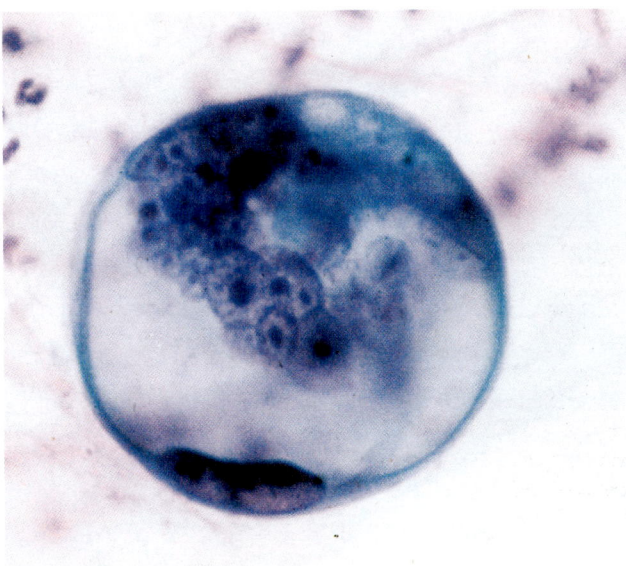

Figure 3.49 Intracellular tumor growth. This is an uncommon occurrence. Tumorlets are growing within a cytoplasmic vacuole of a malignant cell. Sputum, adenocarcinoma lung, Pap stain.

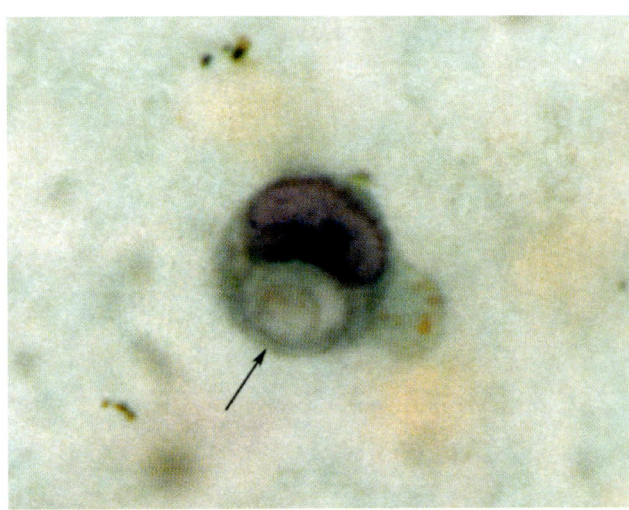

Figure 3.50 Intracytoplasmic ingested red blood cell (arrow) in an endothelial cell. Pleural fluid specimen, Kaposi's sarcoma. Intracytoplasmic lumina appearing as vacuoles may be seen in breast (lobular) adenocarcinoma and other tumors. Millipore filter, Pap stain.

modified in liquid-based preparations and are often of limited diagnostic value.

OLD BLOOD

The presence of "old" blood, often seen as fibrin threads which have uniform thickness and a beaded appearance, or fragments of red blood cells or hemosiderin-laden macrophages should all suggest a bleeding chronic lesion such as malignancy (Figure 3.55).

Hemosiderin-laden macrophages occur commonly in bronchoalveolar lavage (BAL) specimens with intra-alveolar hemorrhage, which is often observed in immuno-compromised patients. These can be stained with Prussian blue reaction. Pigment may appear similar to foreign particles such as carbon and silica, a common occurrence in pulmonary specimens. Certain pulmonary and hepatic aspirations may represent an infarct and specimens may be laden with old bleeding (Figure 3.56).

HEAVY INFLAMMATION

This may occur in the presence of invasive tumors, and malignant cells may be obscured. Necrotic malignant

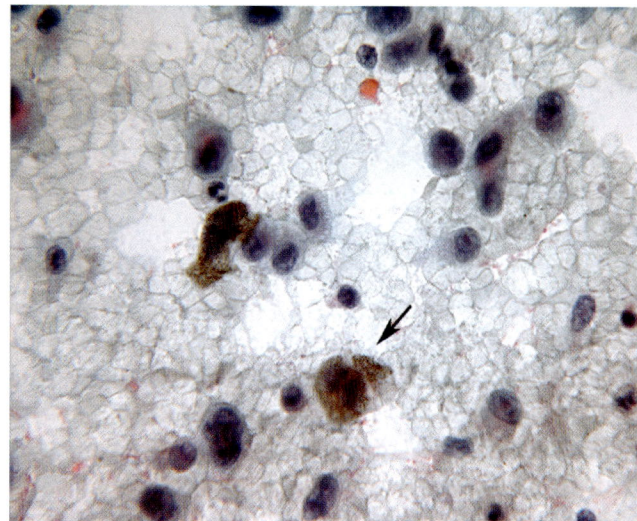

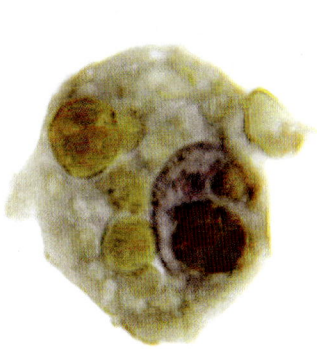

Figure 3.51 Malignant epithelial cell with bile pigment. Pleural effusion, metastatic hepatoma. This pigment needs to be distinguished from similar pigments, including hemosiderin and melanin. Millipore filter, Pap stain.

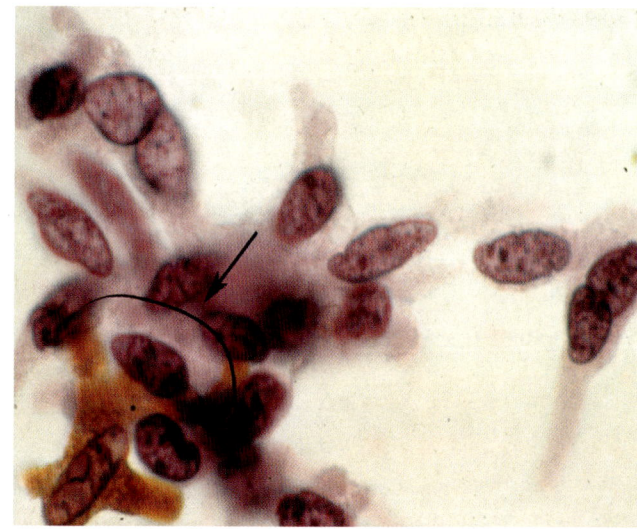

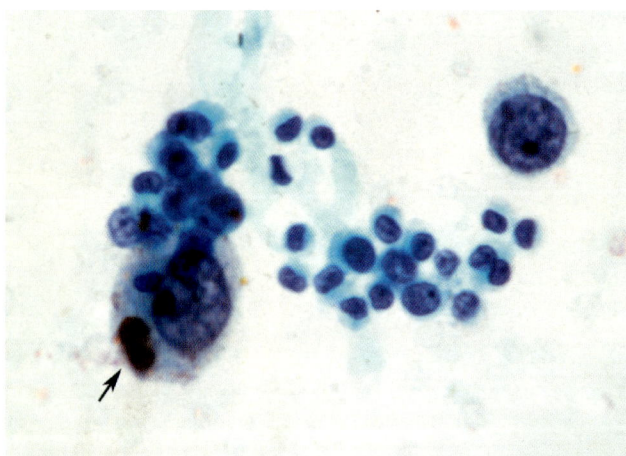

Figure 3.52 Malignant epithelial cell with melanin pigment (arrow). CSF, Millipore filter, Pap stain.

squamous and adenocarcinomas, and urothelial tumors especially following treatment, often may be dominated by acute inflammation (Figure 3.57). Such background findings require a careful examination of the slide. The inflammatory component is reduced considerably in liquid-based preparations. However, this continues to be an important finding in FNA smears.

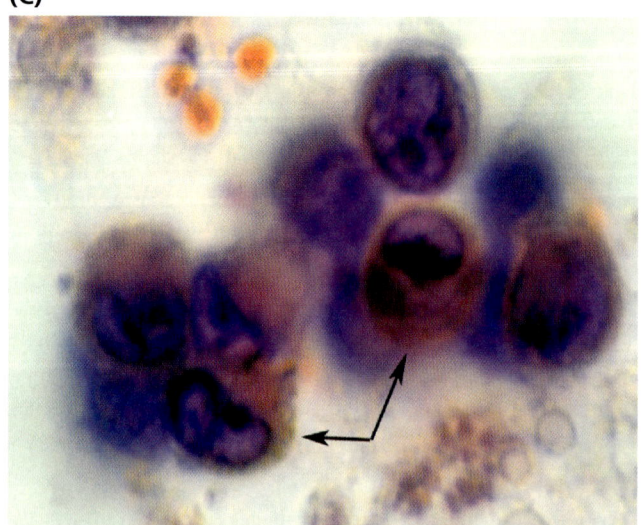

Figure 3.53 Melanin pigment (arrows) containing malignant cells. (A) axillary lymph node, (B) anterior chamber of the eye, (C) pleural fluid specimen, metastatic melanoma. Millipore filter, Pap stain.

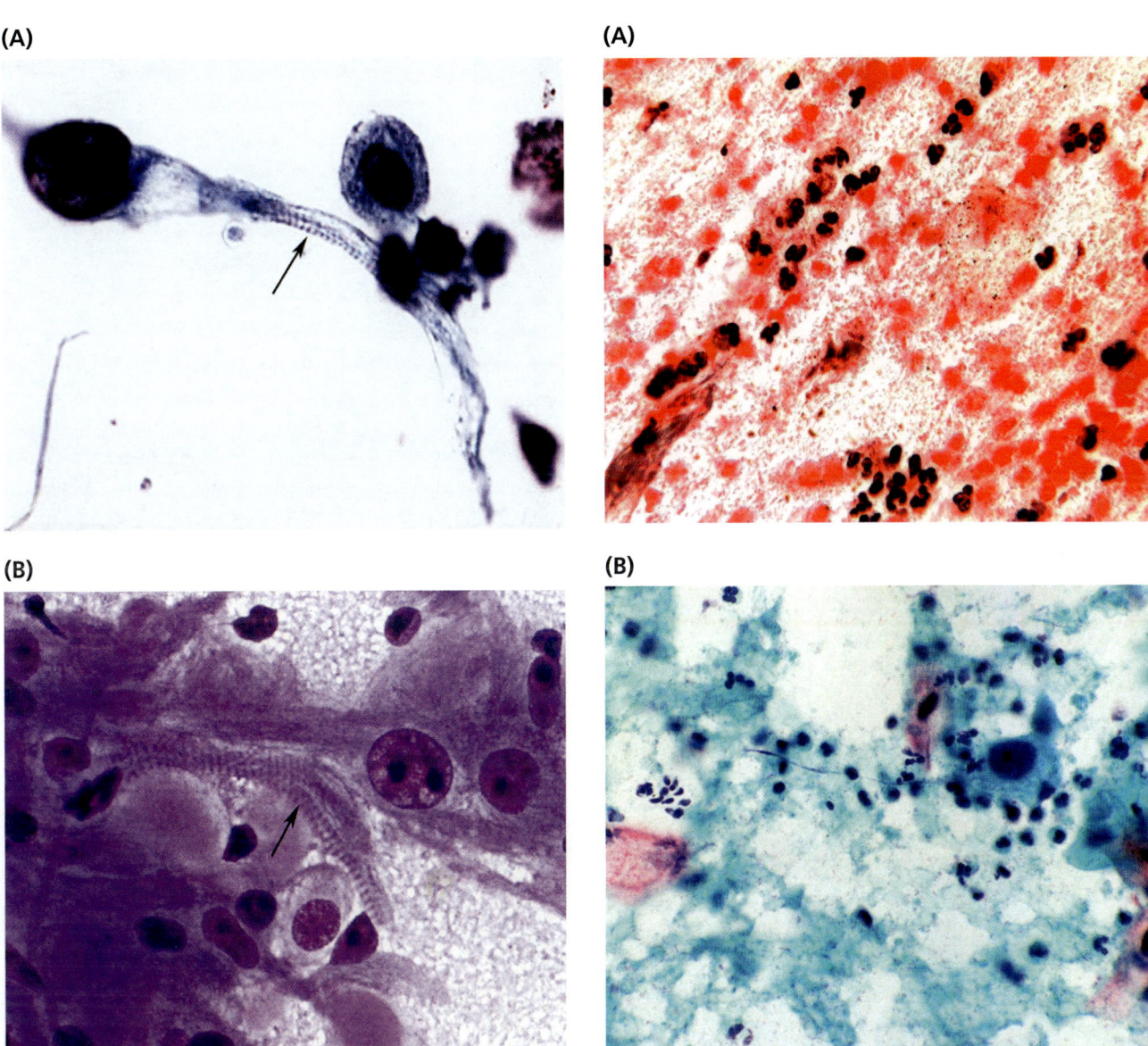

(A)

(B)

Figure 3.54 Malignant mesenchymal tumor cell with cross striations (arrows). (A) Embryonal rhabdomyosarcoma metastatic abdominal fluid. Primary tumor urinary bladder. Abdominal fluid, Millipore filter, Pap stain. (B) Intraoperative FNA, right auricular mass, rhabdomyoma heart. Patient had an adenocarcinoma of the colon. Diff-Quik stain.

Figure 3.55 (A, B) Old blood in direct smears appears as granular and beaded (A). A similar appearance may occur in certain ultrasound-guided fine needle aspirations and results from the mixing of fresh blood and Aqua gel material. Old blood appears as finely granular cobweb-like material in the background (B). LBP.

GHOST CELLS

Infarction of the tumor may occur naturally or as result of intervention such as FNA. Numerous "ghost" tumor cells may be present in the background. This may be seen in squamous and adenocarcinoma and occurs commonly following treatment or interventional procedures such an FNA (Figures 3.58 and 3.59).

CALCIFICATION

Most often, calcification is dystrophic and occurs in the connective tissue. Certain tumors (renal, carcinoid) and secretory products (mucus, colloid) may undergo calcification that may be seen in cytopreparations. Calcipherules, to be distinguished from psamomma bodies, may be seen in pulmonary material, and some crystals may appear as calcified structures (Figures 3.60 and 3.61).

TIGROID BACKGROUND

This is commonly seen in seminoma and germ cell tumors, but can occur in a number of malignant tumors. This feature is best recognized in Diff Quik-stained slides. This

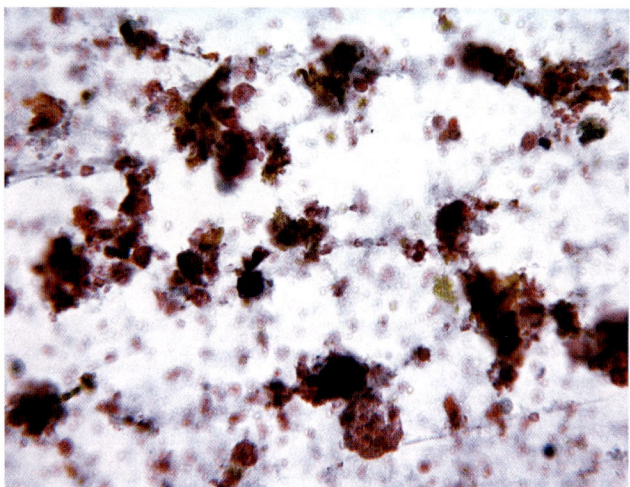

Figure 3.56 Old blood, sputum smear, case of pulmonary infarct. Old blood has been ingested by the pulmonary macrophages. FNA lung, Pap stain.

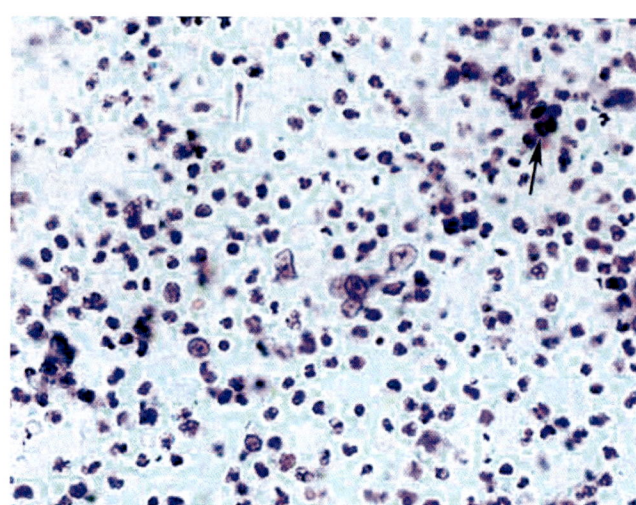

Figure 3.57 Heavy acute inflammation dominating this slide. A single group of tumor cells (arrow) is present but requires careful examination of the preparation. Lung FNA, direct smear, Pap stain.

(A)

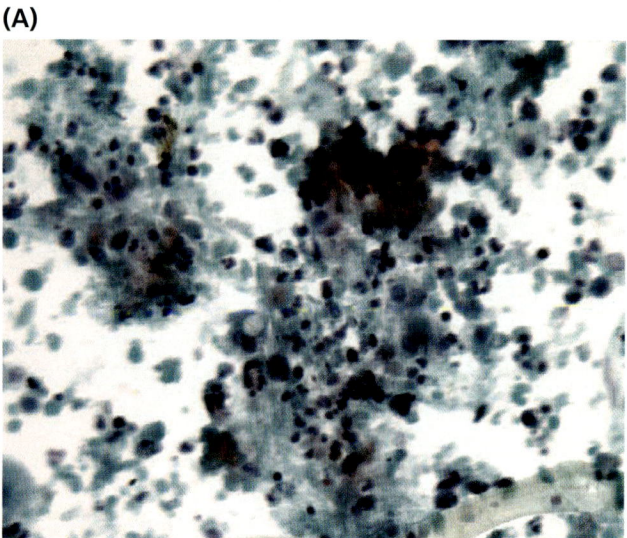

(B)

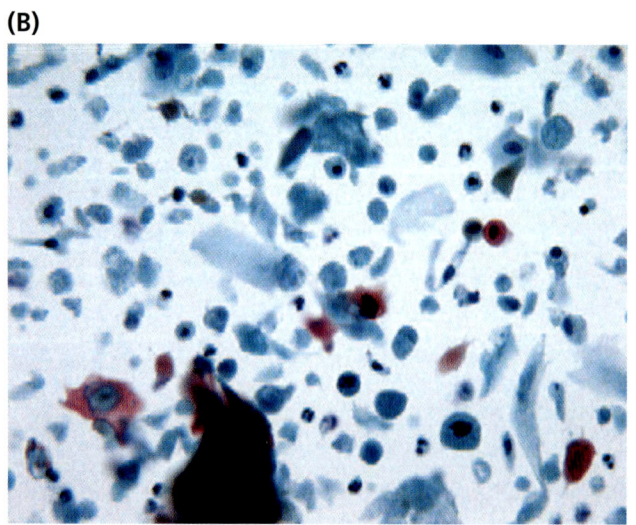

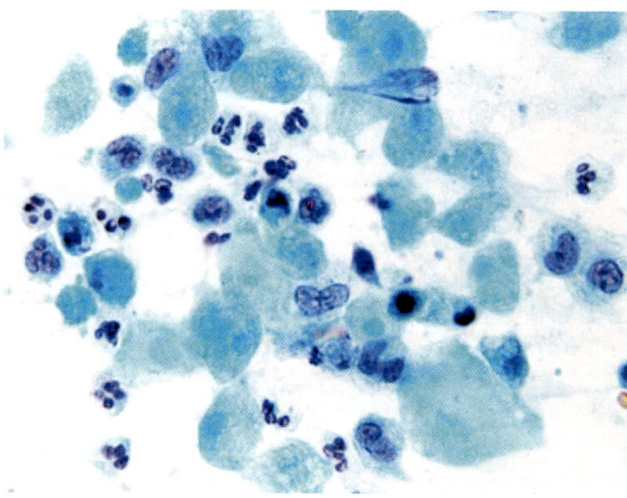

Figure 3.59 Oncocytic (Hurthle) cell infarction following FNA of the thyroid gland. Small thyroid nodules can be easily destroyed by repeated aspirations, and more commonly by the use of large bore needle and core biopsy, Pap stain.

probably reflects cytoplasmic components and smearing artifacts (Figure 3.62).

MUCOPOLYSACCHARIDE-RICH BACKGROUND

This stains metachromatically with Diff Quik and similar basic dyes. It is often seen in various types of mucus, myxoid, and chonodromyxoid material. This can occur in epithelial tumors and mesenchymal tumors as well as benign lesions. Such as chordoma and pleomorphic adenoma (Figure 3.63).

Figure 3.58 Single cell necrosis. (A) liver aspiration from a patient with adenocarcinoma of the colon metastatic to the liver. Notice the background containing numerous ghosts of tumor cells. (B) Squamous cell carcinoma cervical lymph node FNA; notice the ghost tumor cells. Pap stain.

(A)

(B)

(C)

(D)

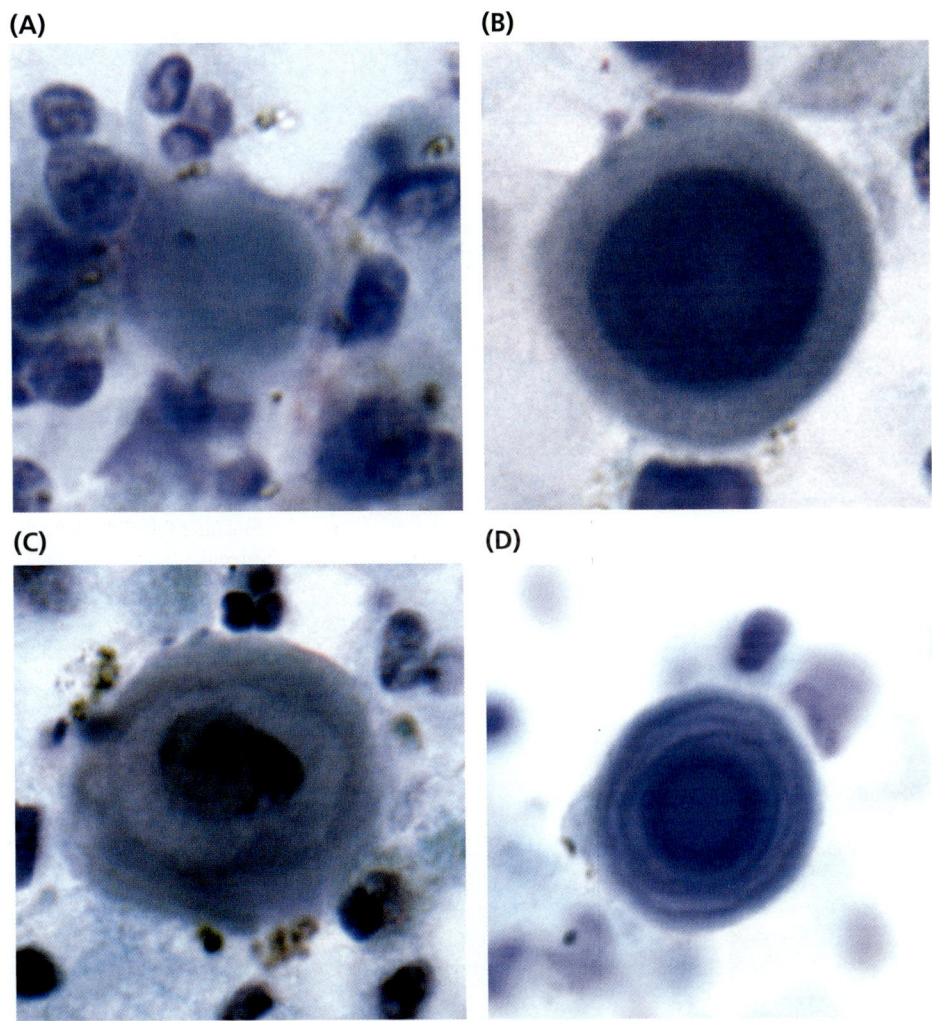

Figure 3.60 Calcipherules seen in sputum specimen. This photomicrograph depicts the various stages of development of Calcipherules. These usually occur in older (>60 years) individuals and especially those with cardiopulmonary diseases. Accumulation of proteinaceous material (A), precipitation of calcium salts (B), early condensation and lamination (C), concentric lamination (D). Sputum specimens, direct smears, Pap stain.

(A)

(B)

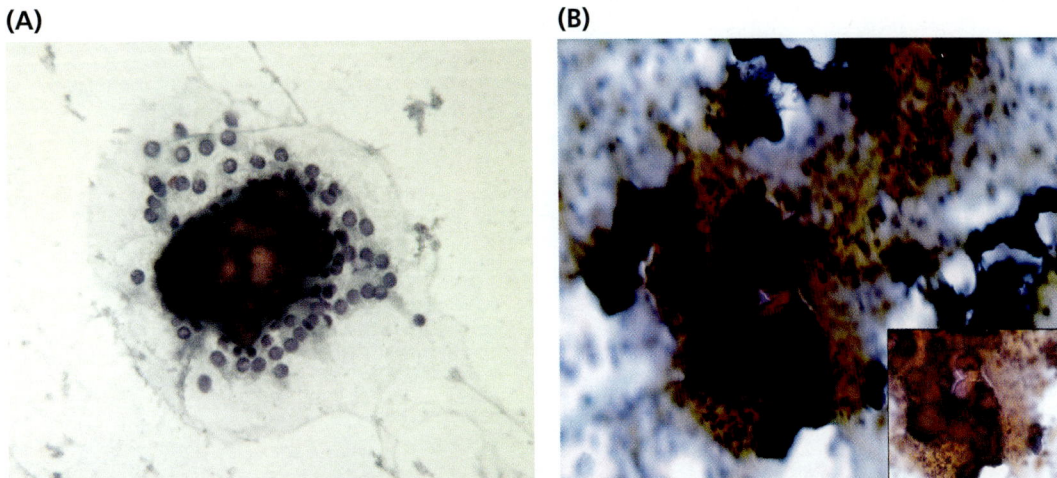

Figure 3.61 Dystrophic calcification (A), thyroid. (B) ascites. Insert shows details of the calcified material. Although laminated, it lacks the malignant cell mantle. This should be distinguished from psammoma bodies even though surrounded by follicular cells (A), Pap stain.

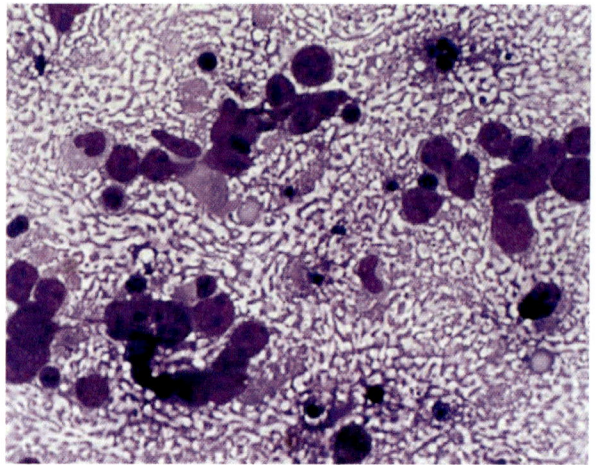

Figure 3.62 "Tigroid" background of germ cell tumor. It occurs in nearly 40% cases of seminoma, but is not specific and may be observed in chordoma and certain sarcomas. Metastatic lung tumor, Diff-Quik stain.

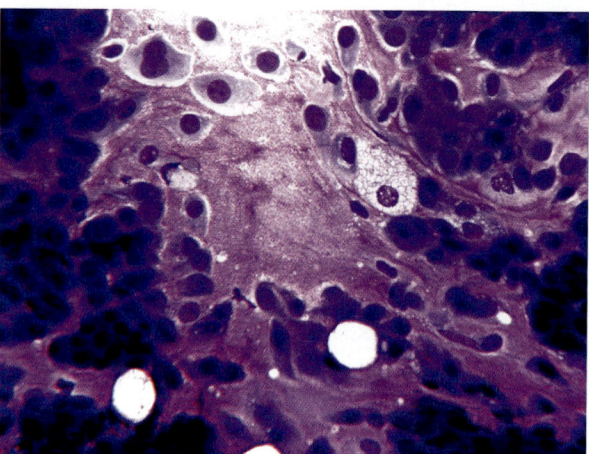

Figure 3.63 Chondoromyxoid background in a fine needle aspiration from a case of pleomorphoic adenoma of parotid gland, Diff-Quik stain.

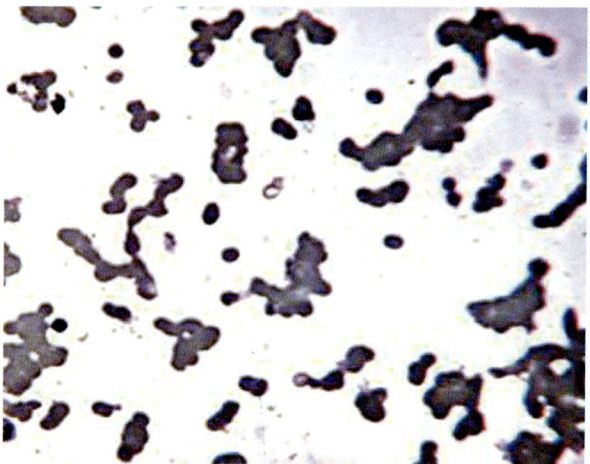

Figure 3.64 Rouleau formation. Often seen in relation to increased proteins including thyroglobins in the blood. Thyroid FNA, Diff-Quik stain.

ROULEAU FORMATION

This is a common occurrence in fresh FNA slides and represents the presence of circulating higher molecular weight proteins such as thyroglobulin and immunoglobulins. The mixing of fresh blood with certain gels used in imaging studies may produce similar appearances (Figure 3.64).

AMYLOID

This may be seen as an acellular, waxy material that often stains metachromatically by Diff Quik dyes. Amyloid material may occur in specimens from deposits and tumors associated with its production, such as medullary thyroid carcinoma (Figure 3.65).

(A)

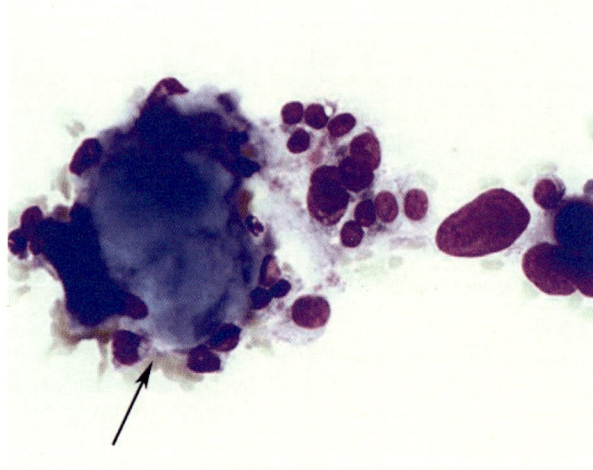

(B)

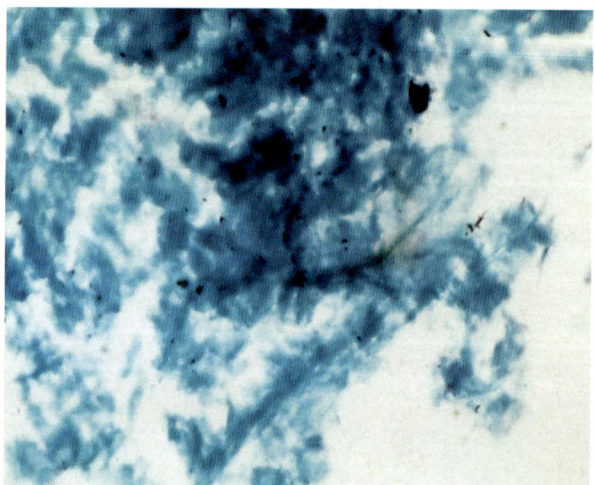

Figure 3.65 Amyloid deposit (A), medullar thyroid carcinoma (arrow), thyroid (B). Lung. (A) This often appears as acellular and waxy. It should be distinguished from mucus, and tumor-type necrosis. (A) Diff-Quik, (B) Pap stain.

LYMPHORRHAGIA

Metastases to the body cavities and pulmonary parenchyma may be preceded by outpouring of mature and immature lymphoid cells and macrophages. This is common in pleural fluids due to blockage of thoracic duct tributaries and leakage of lymphoid cells (Figures 3.66 and 3.67). Tumor cells in such specimens may be few and rare. If such a case is re-examined after a week, invariably frank tumor cells can be observed. Similar cytologic findings may occur among patients with hematopoietic disorders and granulomatous infections such as *Mycobacterium*, and certain viral infections.

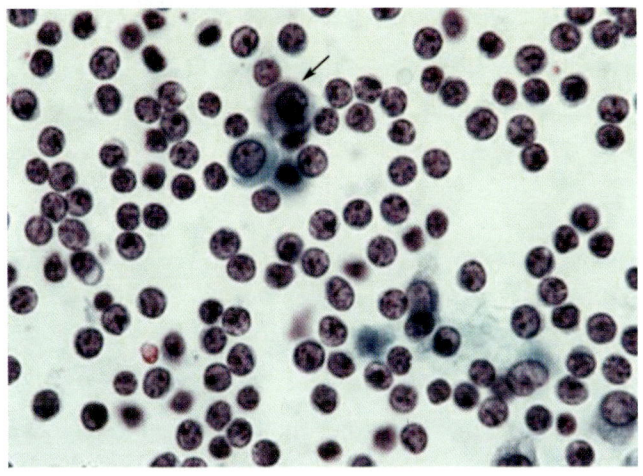

Figure 3.66 Pleural effusion specimen with numerous lymphoid and a rare malignant (arrow) cell. Lung adenocarcinoma, Millipore filter, Pap stain.

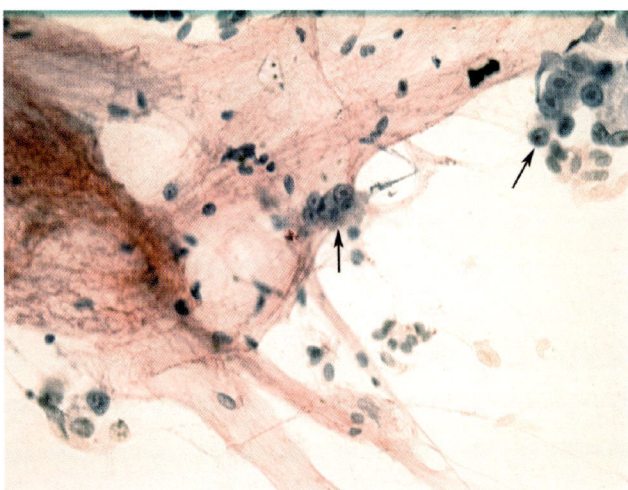

Figure 3.68 Metastatic renal cell carcinoma sputum. Notice the tumor cells embedded in the mucoid material (arrows). Sputum, direct smear, Pap stain.

(A)   **(B)**

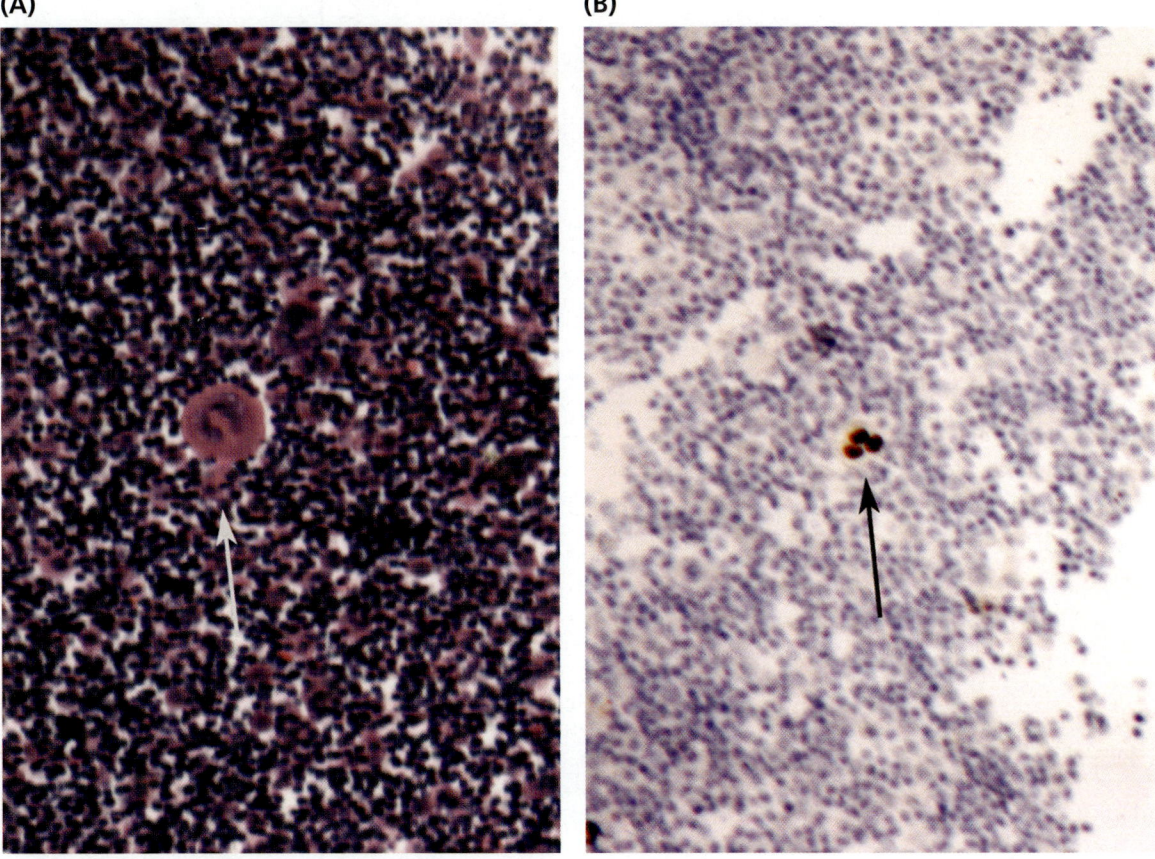

Figure 3.67 Lymphocyte-rich pleural fluid with a single tumor cell (arrow). Cell block H/E (A), TTF-1 (B).

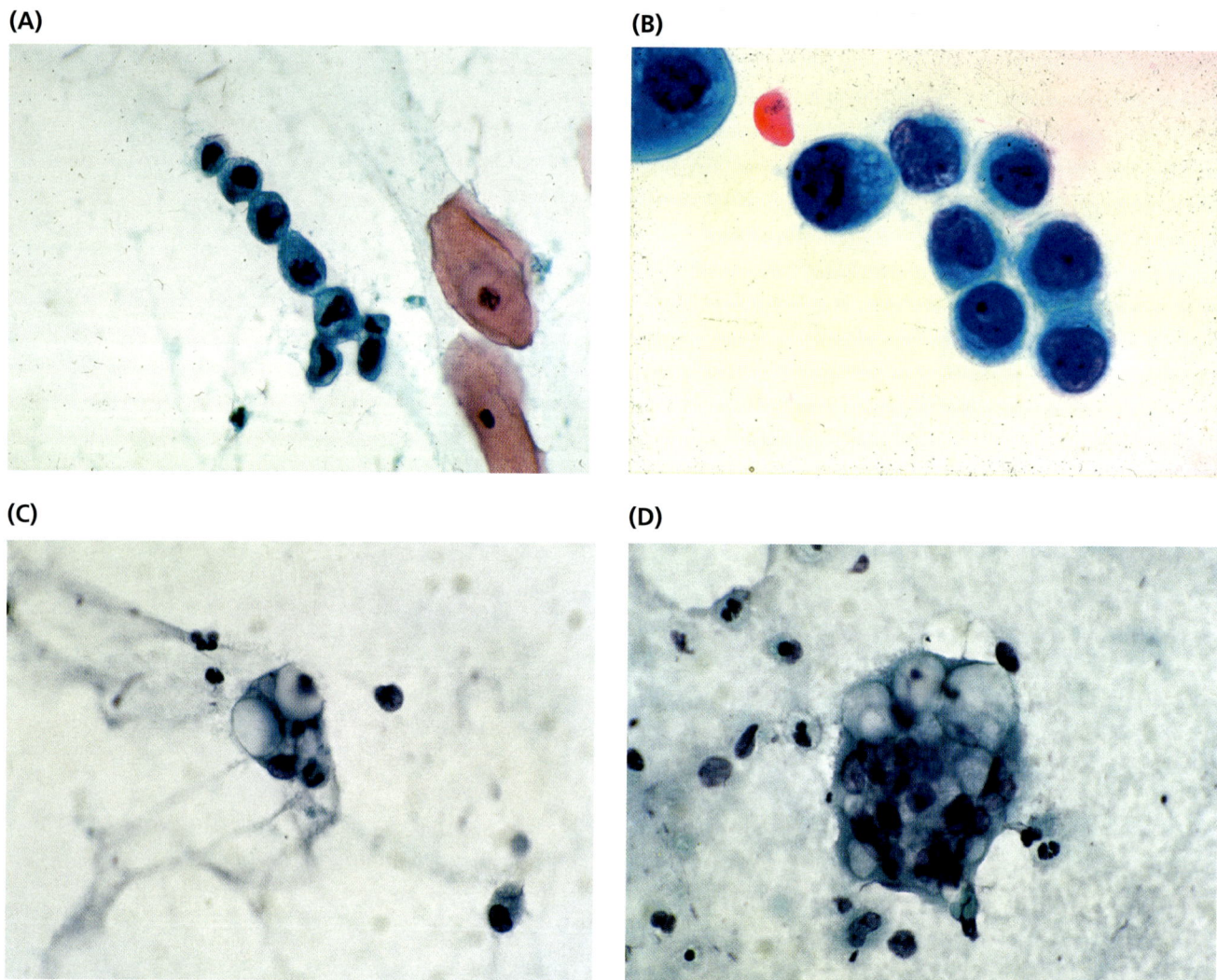

Figure 3.69 (A–D) Metastatic adenocarinoma breast, vaginal smears (A, B). Notice the clean background. Conventional Pap smear. Metastatic adenocarcinoma endometrium. Direct sputum smear (C). Metastatic liposarcoma, direct sputum smear (D), Pap stain.

CLEAN BACKGROUND

On many occasions, metastatic tumor in the pulmonary and gynecologic specimens shed malignant cells in a relatively clean background devoid of much inflammation and tumor cells may appear embedded in the mucus. These appear as "B-B shots" and are often seen with metastatic renal cell, endometrial and ovarian carcinomas and uncommonly with sarcomas (Figures 3.68 and 3.69). It must be appreciated that these background features are considerably modified by the liquid-prepared slides.

FURTHER READING

Abdulla, M., S. Hombal, *et al.* (2000). "Characterizing 'blue blobs'. Immunohistochemical staining and ultrastructural study". *Acta Cytol* **44**(4): 547–50.

Ali, M. A., M. Akhtar, *et al.* (1986). "Morphologic spectrum of hepatocellular carcinoma in fine needle aspiration biopsies". *Acta Cytol* **30**(3): 294–302.

Bayon, M. N. and R. Drut. (1991). "Cytologic diagnosis of adenovirus bronchopneumonia". *Acta Cytol* **35**(2): 181–2.

Bedrossian, C. W. and D. L. Rybka. (1976). "Bronchial brushing during fiberoptic bronchoscopy for the cytodiagnosis of lung cancer: comparison with sputum and bronchial washings". *Acta Cytol* **20**(5): 446–53.

Berthezene, F. and M. A. Greer. (1974). "Studies on the composition of the thyroid psammoma bodies of chronically iodine-deficient rats". *Endocrinology* **95**(3): 651–9.

Bottles, K. and T. Lowhagen. (1985). "Psammoma bodies in the aspiration cytology smears of an acinic-cell tumor". *Acta Cytol* **29**(2): 191–2.

Castro-Gomez, L., S. Cordova-Ramirez, *et al.* (2003). "Cytologic criteria of cystic papillary carcinoma of the thyroid". *Acta Cytol* **47**(4): 590–4.

Chamberlain, D. W., A. C. Braude, *et al.* (1987). "A critical evaluation of bronchoalveolar lavage. Criteria for identifying unsatisfactory specimens". *Acta Cytol* **31**(5): 599–605.

Chang, T. C., S. M. Lai, *et al.* (2004). "Three-dimensional cytomorphology in fine needle aspiration biopsy of subacute thyroiditis". *Acta Cytol* **48**(2): 155–60.

Crabtree, W. N. and W. M. Murphy. (1980). "The value of ethanol as a fixative in urinary cytology". *Acta Cytol* **24**(5): 452–5.

Crapanzano, J. P. and M. F. Zakowski. (2001). "Diagnostic dilemmas in pulmonary cytology". *Cancer* **93**(6): 364–75.

Das, D. K. (2004). "Fine-needle aspiration (FNA) cytology diagnosis of small round cell tumors: value and limitations". *Indian J Pathol Microbiol* **47**(3): 309–18.

Das, D. K. (2005). "Intranuclear cytoplasmic inclusions in fine-needle aspiration smears of papillary thyroid carcinoma: a study of its morphological forms, association with nuclear grooves, and mode of formation". *Diagn Cytopathol* **32**(5): 264–8.

De Las Casas, L. E., H. D. Hoerl, *et al.* (2001). "Utility of urinary cytology for diagnosing human polyoma virus infection in transplant recipients: a study of 37 cases with electron microscopic analysis". *Diagn Cytopathol* **25**(6): 376–81.

Dreyer, T., I. Knoblauch, *et al.* (2001). "Nuclear texture features for classifying benign vs. dysplastic or malignant squamous epithelium of the larynx". *Anal Quant Cytol Histol* **23**(3): 193–200.

Goellner, J. R. and D. A. Johnson. (1982). "Cytology of cystic papillary carcinoma of the thyroid". *Acta Cytol* **26**(6): 797–808.

Gondos, B. (1974). "Cell degeneration: light and electron microscopic study of ovarian germ cells". *Acta Cytol* **18**(6): 504–09.

Gupta, S. K., A. K. Rajwanshi, *et al.* (1985). "Fine needle aspiration cytology smear patterns of malignant melanoma". *Acta Cytol* **29**(6): 983–8.

Hashi, A., T. Yuminamochi, *et al.* (2008). "Intranuclear cytoplasmic inclusion is a significant diagnostic feature for the differentiation of lobular endocervical glandular hyperplasia from minimal deviation adenocarcinoma of the cervix". *Diagn Cytopathol* **36**(8): 535–44.

Hsu, C., Y. C. Choo, *et al.* (1984). "Exfoliative cytology in the evaluation of interferon treatment of cervical intraepithelial neoplasia". *Acta Cytol* **28**(2): 111–7.

Hunt, J. L. and E. L. Barnes. (2003). "Non-tumor-associated psammoma bodies in the thyroid". *Am J Clin Pathol* **119**(1): 90–4.

Jenkins, D. M. and R. Goulden. (1977). "Psammoma bodies in cervical cytology smears". *Acta Cytol* **21**(1): 112–3.

Kaneko, C., M. Shamoto, *et al.* (1996). "Studies on intranuclear inclusions and nuclear grooves in papillary thyroid cancer by light, scanning electron and transmission electron microscopy". *Acta Cytol* **40**(3): 417–22.

Kim, K., C. Mah, *et al.* (1986). "Carcinoid tumors of the lung: cytologic differential diagnosis in fine-needle aspirates". *Diagn Cytopathol* **2**(4): 343–6.

Kini, S. R., J. M. Miller, *et al.* (1980). "Cytopathology of papillary carcinoma of the thyroid by fine needle aspiration". *Acta Cytol* **24**(6): 511–21.

Koss, L. G. (2000). "Utility of liquid-based cytology for cervical carcinoma screening". *Cancer* **90**(1): 67–9.

Koss, L. G., M. R. Melamed, *et al.* (2006). *Koss' Diagnostic Cytology and its Histopathologic Bases.* Philadelphia, PA, Lippincott Williams & Wilkins.

Koukoulaki, M., M. O'Donovan, *et al.* (2008). "Prospective study of urine cytology screening for BK polyoma virus replication in renal transplant recipients". *Cytopathology* **19**(6): 385–8.

Lapkus, O., T. M. Elsheikh, *et al.* (2006). "Pitfalls in the diagnosis of herpes simplex infection in respiratory cytology". *Acta Cytol* **50**(6): 617–20.

LiVolsi, V. A. and P. K. Gupta. (1992). "Thyroid fine-needle aspiration: intranuclear inclusions, nuclear grooves and psammoma bodies – paraganglioma-like adenoma of the thyroid". *Diagn Cytopathol* **8**(1): 82–3; discussion 83–4.

Lozowski, W. and S. I. Hajdu. (1987). "Cytology and immunocytochemistry of bronchioloalveolar carcinoma". *Acta Cytol* **31**(6): 717–25.

Morimura, Y., H. Nishiyama, *et al.* (2002). "Diagnosing endometrial carcinoma with cervical involvement by cervical cytology". *Acta Cytol* **46**(2): 284–90.

Nagy, G. K., J. B. Jacobs, *et al.* (1989). "Intracytoplasmic eosinophilic inclusion bodies in breast cyst fluids are giant lysosomes". *Acta Cytol* **33**(1): 99–103.

Pearson, J. C., L. Kromhout, *et al.* (1981). "Evaluation of collection and preservation techniques for urinary cytology". *Acta Cytol* **25**(3): 327–33.

Pettinato, G., P. E. Swanson, *et al.* (1989). "Undifferentiated small round-cell tumors of childhood: the immunocytochemical demonstration of myogenic differentiation in fine-needle aspirates". *Diagn Cytopathol* **5**(2): 194–9.

Romagosa, C., V. Morente, *et al.* (2002). "Intranuclear inclusions in fine needle aspirates of bronchial low grade mucoepidermoid carcinoma with clear cell change: a report of two cases". *Acta Cytol* **46**(1): 57–60.

Russin, V. L., P. T. Valente, *et al.* (1987). "Psammoma bodies in neuroendocrine carcinoma of the uterine cervix". *Acta Cytol* **31**(6): 791–5.

Sagawa, M., Y. Saito, *et al.* (1994). "Localization of double, roentgenographically occult lung cancer. Cytologic findings from selective brushing of all segmental and subsegmental bronchi". *Acta Cytol* **38**(3): 392–7.

Shet, T. and J. Rege. (2000). "Cystic degeneration in phyllodes tumor. A source of error in cytologic interpretation". *Acta Cytol* **44**(2): 163–8.

Sidawy, M. K. and M. Costa. (1989). "The significance of paravacuolar granules of the thyroid. A histologic, cytologic and ultrastructural study". *Acta Cytol* **33**(6): 929–33.

Silverman, J. F., F. D. Jones, *et al.* (1989). "Cytopathology of neoplasms of the central nervous system in specimens obtained by the Cavitron Ultrasonic Surgical Aspirator". *Acta Cytol* **33**(5): 576–82.

Simmons, T. J. and S. E. Martin. (1991). "Fine-needle aspiration biopsy of malignant melanoma: a cytologic and immunocytochemical analysis". *Diagn Cytopathol* **7**(4): 380–6.

Sinner, W. N. and B. Sandstedt. (1976). "Small-cell carcinoma of the lung. Cytological, roentgenologic, and clinical findings in a consecutive series diagnosed by fine-needle aspiration biopsy". *Radiology* **121**(2): 269–74.

Sironi, M., R. Claren, *et al.* (1999). "Intranuclear cytoplasmic inclusions and nuclear grooves in pleomorphic adenoma of parotid gland". *Diagn Cytopathol* **21**(6): 435–6.

Soyuer, I., C. Ekinci, *et al.* (2003). "Diagnosis of hepatocellular carcinoma by fine needle aspiration cytology. Cellular features". *Acta Cytol* **47**(4): 581–9.

Sprenger, E., H. Ulrich, *et al.* (1979). "The diagnostic value of cell-nuclear DNA determination in aspiration cytology of benign and malignant lesions of the breast". *Anal Quant Cytol* **1**(1): 29–36.

Sun, L., S. Sakurai, *et al.* (2009). "High-grade neuroendocrine carcinoma of the lung: comparative clinicopathological study of large cell neuroendocrine carcinoma and small cell lung carcinoma". *Pathol Int* **59**(8): 522–9.

Szpak, C. A., E. H. Bossen, *et al.* (1984). "Cytomorphology of primary small-cell (Merkel-cell) carcinoma of the skin in fine needle aspirates". *Acta Cytol* **28**(3): 290–6.

Szyfelbein, W. M. and J. S. Ross. (1988). "Carcinoids, atypical carcinoids, and small-cell carcinomas of the lung: differential diagnosis of fine-needle aspiration biopsy specimens". *Diagn Cytopathol* **4**(1): 1–8.

Tanida, O., S. Kaneshima, *et al.* (1982). "Viability of intraperitoneal free cancer cells in patients with gastric cancer". *Acta Cytol* **26**(5): 681–7.

Tao, L. C., G. L. Weisbrod, *et al.* (1986). "Cytologic diagnosis of bronchioloalveolar carcinoma by fine-needle aspiration biopsy". *Cancer* **57**(8): 1565–70.

Taskinen, E., P. Tukiainen, *et al.* (1992). "Bronchoalveolar lavage. Influence of cytologic methods on the cellular picture". *Acta Cytol* **36**(5): 680–6.

Triggiani, V., E. Guastamacchia, *et al.* (2008). "Microcalcifications and psammoma bodies in thyroid tumors". *Thyroid* **18**(9): 1017–8.

Tseng, F. Y., Y. L. Hsiao, *et al.* (2002). "Cytologic features of metastatic papillary thyroid carcinoma in cervical lymph nodes". *Acta Cytol* **46**(6): 1043–8.

Valicenti, J. F., J r. and S. K. Priester. (1977). "Psammoma bodies of benign endometrial origin in cervicovaginal cytology". *Acta Cytol* **21**(4): 550–2.

Wied, G. L. and L. G. Koss. (1984). "Aspiration biopsy cytology". *Acta Cytol* **28**(3): 195–7.

Wolberg, W. H., W. N. Street, *et al.* (1995). "Computer-derived nuclear features distinguish malignant from benign breast cytology". *Hum Pathol* **26**(7): 792–6.

Yang, G. C. (1995). "Mixed small cell/large cell carcinoma of the lung. Report of a case with cytologic features and ultrastructural correlation". *Acta Cytol* **39**(6): 1175–81.

Yoshimura, S., T. Nishimura, *et al.* (1980). "The morphometry of the Sudan-III-positive granules in the cytoplasm of the human amniotic epithelium". *Acta Cytol* **24**(1): 44–8.

Zaharopoulos, P. (2004). "Viral cytopathic changes in urine cytology of ileal conduit attributed to adenovirus: report of a case". *Diagn Cytopathol* **30**(4): 284–7.

Ziabkowski, T. A. and B. Naylor. (1976). "Cyanophilic bodies in cervico-vaginal smears". *Acta Cytol* **20**(4): 340–2.

4 FUNCTIONAL DIFFERENTIATION CHARACTERISTICS IN CANCER

GENERAL FEATURES

Most of the functional differentiation characteristics in malignant neoplasia are atypical, while most in euplasia are typical. The same atypical characteristics can be found in retroplasia and proplasia, but usually less often than in malignant neoplasia. Thus these are *not* malignant criteria, but characteristics indicating differentiation of cancer cells to perform functions. Those cytoplasmic features should be applied only to cells which, primarily, one knows are cancers by virtue of their malignant criteria patterns and, secondarily, have these characteristics of cells differentiating toward a certain type of malignancy.

Cytoplasmic differentiation of a neoplastic cell is an attempt at maturation and to replicate the cell and tissue of origin. While most malignant criteria are represented in the nucleus, tissue differentiating characteristics are manifested within the cytoplasm.

SQUAMOUS CELL CARCINOMA

The cells from squamous cells carcinoma tend to be shed singly; however, in FNA specimens and specimens obtained by scraping, or processed by liquid concentration techniques, small tissue fragments of squamous cell carcinoma may be observed. In the original description, Papanicolaou observed and described two types of cells – tadpole and fiber associated with invasive squamous cell carcinoma. Dr. Ruth Graham working in his laboratory observed the third type cell in the same smears. These three cell types are the hallmarks of the invasive squamous cell tumors and are depicted in Figures 4.1 and 4.2.

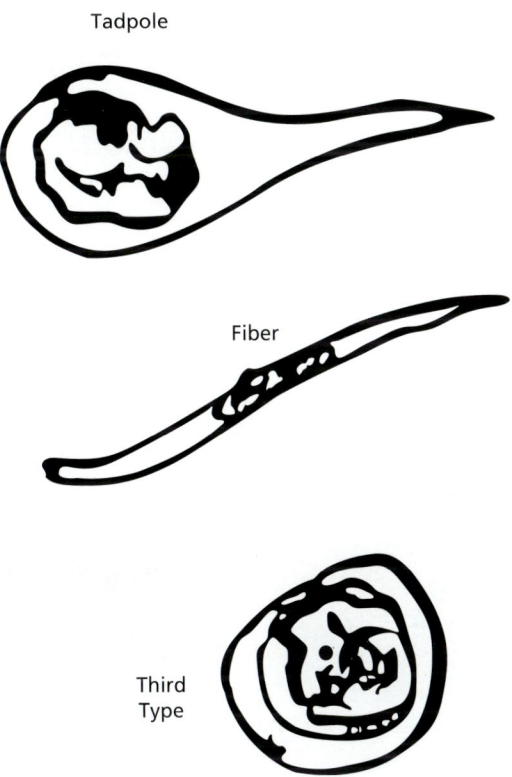

Figure 4.1 Three salient cell types associated with squamous cell carcinoma.

Nucleus

As a normal squamous cell nucleus becomes pyknotic, the same tendency is apparent in malignant squamous cells (Figure 4.3).

This tendency is apparent in malignant squamous cells. With karyopyknosis, however, malignant criteria are obscured, frequently losing the classic diagnostic features. India ink pyknotic nucleus occurring in a large cell should raise the possibility of squamous differentiation (Figure 4.4). These changes are observed commonly among

Cytohistology: Essential and Basic Concepts, Prabodh Gupta and Zubair Baloch. Published by Cambridge University Press. © Cambridge University Press 2011.

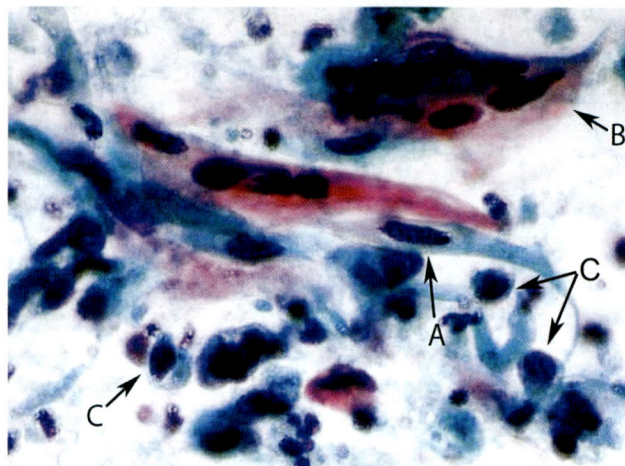

Figure 4.2 Fiber cell (A), tadpole cell (B), and third-type cell (C). Cervicovaginal smear, Pap stain.

(A)

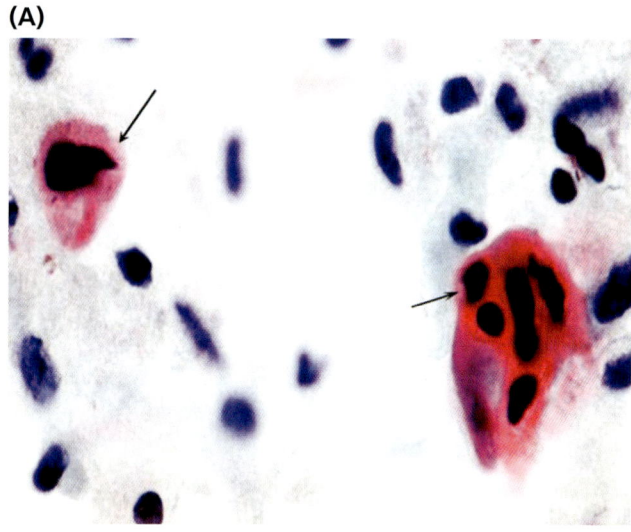

(B)

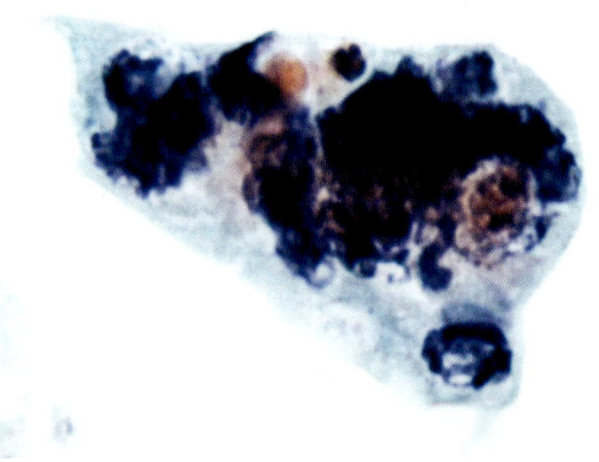

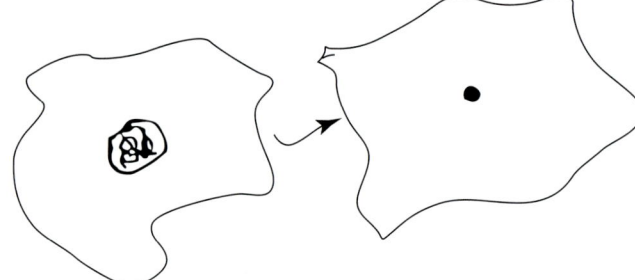

Figure 4.3 The physiologic transition from a vesicular to a pyknotic nucleus in squamous cell.

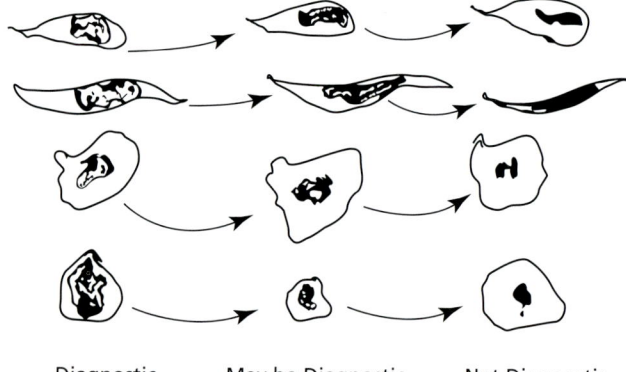

| Diagnostic | May be Diagnostic | Not Diagnostic |

Figure 4.5 Nuclear chromatin condensation. Cellular degeneration may produce similar changes and they should be used to evaluate squamous differentiation.

squamous cells occurring in a cavitary or cystic lesion and on epithelial surfaces exposed to the outside, such as oropharynx and external genital regions.

Independent malignant features should be recognized, and these pyknotic nuclei must not form the basis of squamous cell carcinoma, as these changes often cannot be distinguished from degeneration. Degenerative changes among other epithelial cells including bronchial, urothelial, and hepatobiliary in origin as well as certain mesenchymal and macrophage cells should be distinguished from nuclear chromatin condensation and pyknosis observed in squamous carcinoma cells (Figures 4.4–4.7).

Some malignant squamous nuclei may have limited or variable karyopyknosis, and may retain sufficient malignant criteria to be diagnostic (Figure 4.8).

Figure 4.4 Squamous cell carcinoma showing condensed, dark, pyknotic (India ink) nuclei (A) (arrows). In large cells, such changes should raise the possibility of squamous cell carcinoma (B). Bronchial wash specimen (A), FNA base of the skull (B). Pap stain.

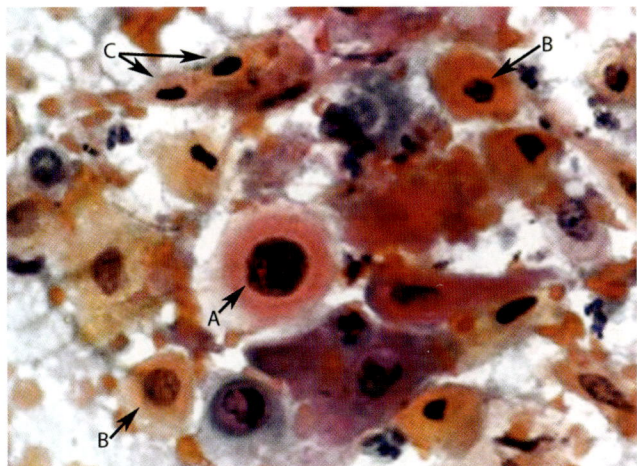

Figure 4.6 Squamous cells nuclear pyknosis. While nucleus (A) is most worrisome for squamous cell carcinoma, nuclei in (B) and (C) should not be diagnosed as representing malignant cells. Lateral neck aspiration, squamous cell carcinoma of the tongue. Conventional smear, Pap stain.

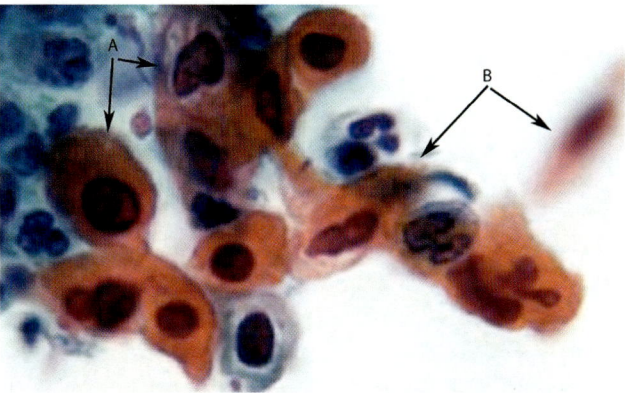

Figure 4.7 Hyperchromatic dysplastic (A) and metaplastic columnar (B) cells. There is also evidence of nuclear degeneration. Such features should not be considered diagnostic for squamous cell carcinoma. Bronchial wash specimen. Early Lung Cancer Project (ELCP), direct smear, Pap stain.

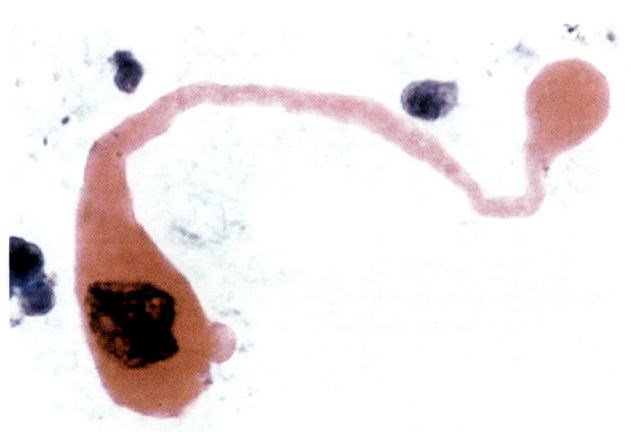

Figure 4.8 Malignant squamous cell. The pyknotic nucleus still retains sufficient chromatin and membrane abnormalities to be diagnostic. There is also cytoplasmic abnormal thinning with a bulbous terminal end. Bronchial brush specimen (ELCP), direct smear, Pap stain.

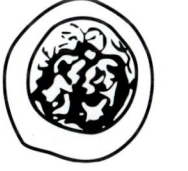 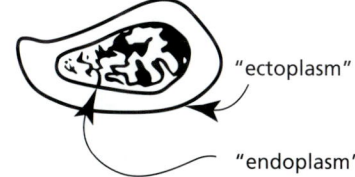

Figure 4.9 Biphasic cytoplasm. Such changes may be observed in well-differentiated squamous cell carcinoma. These alterations appear degenerative in origin and may be seen in mesothelial cells.

Cytoplasm

Cytoplasm often provides good characteristics to suggest squamous differentiation. These include the following.

Keratinization cell border

A sharp, crisp, "hard" cell border is often seen in squamous cells with keratinizing cytoplasm.

"*Endoplasm/ectoplasm*": the cytoplasm separates into two distinct types: the outer (ectoplasm) becomes a hyaline shell, while the inner (endoplasm) remains amorphous and always contains the nucleus (Figures 4.9 and 4.10). The endo-ectoplasmic border is sharp. Care needs to be exercised in the interpretation of these changes in body cavity fluids: mesothelial cells may exhibit similar cytoplasmic attributes.

Keratinizing clumps: irregular aggregates of keratinizing material appear within the cytoplasm, usually very orange, and hyaline – as in the Papanicolaou-stained preparations (Figures 4.11–4.13).

Hyalinization: the cell ectoplasm becomes very dense hyalin or glassy – like a church window-glass. This has nothing to do with color (which can be of any cytoplasmic hue) and concerns only the highly refractile appearance of glass. It may be intensely organophilic giving a "Halloween orange" or pumpkin-colored appearance (Figures 4.14 and 4.15).

Ringing: refractile rings or lamination appear in the hyaline outer cytoplasm, best seen by focusing up and down through the cell. They appear to represent interfaces of progressive shells, or rims, laid down in the hyaline formation as if by successive gelation or layering (Figures 4.16 and 4.17).

Color: artifactual acidophilia due to drying, improper fixation, pH change in the centers of cell clumps and mucopolysaccharides may occur among malignant cells. A brilliant "Halloween orange" best suggests keratinization.

(A)

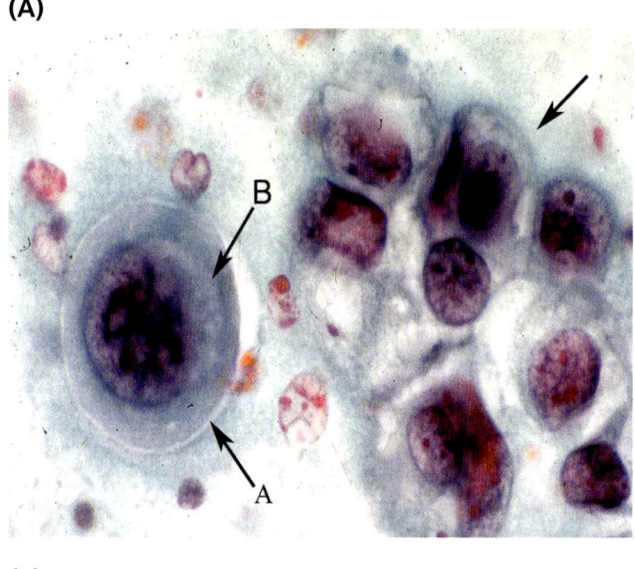

(B)

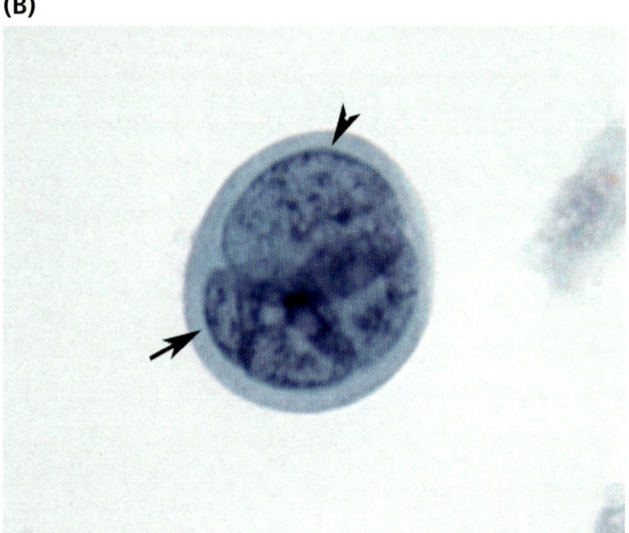

Figure 4.10 Squamous cell carcinoma with biphasic cytoplasm. Poorly differentiated carcinoma (A) (arrow) with single cell demonstrating a biphasic (ectoplasmic (arrow A) and endoplasmic (arrow B)) cytoplasm as an evidence of squamous differentiation. Cervicovaginal conventional smear, Pap stain. Ecto/endoplasmic differentiation (B), notice the variation in the nuclear size; small (arrow), large (arrowhead). FNA, neck mass, LBP.

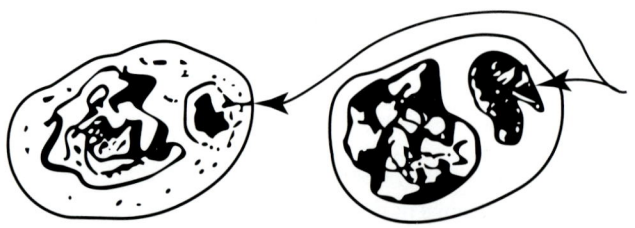

Figure 4.11 Occurrence of irregular orangophilic aggregates (arrow) in cases of squamous differentiation.

(A)

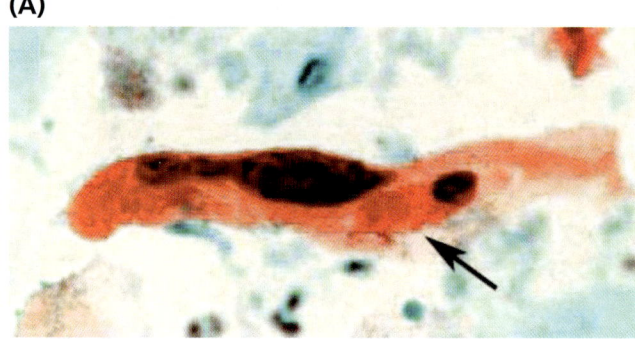

(B)

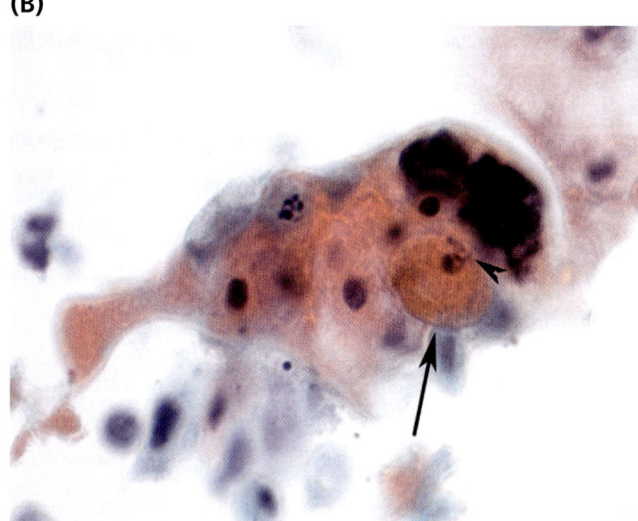

Figure 4.12 Malignant squamous cell with an orangophilic aggregate of keratin within the cytoplasm (arrows). There is a nuclear tag (arrowhead). (B) In well-stained cells these often appear as "Halloween Orange." ELCP, direct smear, Pap stain (A), base of the skull FNA (B), LBP.

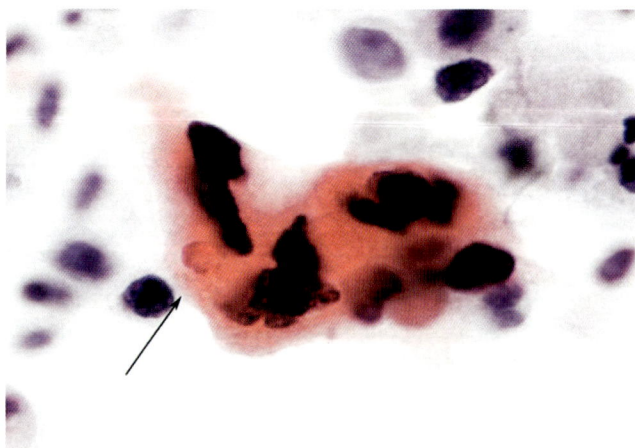

Figure 4.13 A group of atypical but degenerated cells in a pulmonary specimen showing an orangophilic intracytoplasmic clump (arrow). This is evidence of cytoplasm differentiation and not of malignancy. Bronchial wash specimen, Pap stain.

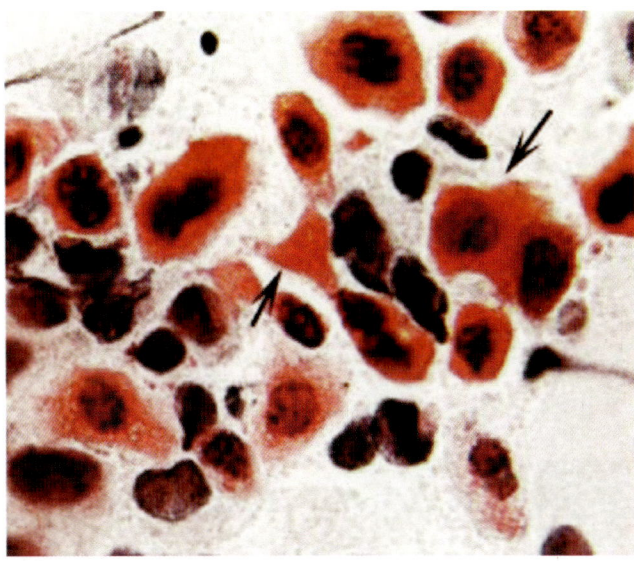

Figure 4.14 Squamous cell carcinoma lung. Notice a number of intensely hyaline, orangophilic (arrows) cells. The nuclei of most cells are degenerated, dark, and pyknotic. Sputum specimen, conventional smear, Pap stain.

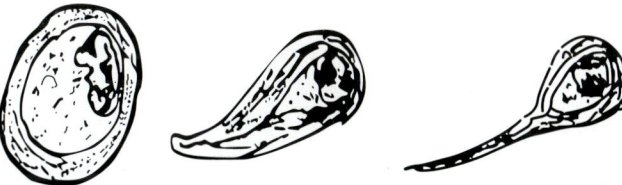

Figure 4.16 "Ringing" or lamination of the dense cytoplasm seen in squamous cell carcinoma cells.

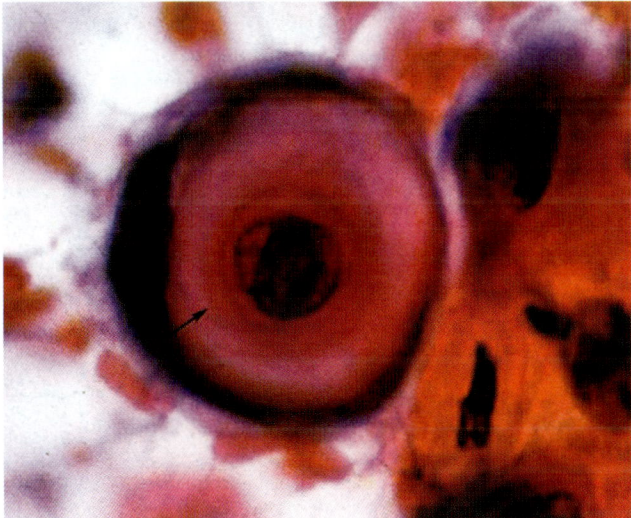

Figure 4.17 Malignant squamous cell with cytoplasmic concentric lamination (arrow). Oral smear, Pap stain.

As mentioned earlier, cytoplasmic color must not be a diagnostic criterion (Figure 4.18). In body cavity specimens, keratinzation may occur in metaplastic tumors and benign mesothlial cells.

(A)

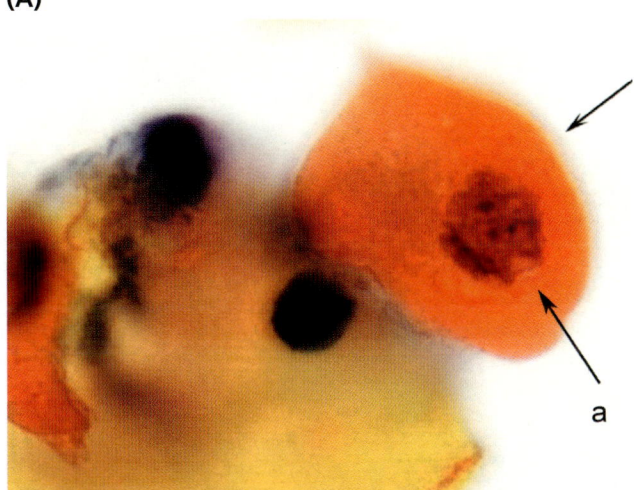

(B)

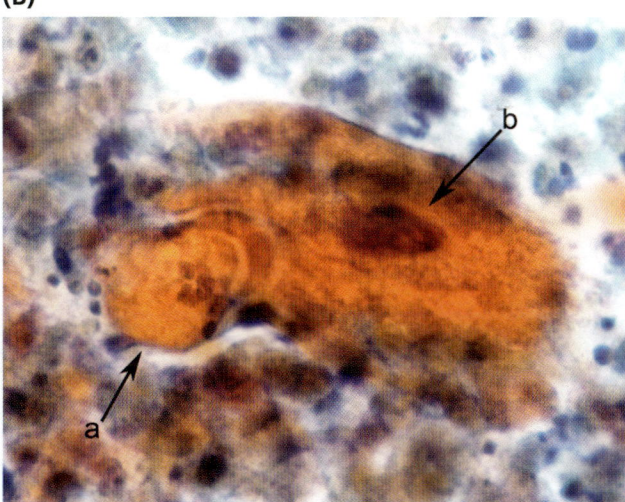

Figure 4.15 (A, B) Hyalinization in squamous cell carcinoma (A) (arrow). Notice the nuclear membrane bite, (a) in an otherwise vesicular and unremarkable nucleus. (B) Hyalinization (a), notice the unremarkable nucleus (b). Sputum specimens, direct smear, Pap stain.

Atypical thinning

Cytoplasmic thinning (tail formations): a maturing normal squamous cell typically thins to wafer-thickness (Figure 4.19). A malignant or dysplastic squamous cell thins either typically as a squamous flake or atypically in an elongated spindloid fashion (Figures 4.20–4.22).

Caudate (tail) formation

Sometimes, squamous cell cytoplasm may not thin and indeed may condense and thicken. This atypical thinning occurs frequently and is best developed in the "tadpole" and "spindle" cells.

As the squamous cells become malignant, the cytoplasmic thinning becomes atypical. The best examples include the tadpole and fiber cells. Also, the elongated cells may develop

(A)

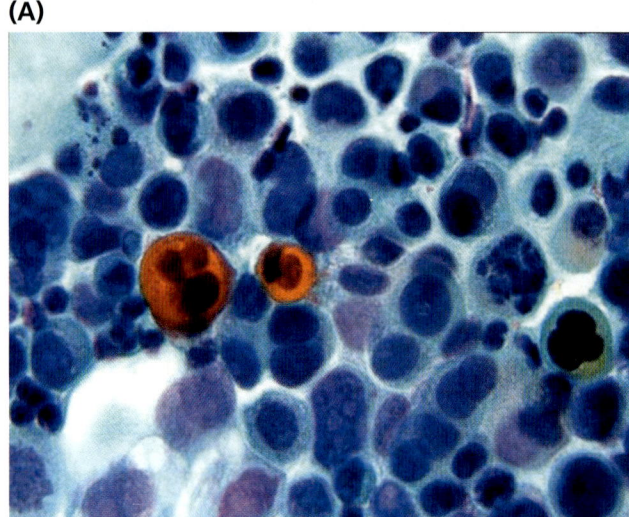

(B)

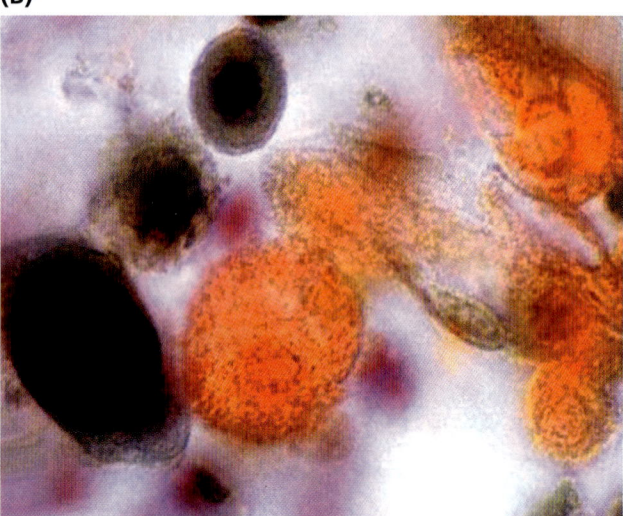

Figure 4.18 Bright orange tumor cells in a pleural fluid specimen from a patient with colon adenocarcinoma (A). Degenerated cells with cytoplasmic orangophilia. Gastric adenocarcinoma metastatic to the brain. CSF specimen, ventricular tap (B). Millipore filter, Pap stain.

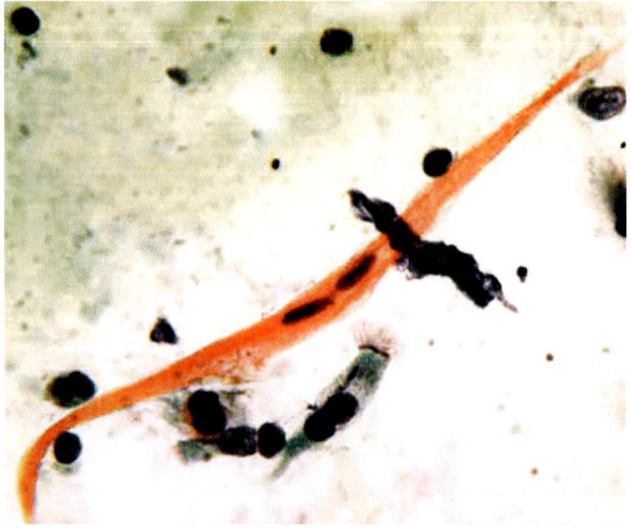

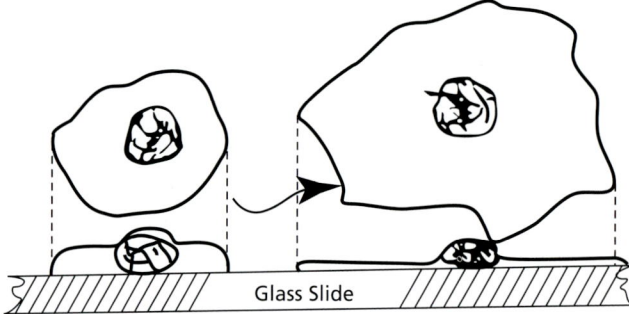

Figure 4.19 Thinning of maturing squamous cells.

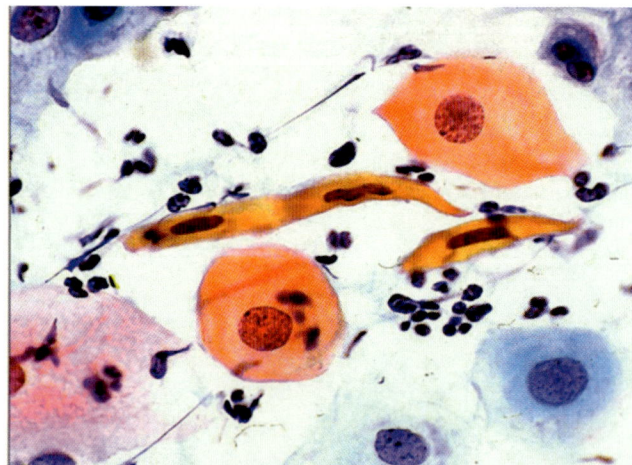

Figure 4.21 Atypical cytoplasmic thinning. Squamous cells appear to have cytoplasmic condensation and thickening at the edges. Such changes occur in HPV-infected cells and a koilocyte is an extreme example of peripheral cytoplasm condensation. Cervicovaginal smear, Pap stain.

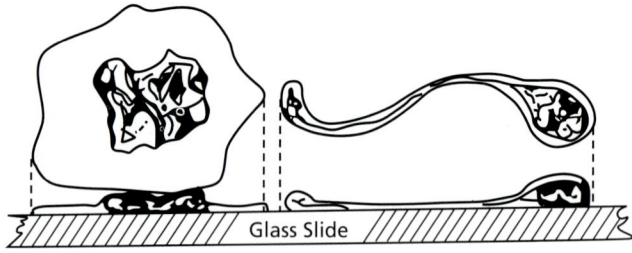

Figure 4.22 Atypical cytoplasm thinning. There is a terminal bulbous condensation that may contain another nucleus or some cytoplasm organelle.

Figure 4.20 Atypical cytoplasmic thinning of a squamous cell; it is uneven, being tapered at one end and bulbous at the other. There is an abnormal nucleus. Dysplastic squamous cell. Bronchial wash specimen, Pap stain.

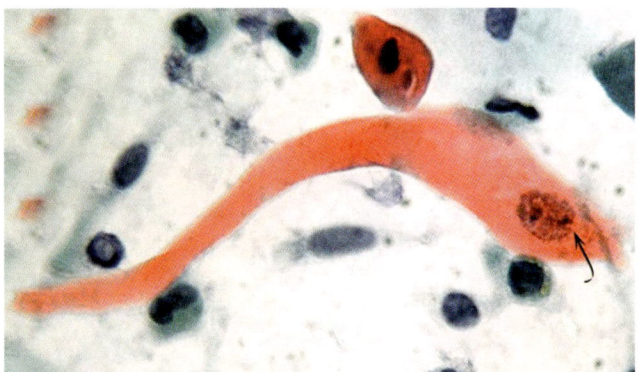

Figure 4.23 Atypical cytoplasmic thinning with tadpole cell formation. Notice the nuclear membrane irregularity (arrow). Bronchial wash, ELCP, Pap stain.

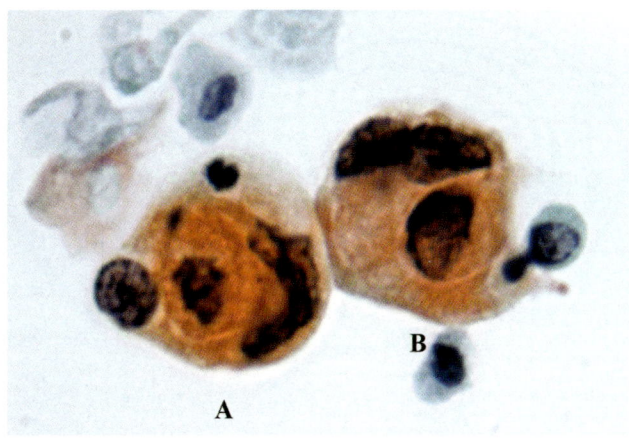

Figure 4.24 (A) Malignant pearl formation. Notice the nuclear malignant features (B). Sputum, LBP, Pap stain.

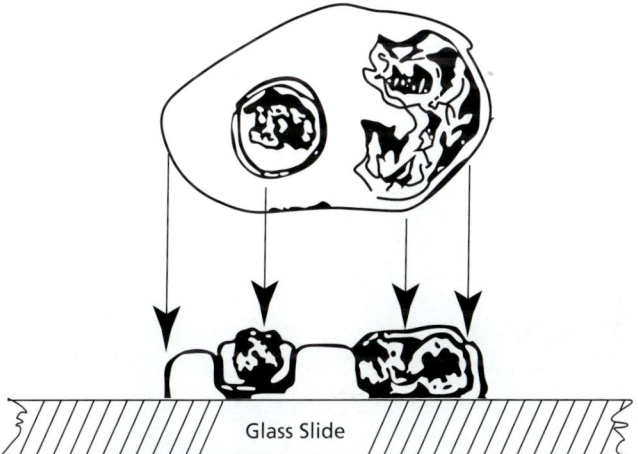

Figure 4.25 Depiction of the need to focus up and down to appreciate the cell-in-cell arrangement.

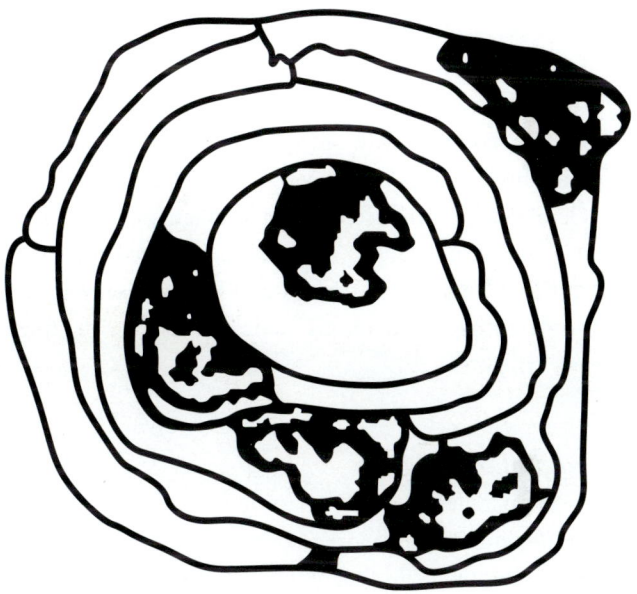

Figure 4.26 Nuclear features of a malignant pearl.

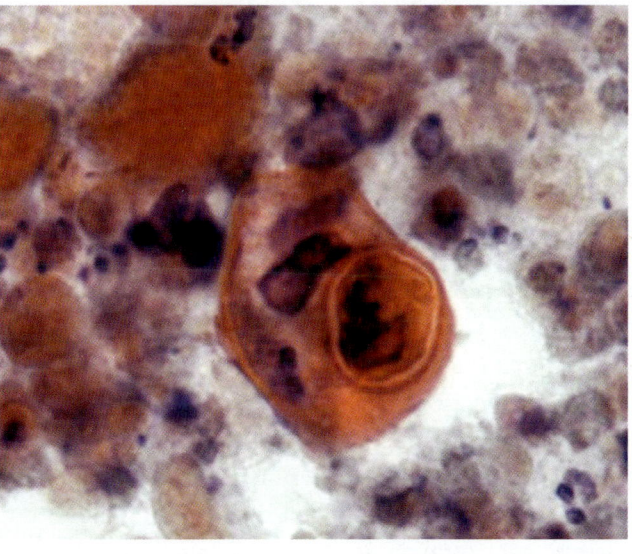

Figure 4.27 Cell-in-cell arrangement, squamous cell carcinoma lung, notice the malignant nuclear features, sputum specimen, Pap stain. Similar changes are also seen in Figure 4.24B.

bulbous ends that may contain a fibrillary structure (Figures 4.22 and 4.23). Similar changes can be seen in benign cells.

"Pearl" formation

The same tendency (described earlier) to exfoliate rounded stratified structures of multiple squames as "pearly bodies" is carried over into the malignant cell trying to differentiate toward squamous. It is composed of malignant squamous cells (by malignant nuclear criteria pattern) primarily, then a pearl formation secondarily, which gives it the connotation of a "malignant pearl" – not vice versa. When only two cells are involved, the first impulse is to call it "cannibalism". Fine focusing up and down will point out the layering – stratification with the upper cell lying within a pit on the lower cell's upper surface (Figures 4.24–4.27).

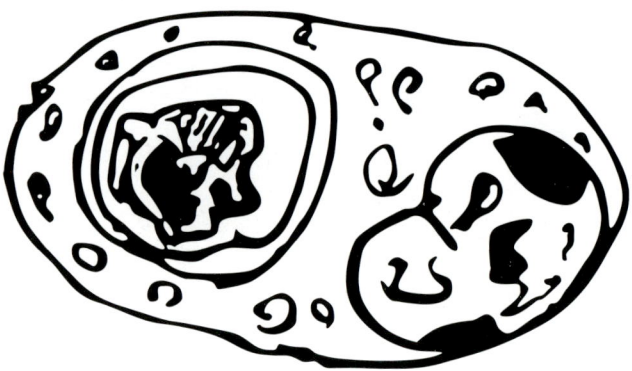

Figure 4.28 Phagocytosis of a tumor cell by a macrophage.

At times an outside cell will simply ring the inner cell, without stratification. Such appearances can be misdiagnosed as pearl and thus a squamous lesion.

Frequently, an "active" histiocyte may engulf another cell which may be benign or malignant, and their close association coupled with interpretative enthusiasm may label the histiocyte as malignant (Figures 4.28 and 4.29).

Occasionally, undifferentiated malignant cells may truly phagocytose. This is more often observed in poorly differentiated malignant tumors and uncommonly in the well-differentiated squamous cancer cells which form "pearls" (Figure 4.29).

Intercellular bridges

These are parallel linear cytoplasmic connections. In cases of undifferentiated or poorly differentiated malignant epithelial carcinoma, a finding of intercellular bridges helps in correctly diagnosing the functional differentiation of the malignancy (Figure 4.30). Care must be exercised in proper identification of the intercellular bridges; intercellular secretions and degeneration can produce similar structures (Figure 4.30).

Cell as a whole

Some of the above characteristics are found together consistently in patterns, and are conveniently recognized as "cell types." When these cells are shed from cancer, they ought to be recognized as malignant by the nuclear patterns of malignant criteria and not by virtue of their "cell type." Benign cells appearing as "tadpole", "spindle", and "third-type" cell forms may be observed in irritation, repair, atypias, and other retroplastic and proplastic states.

(A)

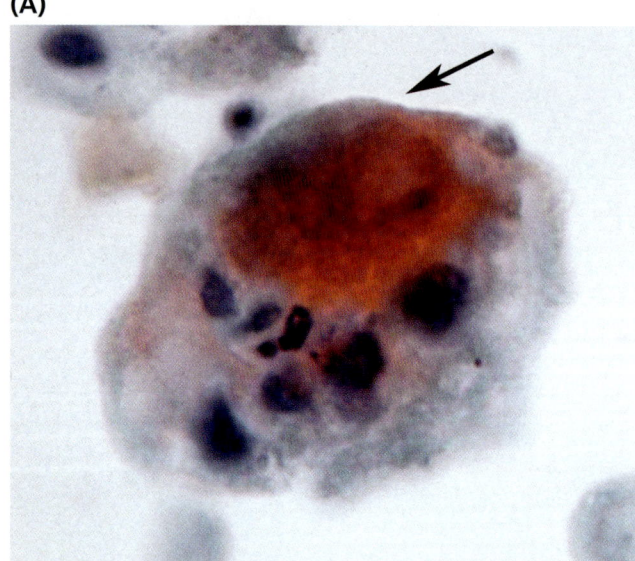

(B)

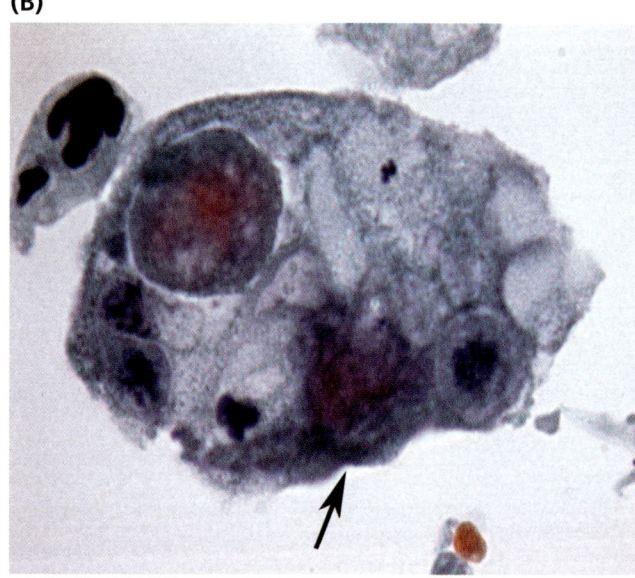

Figure 4.29 Squamous cell carcinoma with intracytoplasmic ingestion of cells, epithelial cells. Malignant nuclei (arrow) (A), leucocytes (B). Degenerated tumor cells. FNA base of the skull lesion, LBP, Pap stain.

"Tadpole" cell

This unilaterally elongated cell has its nucleus at the "head end," with a cytoplasmic tail streaming out – distinctively different from a columnar cell, whose nucleus is near the tail. The nucleus is rounded and may lie in an amorphous endoplasm within an ectoplasmic rim. The ectoplasmic rim extends down the tail, with the remaining thin endoplasmic core forming an apparent "spiral" (of Herxheimer), which is the refractile endo-ectoplasm interface, not an actual fiber. The tip of the tail is frequently bulbous.

(A)

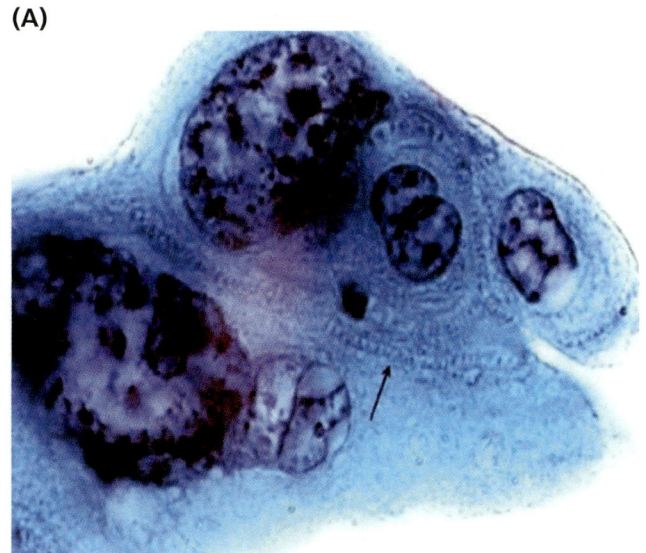

(B)

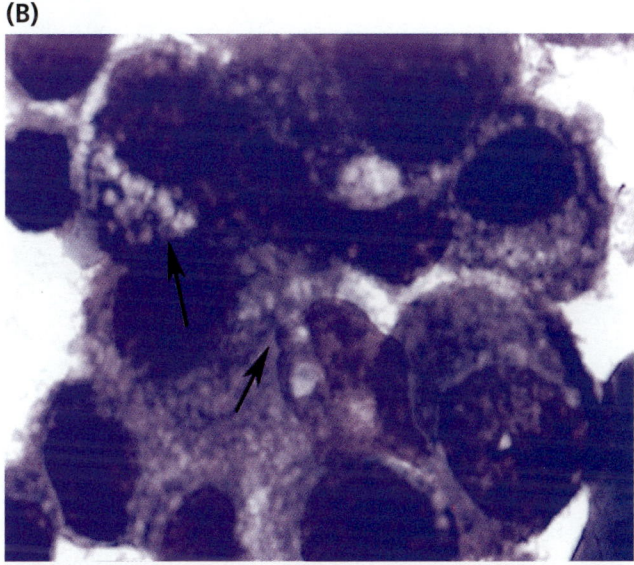

Figure 4.30 (A) Intercellular bridges (arrow) at the margins of malignant cells. These establish squamous differentiation of the other wise undifferentiated tumor. (B) Thyroid follicular cells with intercellular secretory vacuoles simulating intercellular bridges (arrows). Fine needle aspiration. (A) Lung FNA, Pap stain; (B) Diff-Quik stain.

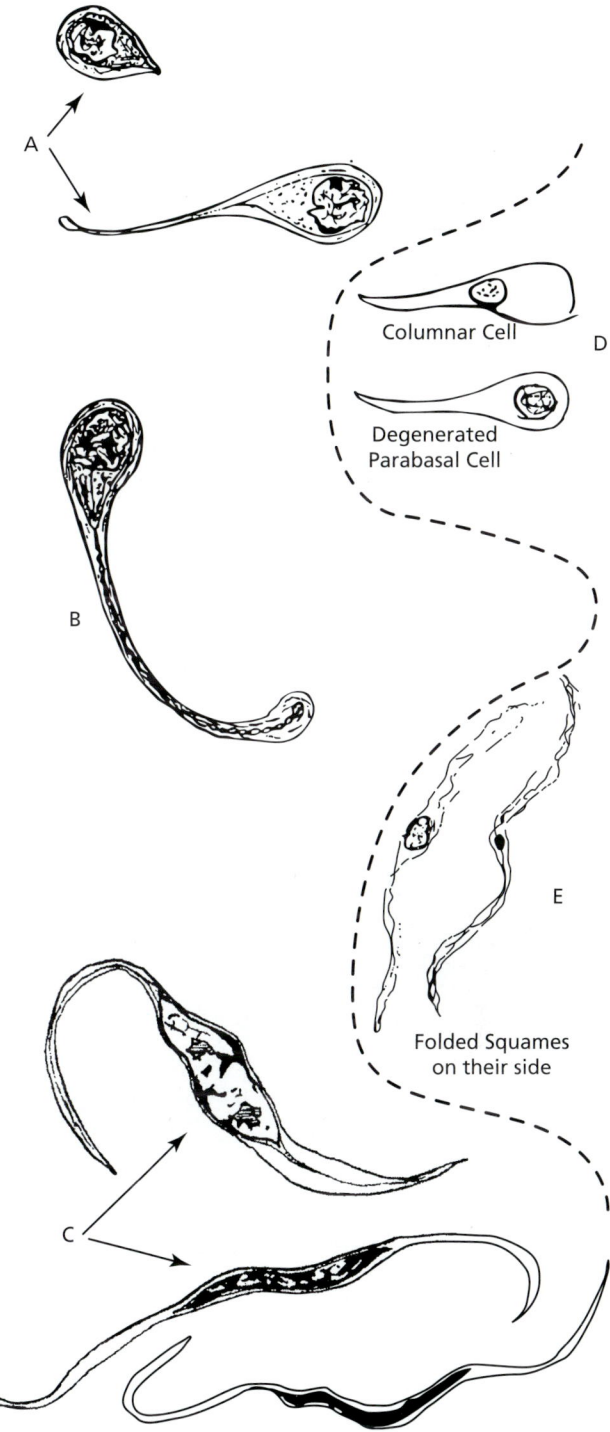

Figure 4.31 Salient characteristics of tadpole and fiber cells. Variable amount of cytoplasm with abnormal nucleus is seen in the two cells (A). A tadpole cell with intracytoplasmic fibrillary structure is shown in (B). Fiber cells with bipolar cytoplasmic thinning and nuclear transgression in to the cytoplasm (C). Similar appearing cells include columnar (D) and folded and degenerated squamous (E) cells.

The total amount of cytoplasm is abundant, giving a normal N:C ratio (Figures 4.31–4.35).

Fiber cell

The nucleus is usually elongated, thinned, and pointed at both ends. Varying degrees of pyknosis frequently obliterates malignant criteria. The cytoplasmic rim is generally thinned and extremely molded as it extends past the nucleus. It rarely shows an ectoplasm–endoplasm differentiation. The cytoplasm is abundant, usually giving a normal N:C ratio.

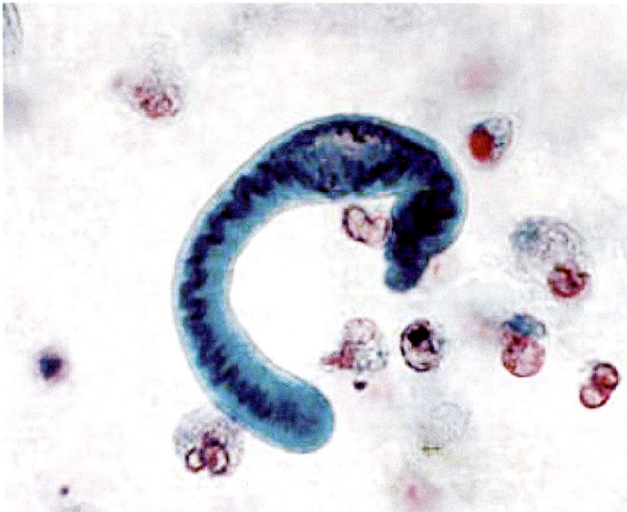

Figure 4.32 Tadpole cell with intracytoplasmic Herxheimer spiral extending into the tail, pulmonary specimen. Similar appearing spiral structure around parabasal cells – fibrils of Eberth may be seen in cervical squamous cells. These changes often suggest an abnormal squamous differentiation and an underlying epithelial abnormality. Sputum, Pap stain.

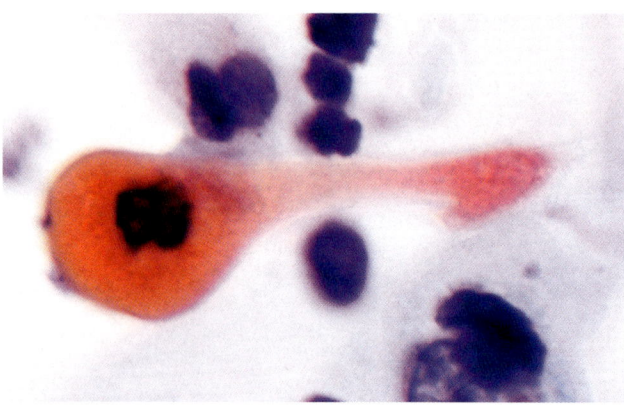

Figure 4.33 Tadpole cell with an abnormal nucleus and a tail formation containing a small bulbous tip. Cytoplasm appears biphasic; this has limited diagnostic value; the terminal tail enlargement is a worrisome feature. Sputum, Pap stain.

Both in the tadpole and spindle malignant cells, one may observe a bulbous enlargement at the tail end of the cell. Finding a nucleus that may be degenerated in such an elongated cell is often a good indicator of malignancy with squamous differentiation (Figures 4.36 and 4.37).

Carcinoma in situ (third-type) cell

Ruth Graham describes this (third-type) cell that may occur in squamous cell carcinoma (tadpole and fiber cells described earlier being the other two types of cells). This cell is the hallmark of carcinoma in situ (CIS), a lesion invariably associated with invasive squamous cancer.

(A)

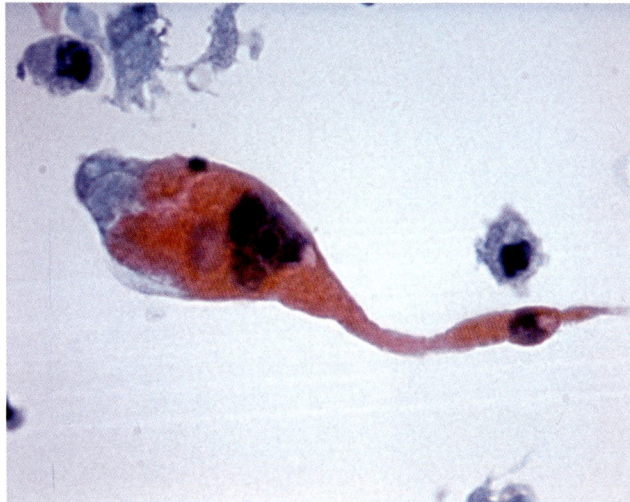

(B)

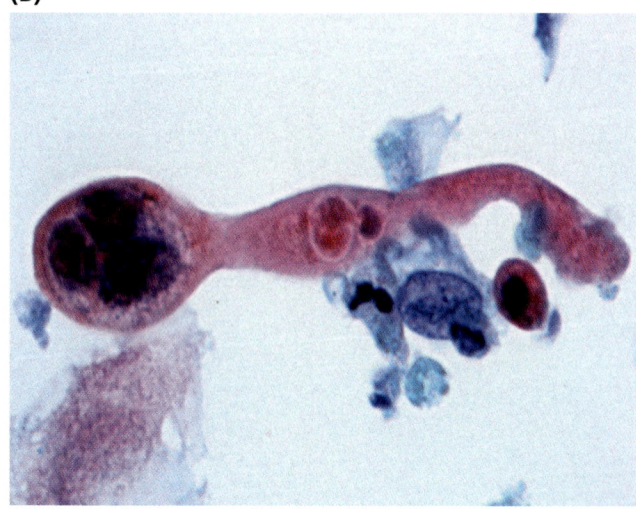

Figure 4.34 Tadpole cell with a malignant (dark, pyknotic India ink) nucleus situated at the head (A) and the body (B). Cytoplasmic thinning is abnormal, tapering (A) and bulbous (B). Tongue squamous cell carcinoma. Neck lymph node FNA, LBP, Pap stain.

The "third-type" cell is round and symmetrical. Its large nucleus is centrally placed in scanty cytoplasm. The nuclear membrane is wavy or undulated as if due to increased activity (p. 123), in contrast to the wrinkled or shrunken membrane found with degeneration. The nuclear chromatin is finely granular and evenly distributed without any areas of parachromatin clearing. As a rule, nucleoli are not observed in these cells with squamous differentiation (Figures 4.38–4.40).

Carcinoma in situ (CIS): in current practice, CIS is not described as a separate entity, being included in the discussions of CIN III/HSIL and sometimes with the ASCH lesions. Purists still like to identify CIS as a distinct morphologic entity and it may occasionally be possible to make such a diagnosis based upon the criteria discussed here.

(A)

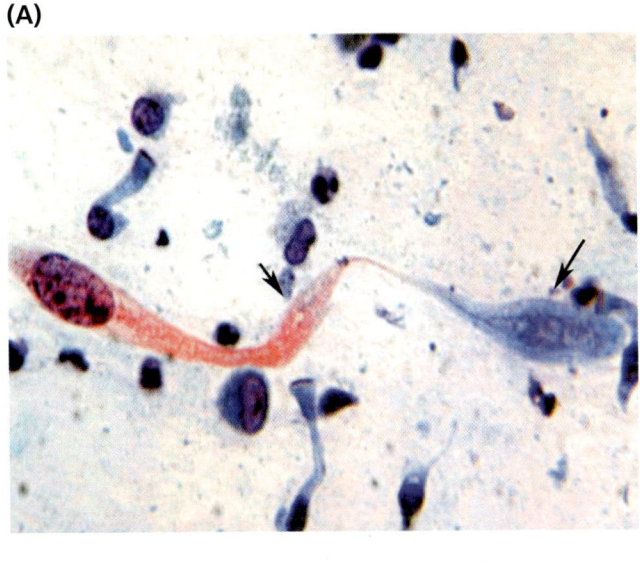

(B)

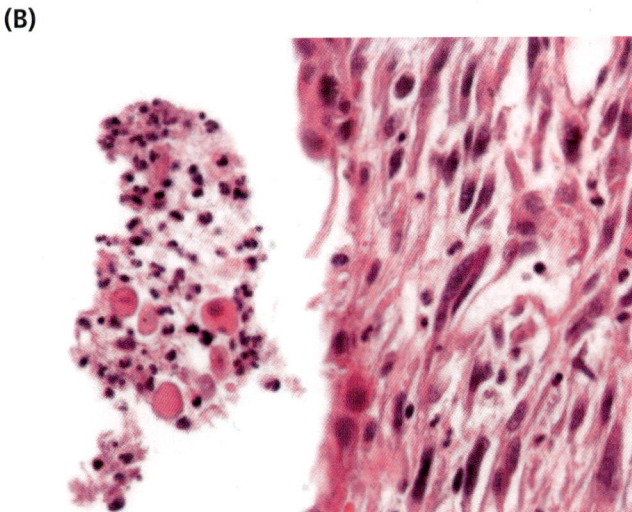

Figure 4.35 (A, B) Tadpole cell with a hyperchromatic nucleus and abnormal cytoplasmic thinning and functional differentiation. There are two ghost nuclei (arrows) and a thin strand of intervening cytoplasm. Bronchial brush specimen, Pap stain (A). Lung biopsy specimen showing well-differentiated squamous cell carcinoma of lung, H/E stain (B).

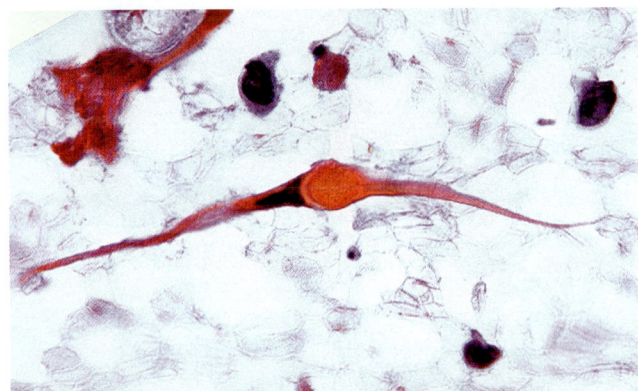

Figure 4.36 Fiber cell. Notice the abnormal nucleus that is spreading into the cytoplasm, a cytoplasmic condensation with nuclear molding and bipolar cytoplasmic tapering. Neck lymph node aspiration, tongue primary. LBP, Pap stain.

(A)

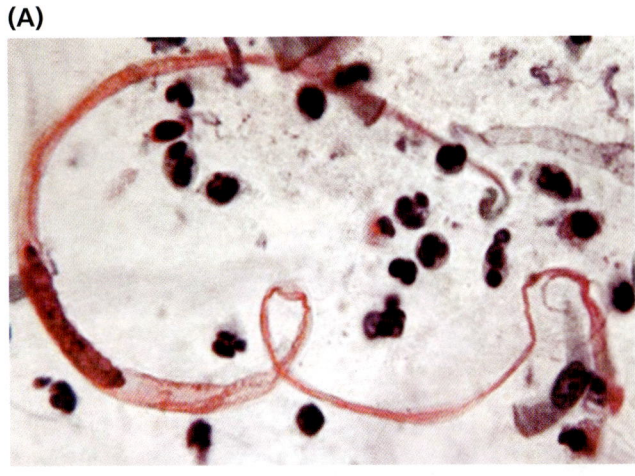

(B)

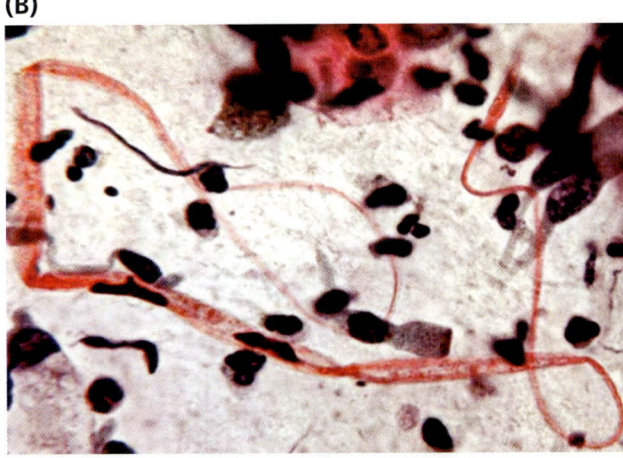

Figure 4.37 (A, B) Fiber cells. Notice the nucleus and extremely abnormal cytoplasm that has a bulbous enlargement at the tip (A). Fiber cell in (B) has two malignant nuclei and variable thinning of the cytoplasm. Such changes occur more commonly in cavitary squamous cell carcinoma. Bronchial brush specimen. Direct smear, Pap stain.

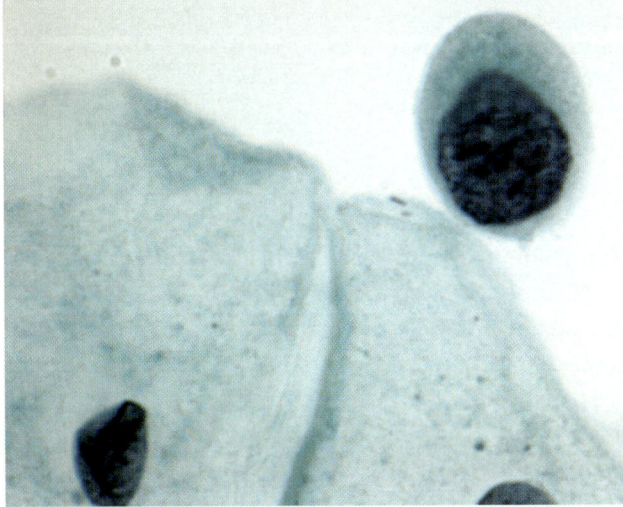

Figure 4.38 Single cell representing a third-type cell. This case was HPV Hi-risk positive. An intermediate cell nucleus is shown for comparison. LBP, Pap stain.

(A)

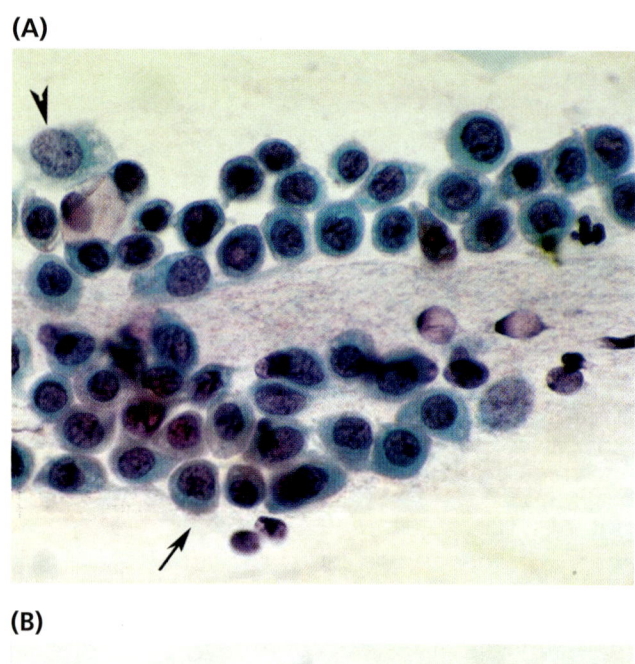

(B)

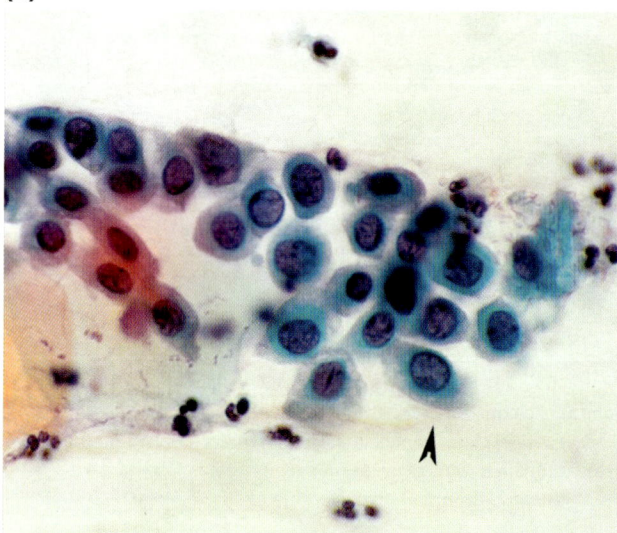

Figure 4.39 (A) Cervical smears diagnosed as HSIL and contain a number of third-type cells (arrow). (B) Notice the morphologic overlap with metaplastic cells; they are intermixed (arrowhead). Vaginocervical smear, Pap stain.

(A)

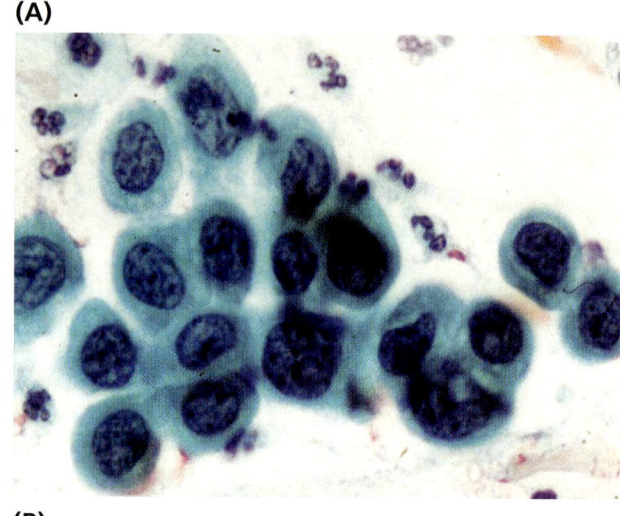

(B)

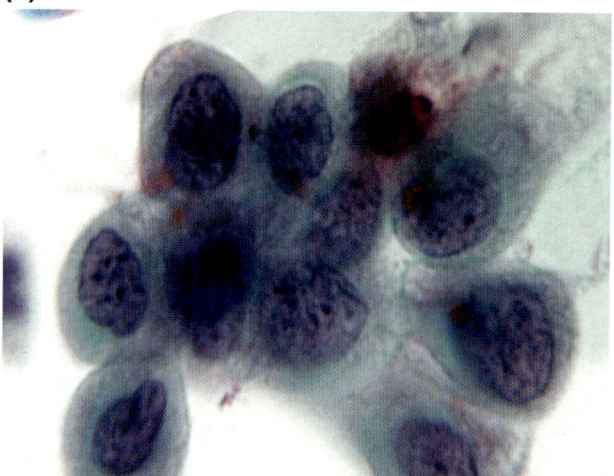

(C)

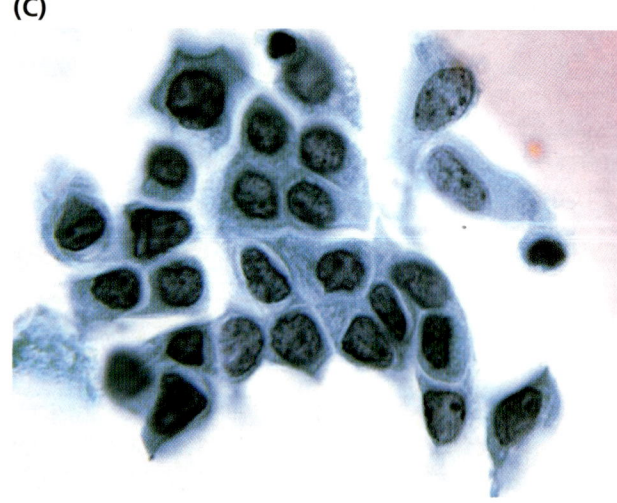

Figure 4.40 Third-type cells. These cells have overlapping morphologic features with ASC-H (A, B) and when originating from the transformation zone, they lack nucleoli (C). Some changes simulate carcinoma in situ cells. Cervical specimen, SurePath slide.

While CIS tends to show a distinctly different morphologic pattern, CIS of the cervix sheds large numbers of dyskaryotic cells. Their nuclei tend to be severely dyskaryotic and, in addition, varying numbers have an extremely scanty, thin rim of cytoplasm.

In the CIS cells, nucleoli are extremely rare (less than 5%). There is hyperchromasia; chromatin is fine, granular, and uniformly dispersed, not aggregated in large irregular and jagged clumps. Parachromatin is usually cleared, but is not found in large irregular areas of extreme clearing. The nuclear membrane is wavy, but not morbidly irregular. It is somewhat

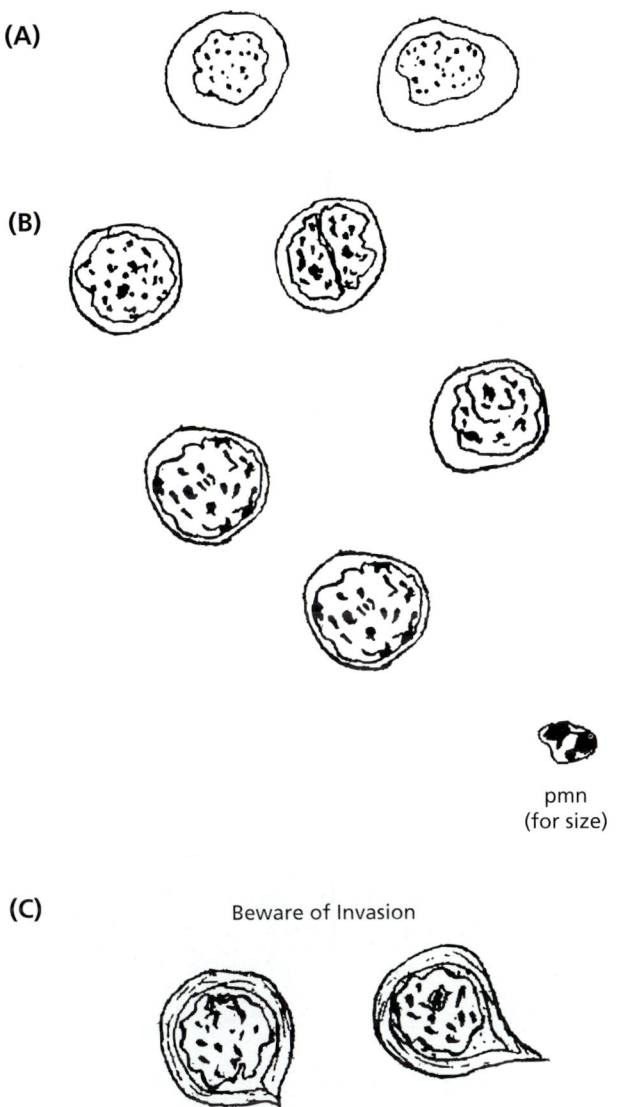

(A)

(B)

pmn
(for size)

(C)

Beware of Invasion

Figure 4.41 Changes included as third-type cells (CIS). Cells in (A) are similar to ASC-H (Figures 4.41–4.43). Cells in (B) are the classic carcinoma in situ, and (C) represents early invasion.

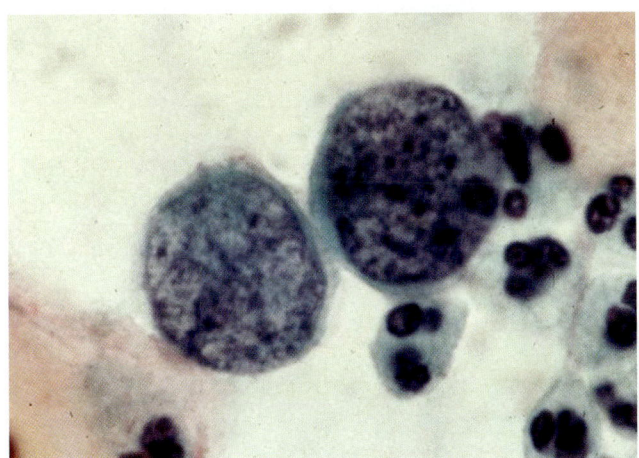

Figure 4.43 Carcinoma in situ cells. Notice the scant cytoplasm and uniformly distributed chromatin. Vaginocervical smear, Pap stain.

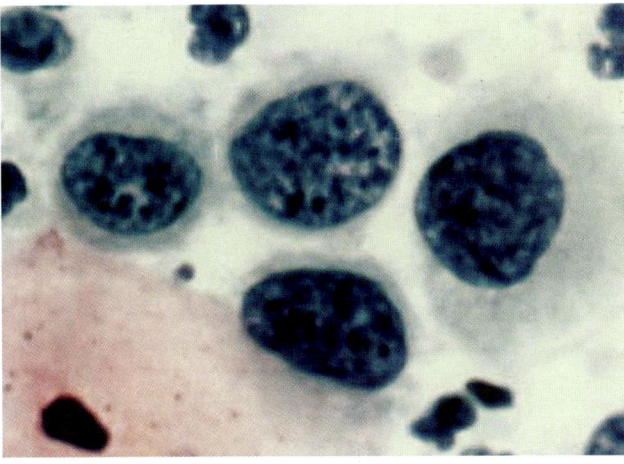

Figure 4.42 Classic carcinoma in situ cell. Notice the uniform chromatin and parachromatin as well as some nuclear membrane changes. Vaginocervical smear, Pap stain.

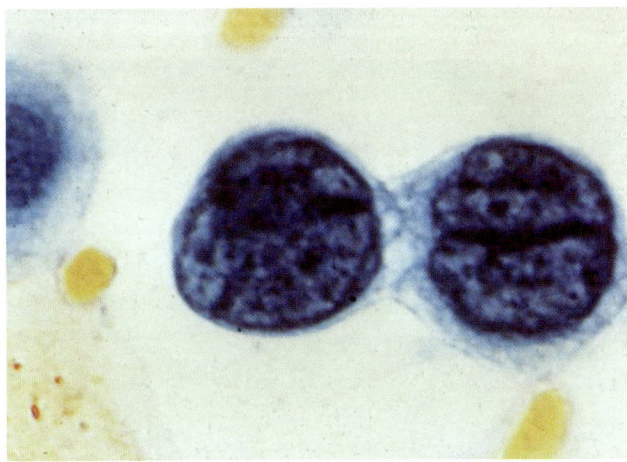

Figure 4.44 Carcinoma in situ cells with nuclear membrane and chromatin changes including abnormal thickening and clearing, respectively. These are bi- and multinucleation also. Such changes may suggest an early invasion. Vaginocervical smear, Pap stain.

thickened and its thickness may vary from cell to cell, but within a cell it tends to be very uniform (Figures 4.41–4.44).

Microinvasive carcinoma

Squamous carcinoma of the cervix as well as bronchial epithelium provides the best example of these transformations. This is rarely diagnosed in cytopathology. In cervical lesions, a suggestion to the probable early or microinvasion can be made based upon the nuclear and cytoplasmic changes. One should be sure of a CIS lesion before a microinvasion is diagnosed. Both cytoplasmic and nuclear alterations and their degree of severity are highly significant (Figure 4.45).

Most cells occur singly, but in liquid-based preparations, small tissue fragments with morphologic features of

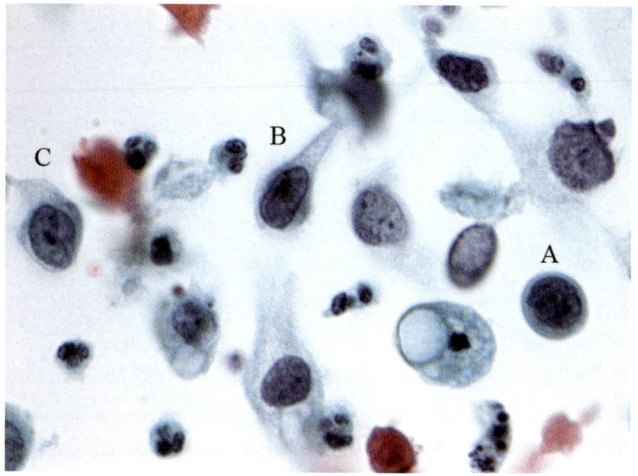

Figure 4.45 Salient features of microinvasive carcinoma. Nuclear membrane changes (A), cytoplasmic elongation (B), and prominent nucleoli (C). Cervical smear, LBP, Pap stain.

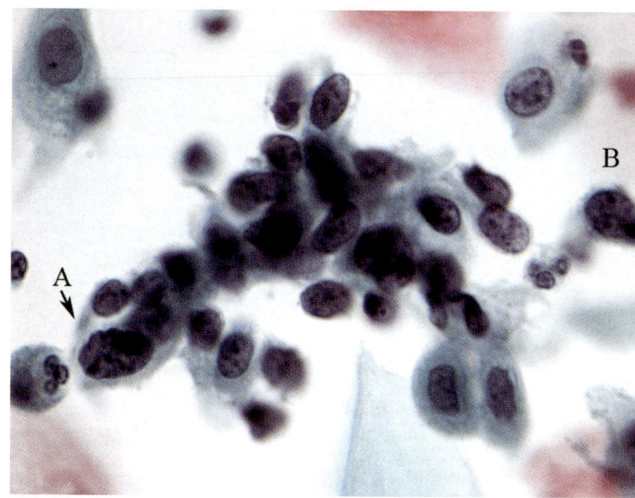

Figure 4.46 Tissue fragment microinvasive carcinoma. Notice that the majority of cells in the middle have the nuclear chromatin pattern of CIS; nuclear elongation is seen in a few cells. Prominent nuclear membrane changes are present in (A) and nucleoli are seen in (B). Cervical smear, LBP, Pap stain.

(A)

(B)

(C)

(D)

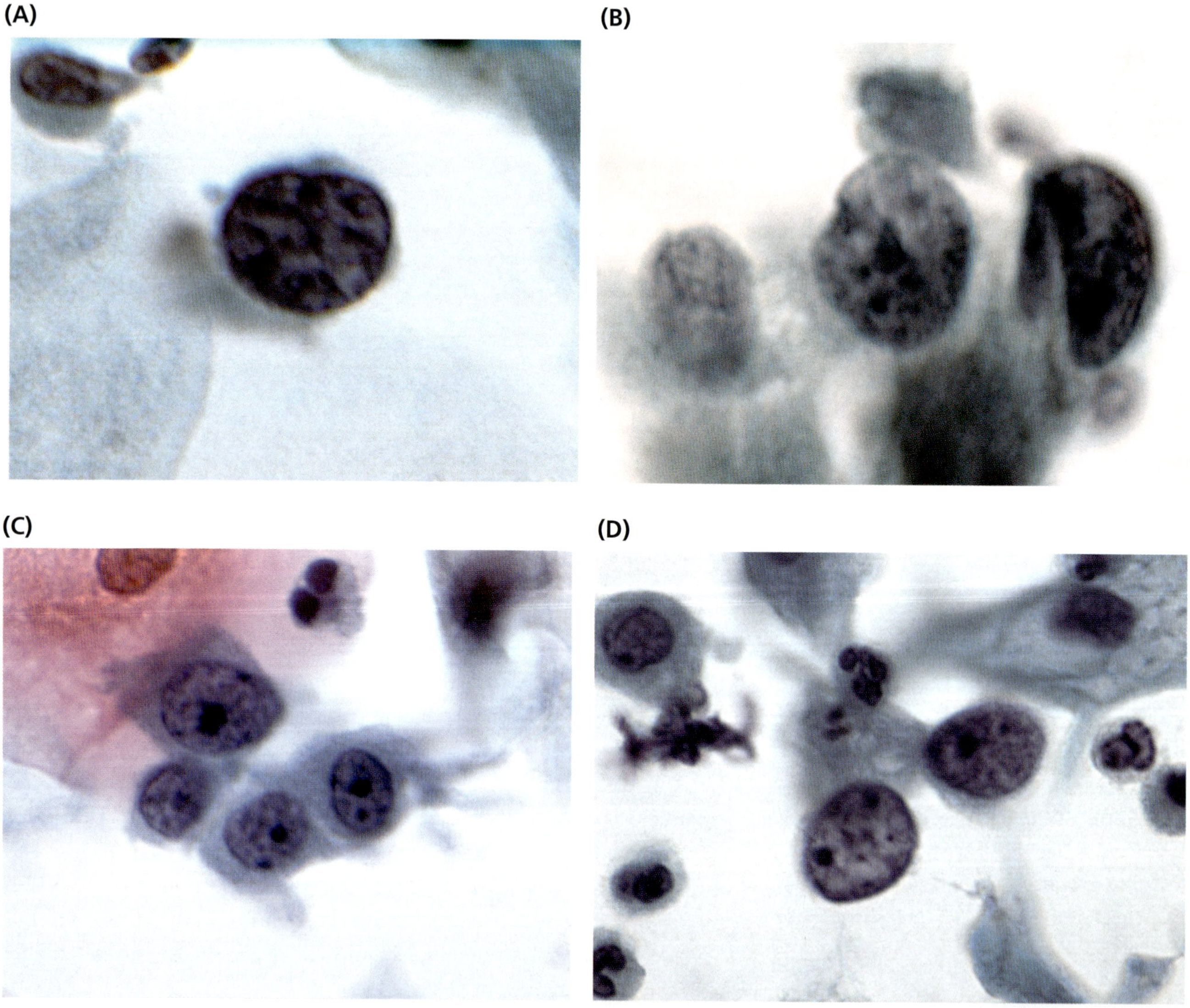

Figure 4.47 Nuclear changes, microinvasion. Chromatin clumping (A–C), parachromatin clearing (A–C), nuclear membrane changes (A, B) and prominent nucleoli (C, D). Cervical LBP, Pap stain.

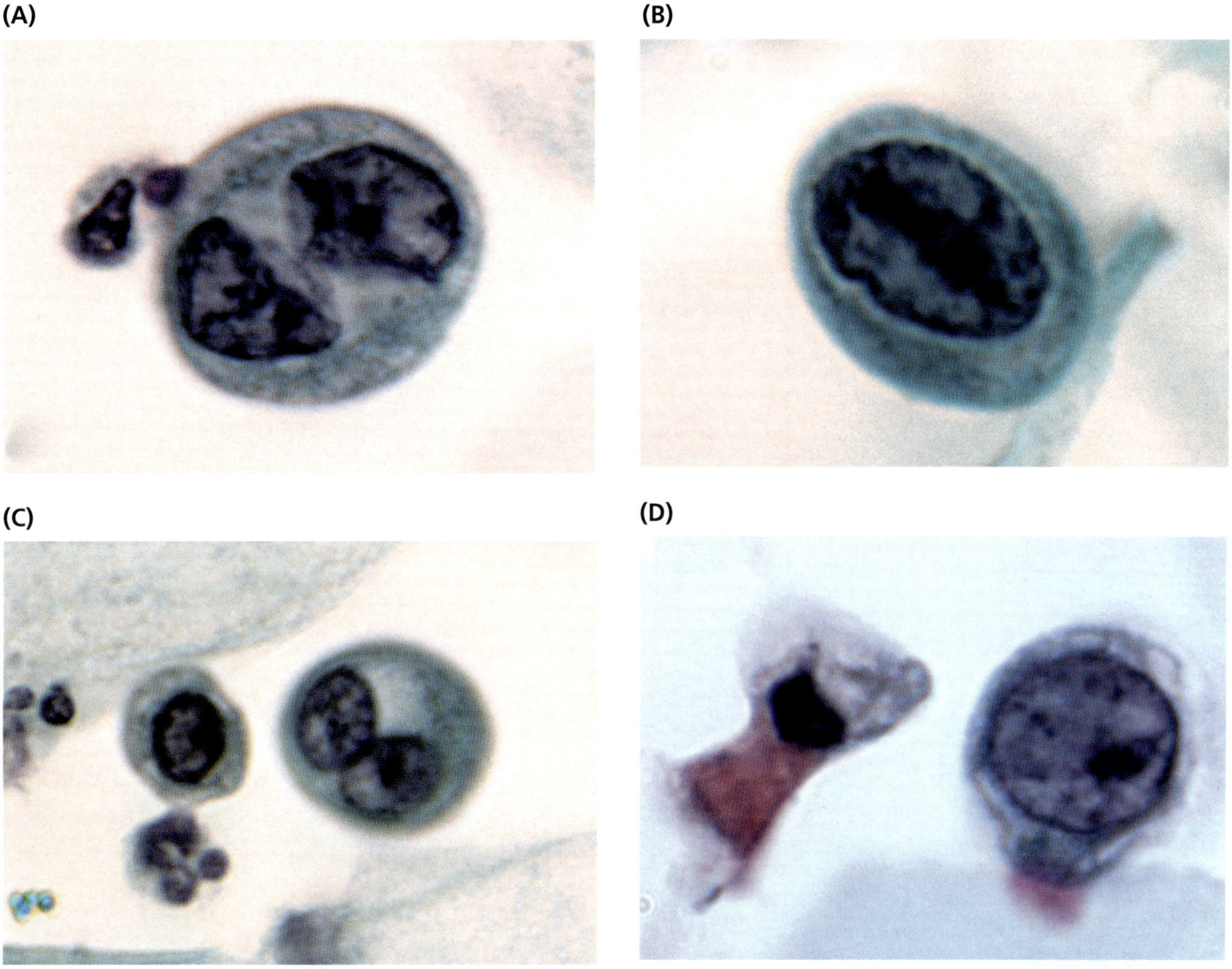

(A)

(B)

(C)

(D)

Figure 4.48 (A–D) Cytoplasmic changes in microinvasive carcinoma in two cases. Nuclear chromatin and membrane changes (A) (compare to Figures 4.43, 4.44). Dense cytoplasm with ecto/endoplasmic differentiation (B), note the nuclear membrane bite. Round cells with nucleoli (C), cytoplasmic changes (D). Cervical specimen, LBP, Pap stain.

microinvasion may occur (Figure 4.46). Cells occur as small fragments with frayed margins, variable cytoplasm that may show condensation, elongation, and other invasion features. Nuclei tend to be rounded with obvious HSIL/CIS changes and additional alterations suggestive of microinvasion.

i. The nuclei tend to elongate and become more asymmetrical. Nucleoli begin to appear and become prominent. Chromatin granules aggregate with the formation of large, irregular pointed chromatin clumps. The parachromatin becomes cleared and irregularly dispersed (Figures 4.47–4.49).

ii. Cytoplasmic keratinization appears with ecto-endoplasmic formation, hyalinization, and orangophilia. Tailing of the cytoplasm appears, at times with a fibrillary apparatus down its core where the endoplasm extends within the outer ectoplasm (Figures 4.48 and 4.49).

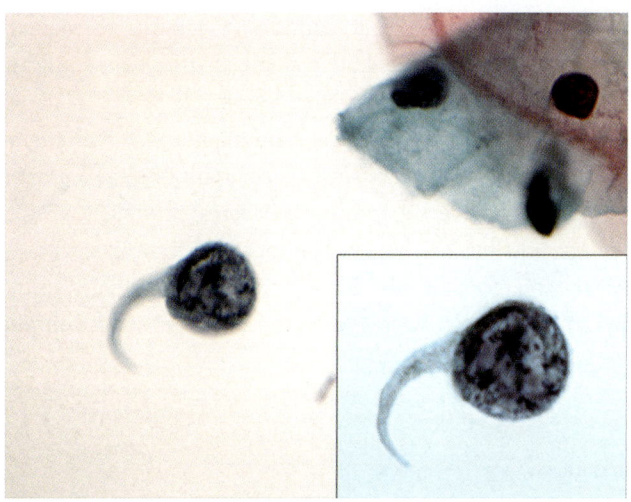

Figure 4.49 Early invasion, squamous cell carcinoma, third case. Notice the cytoplasmic elongation and some chromatin clearing (insert). Cervical specimen, LBP, Pap stain.

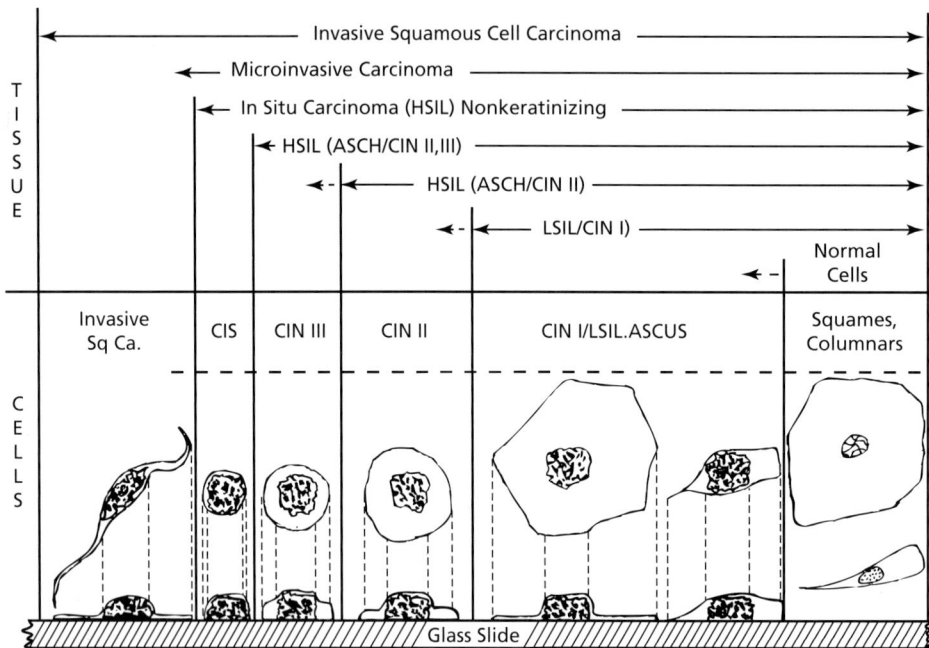

Figure 4.50 Depiction of the development of squamous invasive cancer and cells typically associated with these lesions. It also compares the various common currently used terminologies to identify and report different but continuous developmental stages.

Invasive carcinoma

Most of the changes have already been presented in this chapter. The changes noted in microinvasive lesions become more pronounced and numerous. The classical forms as depicted (see pp. 95–104) include both nuclear and cytoplasmic features and are present in the better differentiated tumors. Virtually only nuclear features of invasion can be all that are present in undifferentiated cancers (i.e. massive chromatin clumps, nucleoli, macabre parachromatin clearing, nuclear elongation, and asymmetry). Since there is a continuous gamut of cellular changes seen in Figure 4.50, a single snapshot may not be representative of the underlying lesion.

It is critical that an independent diagnosis of malignant transformation be established based upon nuclear features before diagnosing squamous invasive carcinoma. It is not always possible to characterize each cell into an accurate diagnostic term. In this regard, the value of ancillary studies (discussed elsewhere) and clinical management implications are critical.

ADENOCARCINOMA

These tumors may have a morphologic and or functional differentiation. Adenocarcinoma generally tends to shed tissue fragments. The cells are basically a "large cell undifferentiated" type with differentiating characteristics present at times (Figure 4.51).

Nucleus

The nucleus may be vesicular with variable malignant criteria varying from the very best sharp chromatin clumping and clearing, nuclear membrane infoldings and out-pouching and jagged nucleoli to extremely bland gray or more typically "ground glass" in appearance. They tend to be rounded with stretched nuclear membranes. The occurrence of intercellular variations such as marked anisocytosis (more than 4 times among cells), nuclear membrane irregularities, nuclear grooves, and aggregation of the cells in tight groups helps in the correct diagnosis of such cells. These features are seen in Figures 4.52–4.54.

Cytoplasm

This can be extremely variable from cell to cell. Cytoplasm may be distributed on one side of the nucleus, or it may be scant or almost imperceptible occurring around or on one side of the malignant nucleus. Various changes may include:

(i) cellular borders, indistinct and hazy (Figure 4.53);

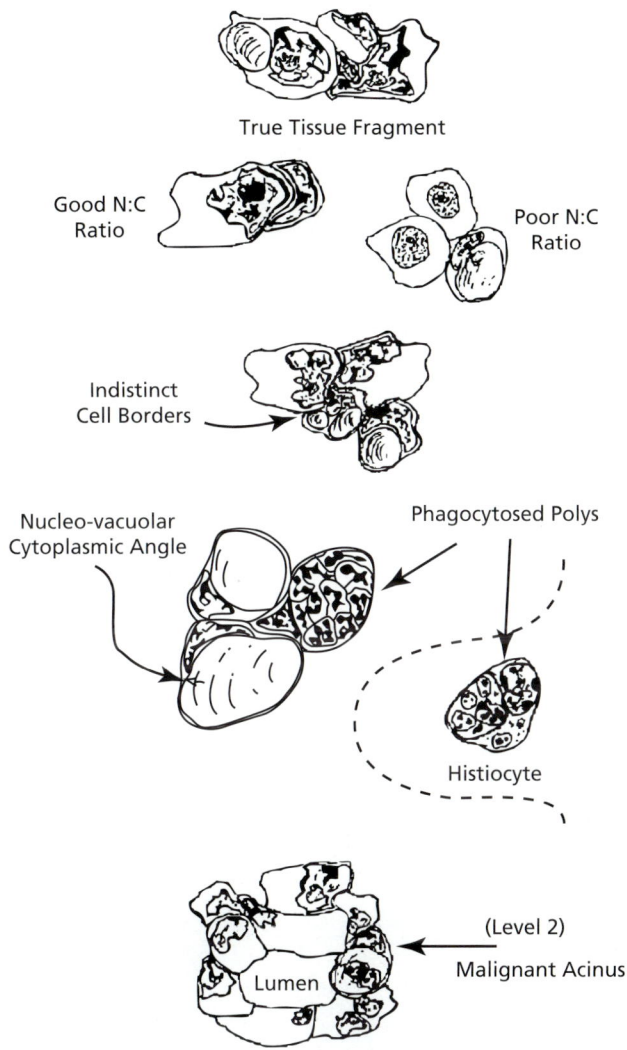

Figure 4.51 Various common nuclear and cytoplasmic patterns seen in adenocarcinoma.

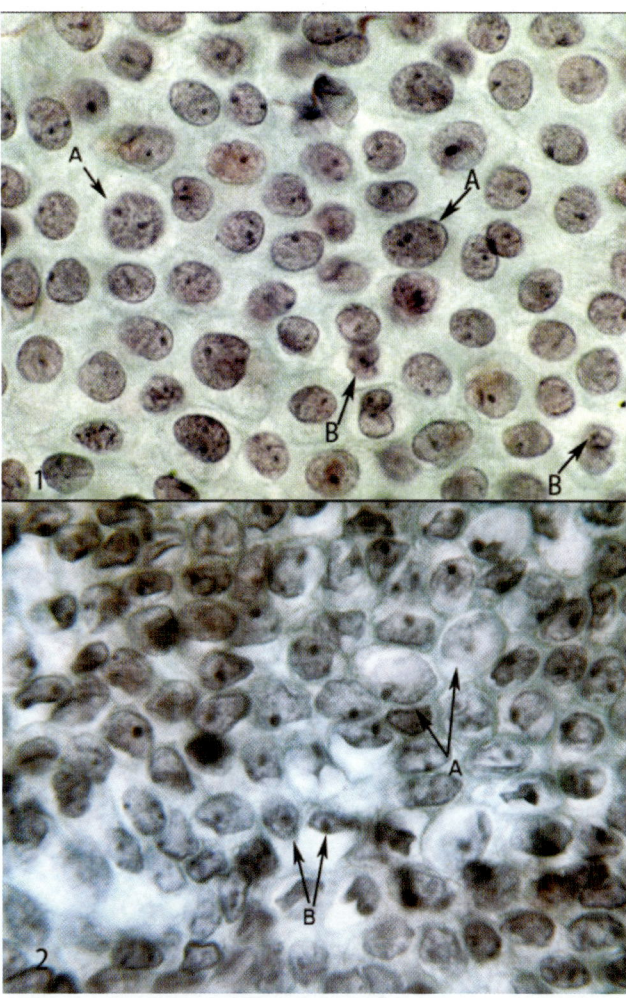

Figure 4.52 Nuclear size variation in adenocarcinoma pancreas. (A) represents the large and (B) the small nuclei. (1) EUS direct smear, (2) EUS LBP, Pap stain. (Same as Figure 3.37.)

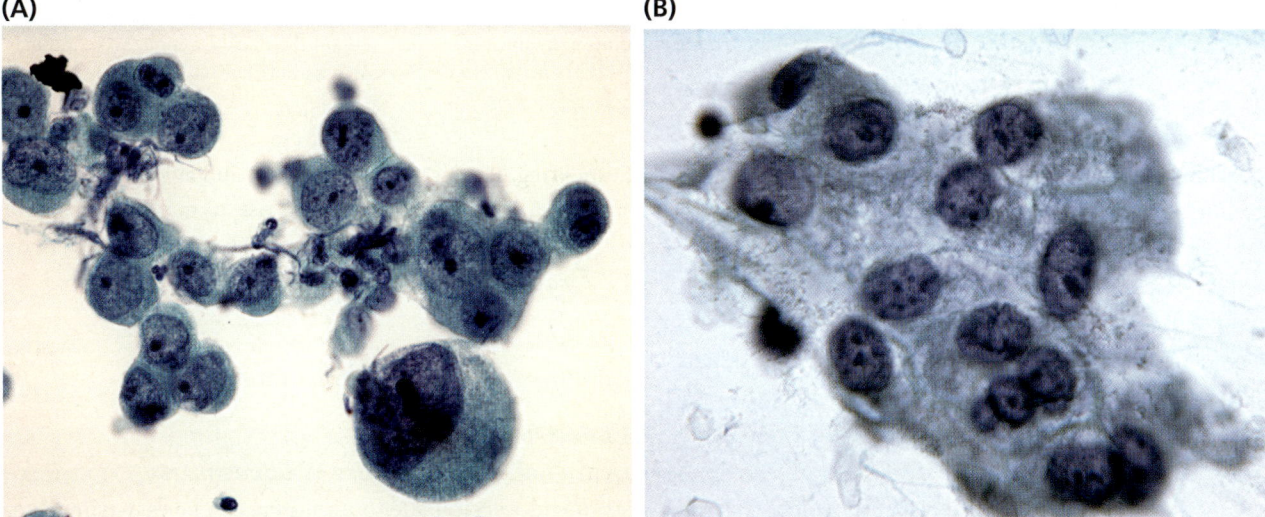

Figure 4.53 Indistinct cell borders adenocarcinoma lung. Notice the nuclear size variation, indistinct cell borders (A), and finely vacuolated abundant columnar cytoplasm, bronchoalveolar carcinoma (B). FNA lung, direct smear (A), ThinPrep (B). (Same as Figure 3.38.)

(A)

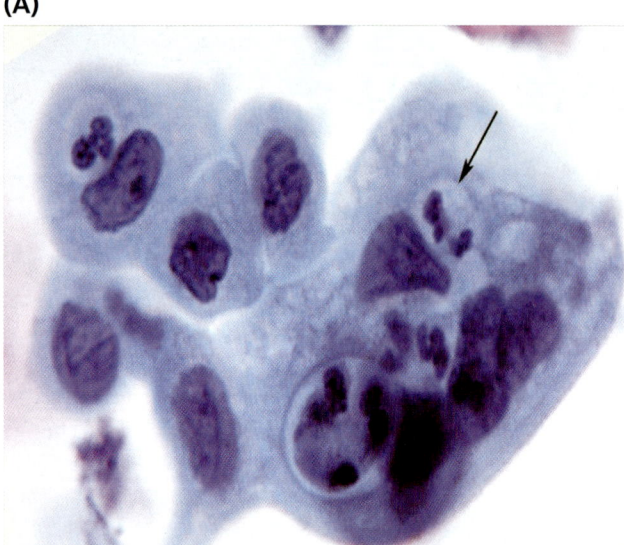

(B)

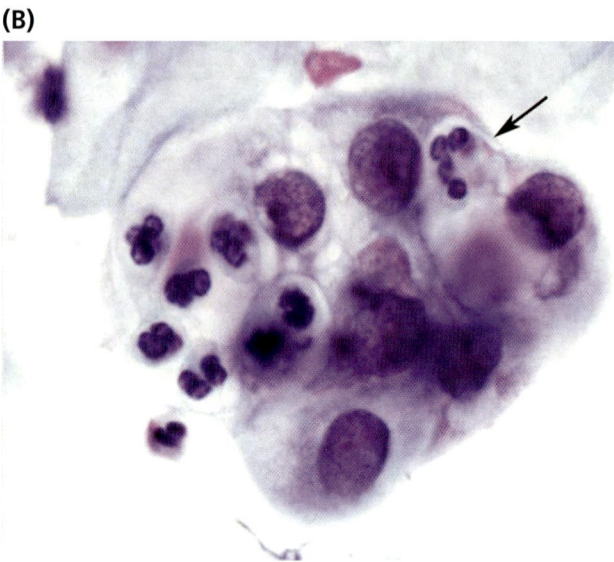

Figure 4.54 Adenocarcinoma endometrium, notice the well-preserved neutrophil within the cytoplasm (arrows). Cervical specimen (A), LBP. Cervicovaginal smear (B), Pap stain.

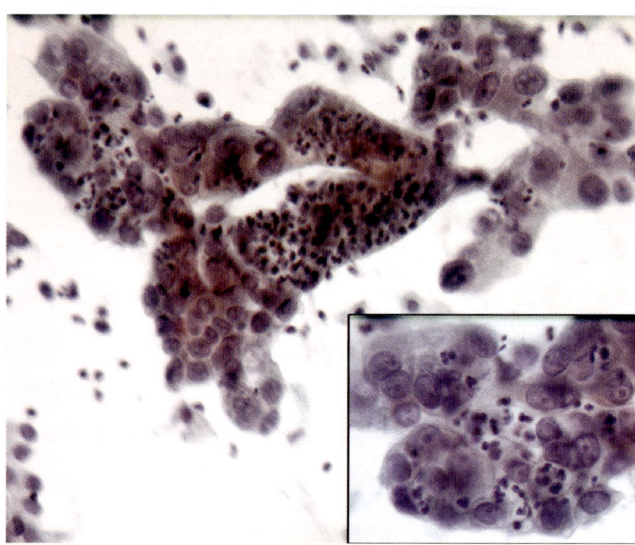

Figure 4.55 Adenocarcinoma lung specimen demonstrating the presence of intracytoplasmic well-preserved neutrophils (insert). Lung FNA, Pap stain.

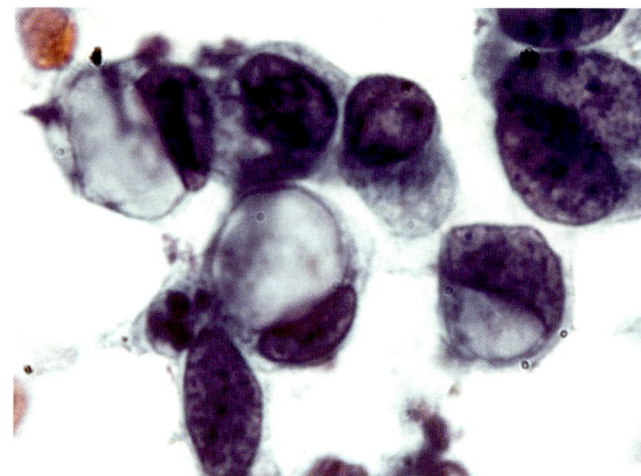

Figure 4.56 Intracytoplasmic secretion, adenocarcinoma stomach. Notice the nuclear molding around the thick secretion. Secretion may be thin and watery or inspissated and opaque. Gastric brush, direct smear, Pap stain.

(ii) secretion may be granular, inspissated, or vacuolated. At times they occur as hyperdistended vacuoles with "out-pouching" and loss of cytoplasm at the nucleo-vacuolar cytoplasmic angle; also with extreme thinning and molding of well-preserved nucleus. Frequently the vacuoles contain many neutrophils which are digesting the mucus and other products and thus appear well-preserved and healthy; they are not degenerated as they would be if they were being phagocytosed and digested by the cancer cell. At times a pouched-out, thin-walled vacuole will be packed with well-preserved polymorphonuclear leucocytes (Figures 4.54–4.56);

(iii) cell groups (acini, polyps, and morula forms). Various adenocarcinomas give rise to acini, polyps, and morula formations especially when occurring in body cavity fluids (Figures 4.57–4.60).

Adenocarcinoma – specific sites

Endocervix

Depending upon the degree of differentiation, cytodiagnosis of endocervical adenocarcinoma can be easy (similar to another adenocarcinoma) or difficult (almost mimicking reactive glandular cells). Tumor cells in classic cases have

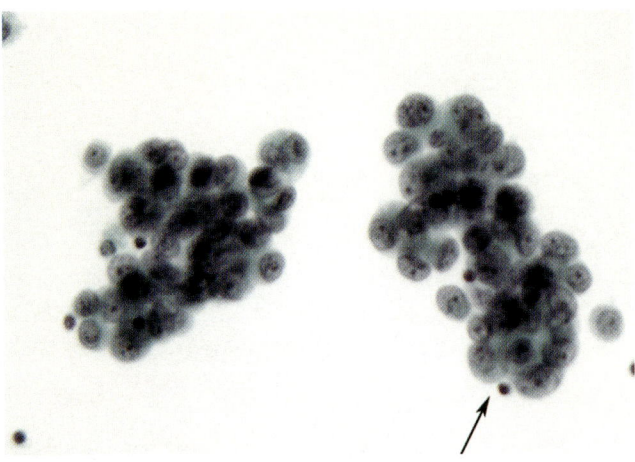

Figure 4.57 Adenocarcinoma breast. Notice the acinic form of tumor cells (arrow). FNA, breast, Thinprep, Pap stain.

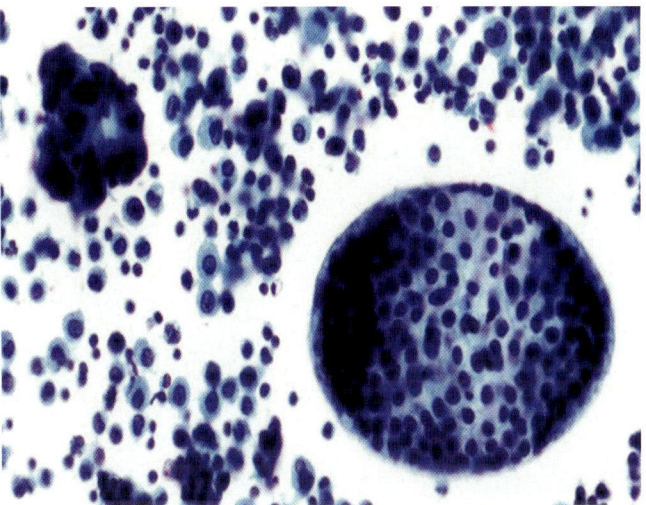

Figure 4.58 Morula formation, breast adenocarcinoma. Such structures represent the terminal cell proliferation in an acinic polypoidal tumor structure. Pleural fluid, Pap stain.

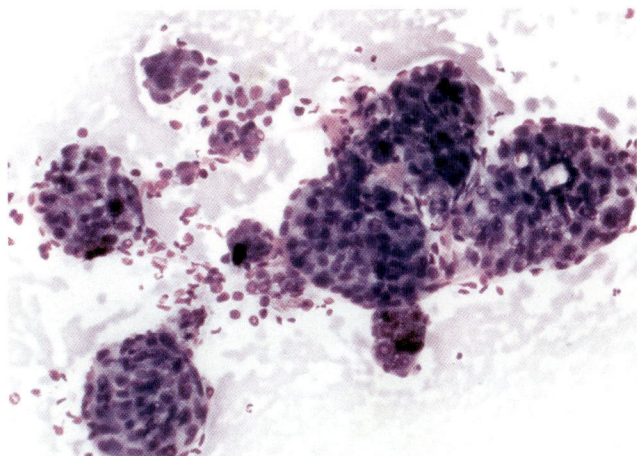

Figure 4.59 Hepatoma, morula formation, fine needle aspiration liver, Diff-Quik stain.

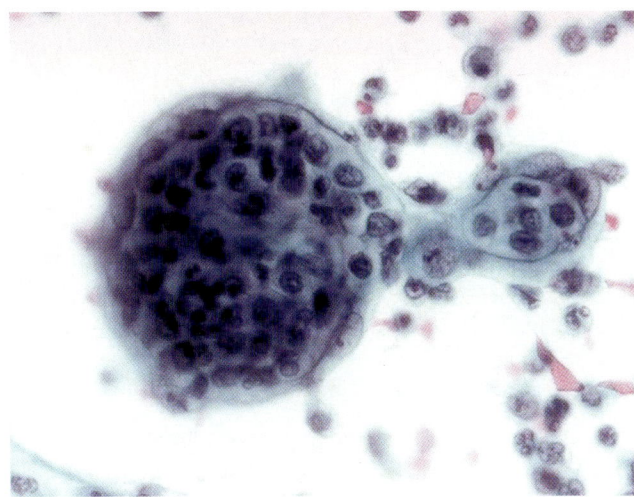

Figure 4.60 Morula formation, adenocarcinoma endometrium. Notice the numerous ingested neutrophils. Abdominal fluid, Millipore filter, Pap stain.

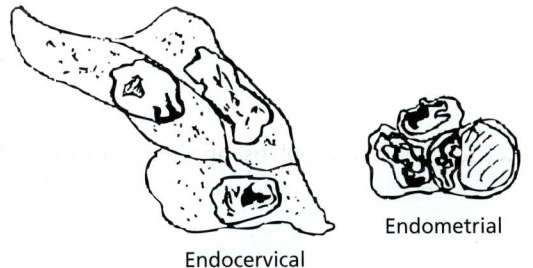

Endometrial

Endocervical

Figure 4.61 Differences in "typical" endocervical and endometrial adenocarcinoma.

columnar appearance; cells are larger than endometrial cells, with some molding and malignant features (Figure 4.61). Endocervical adenocarcinoma nuclei are larger and more vesicular, and frequently contain multiple, prominent nucleoli varying in size and number. The background

can be necrotic, dominated by single tumor cells, or they may occur in tissue fragments (Figures 4.61–4.64).

Early tumors appear in sheets and micro-acinic formations. Some cells retain distinct columnar forms. Palisading is often seen as in feathering (Figure 4.65).

Often it is difficult to separate endocervical lesions from squamous tumors or transformation zone neoplasia involving the endocervical canal. Nuclear apoptosis, although not specific for endocervical and endocrine diagnosis, occurs commonly within the neoplastic cell groups (Figure 4.66a,b). The cytoplasm of adenocarcinoma arising from the endocervix tends to be lavender-colored, textured, and more abundant than the clear, scanty cytoplasm

113

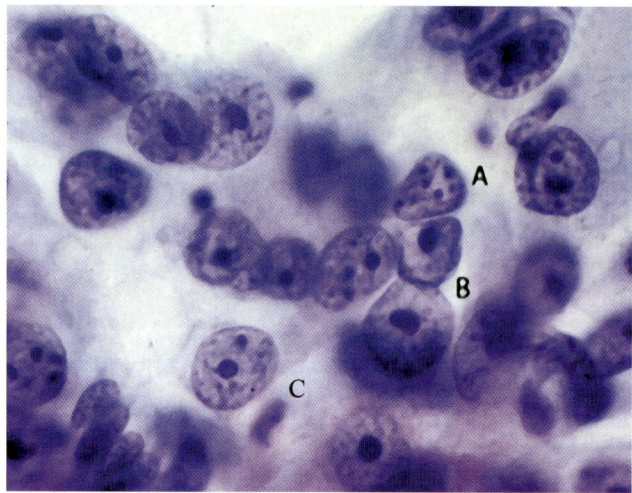

Figure 4.62 Adenocarcinoma endocervix. Notice the nucleoli number variation (A, B) and columnar cytoplasm (C). Vaginocervical smear. Pap stain.

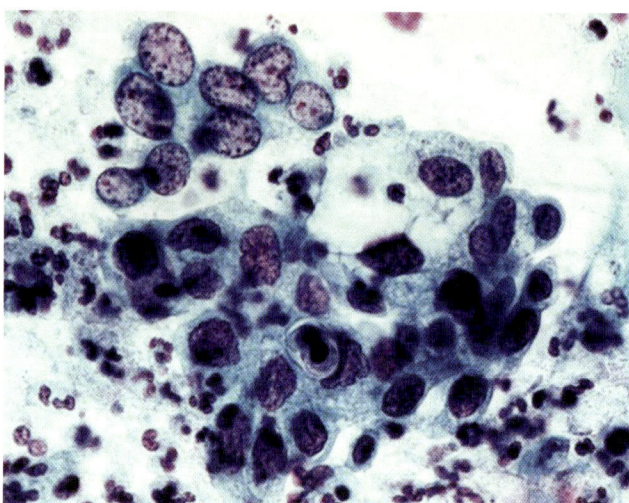

Figure 4.63 Adenocarcinoma endocervix. This represents a rather poorly differentiated tumor and some suggestion of columnar origin in the upper area. Vaginocervical smear, Pap stain.

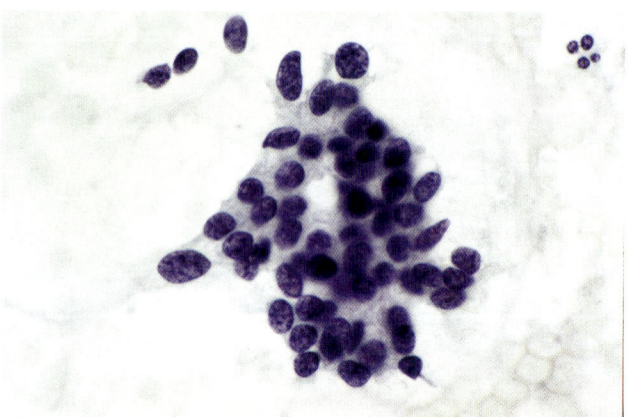

Figure 4.64 Adenocarcinoma endocervix. There is a morphologic overlap with endometrial tumor. Vaginocervical smear, Pap stain.

(A)

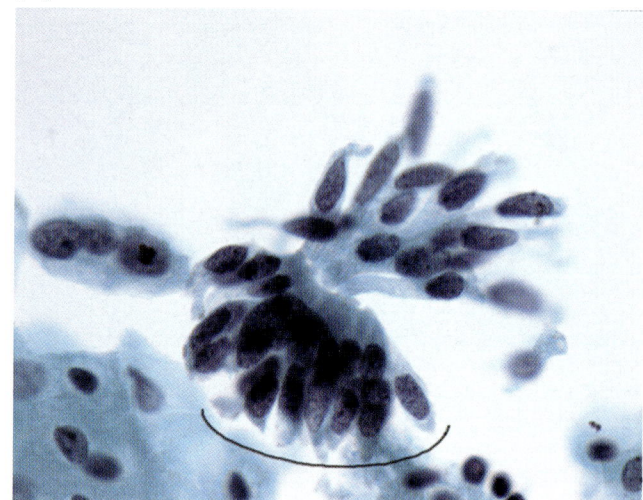

(B)

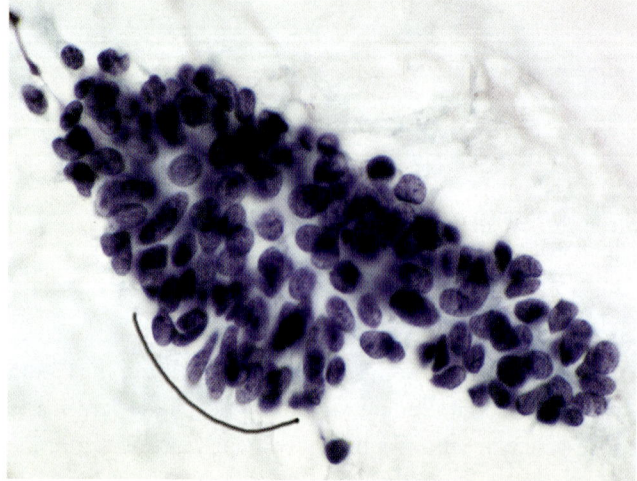

of endometrial adenocarcinoma cells. Endocervical adenocarcinoma nuclei are larger and more vesicular, and frequently contain multiple, prominent nucleoli varying in size and number.

Endometrium

These tumors can be low-grade and extremely well-differentiated or high-grade with poor differentiation. Advanced tumors may have tumor diathesis and old blood in the background. These tumors almost always appear in tissue fragments, they are well preserved in

Figure 4.65 Adenocarcinoma in situ (AIS) of endocervix. Notice the feathering at the edges of tissue fragments of lesional cells (curved line) in two separate cases. Cervical smear (A), LBP (B), Pap stain.

(A)

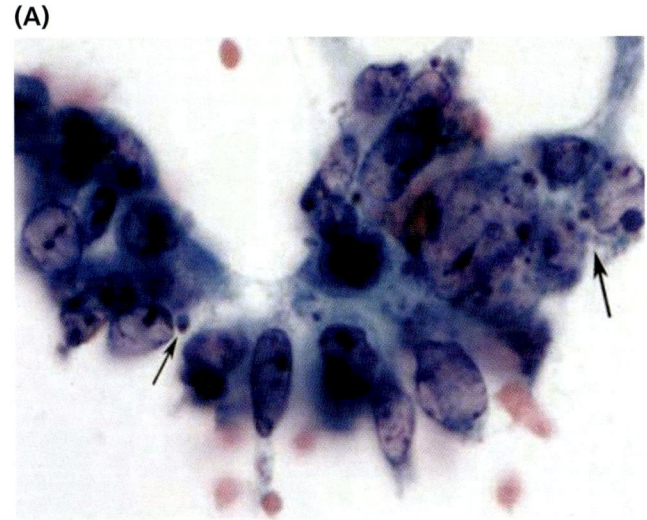

(B)

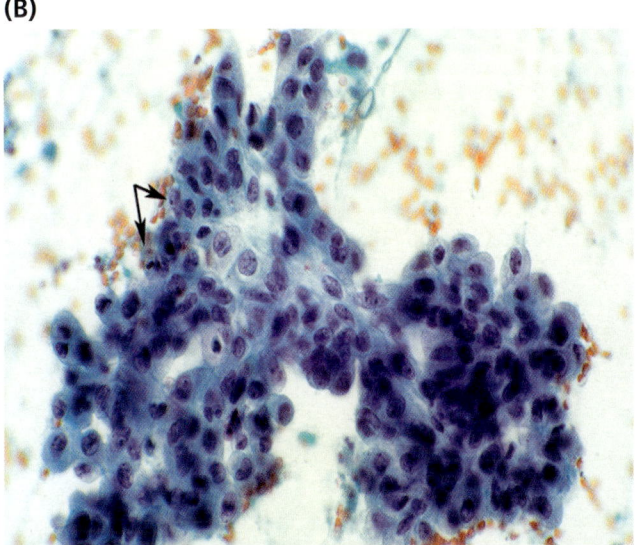

(C)

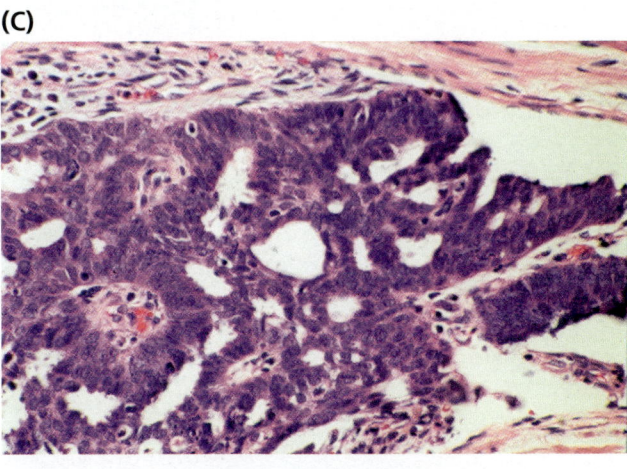

Figure 4.66 Adenocarcinoma, endocervix. Notice the apoptotic change (arrows) and cellular feathering. Nuclei in (A) appear pale and pleomorphic and in (B) are well-differentiated cervical specimens. LBP, Pap stain. Specimen (C) represents an endocervical curettage specimen, H/E stain.

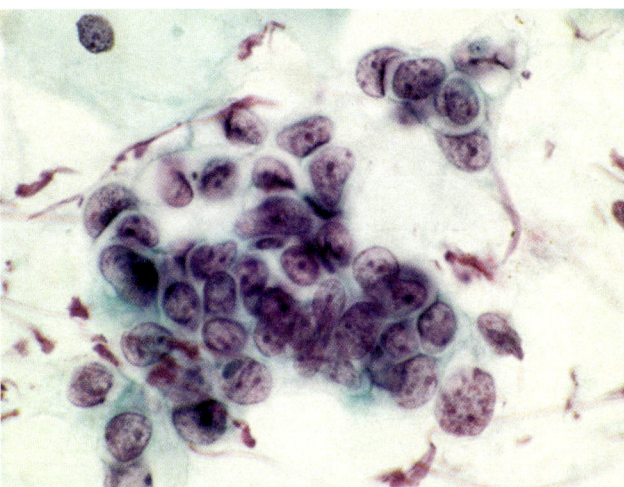

Figure 4.67 Low-grade endometrial adenocarcinoma. Notice the good cellular preservation and prominent nucleoli. Vaginocervical smear, Pap stain.

(A)

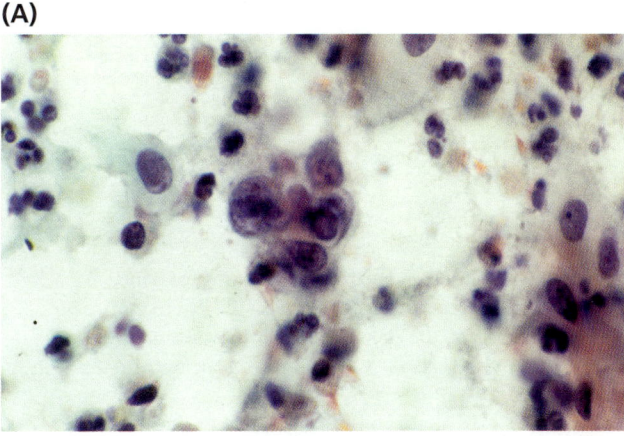

(B)

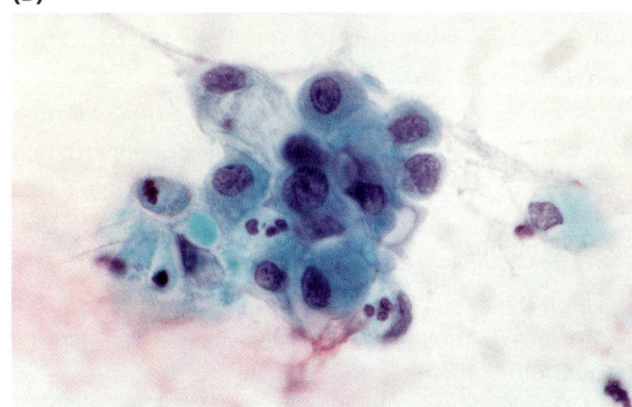

Figure 4.68 Endometrial adenocarcinoma, high grade. Notice the cytoplasmic secretion (B) and pleomorphism (A, B). Vaginocervical smear, Pap stain.

contrast to the cells seen in menstrual specimens. Tumor cells can have variable cytoplasm and generally a single large nucleolus (Figures 4.67 and 4.68). They need to be

(A)

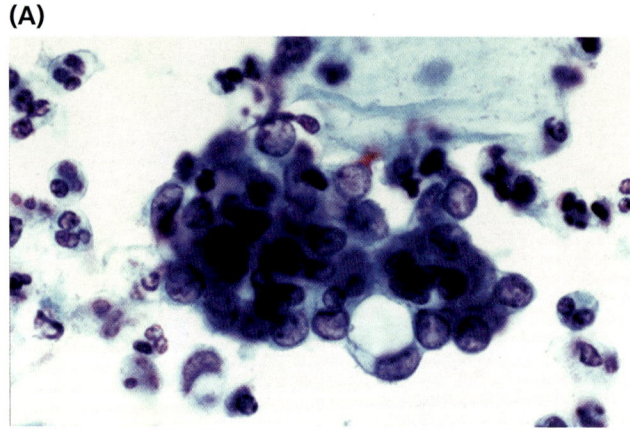

(B)

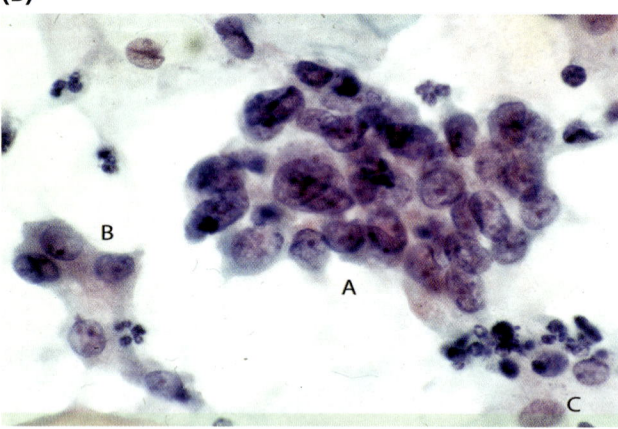

Figure 4.69 Reactive endometrial cells following an abortion (A) and dilation and curettage (D&C) (B) procedure. Notice the mucinous change in the endometrial cells – vacuolation (A), metaplastic and degenerative changes in (B). Vaginocervical smears, Pap stain.

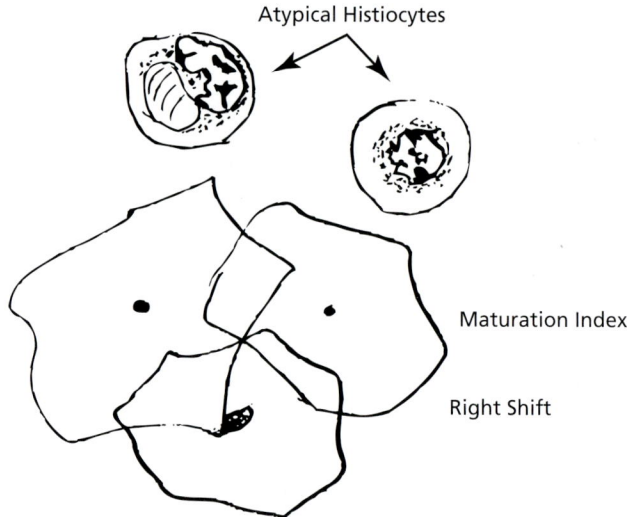

Figure 4.70 Salient features of "early" endometrial carcinoma.

differentiated from extremely atypical and bizarre epithelial cells (Figure 4.69).

"Early" endometrial adenocarcinoma: cells shed from extremely small or "early" carcinoma of the endometrium can appear distinctly different from those of the classic advanced lesions. They usually occur singly with abundant, foamy, basophilic, asymmetrical cytoplasm closely resembling histiocytes. Frequently, the outer portion of the foamy cytoplasm appears as a pale rim falsely suggesting hyalinization. In other early lesions, in the absence of an external source, an abnormal cytohormonal pattern (MI shift to the right) may occur as the only abnormality (Figures 4.70 and 4.71).

Ovarian

Only rarely seen, these tend to occur in papillary fronts in the vaginal material (Figure 4.72).

(A)

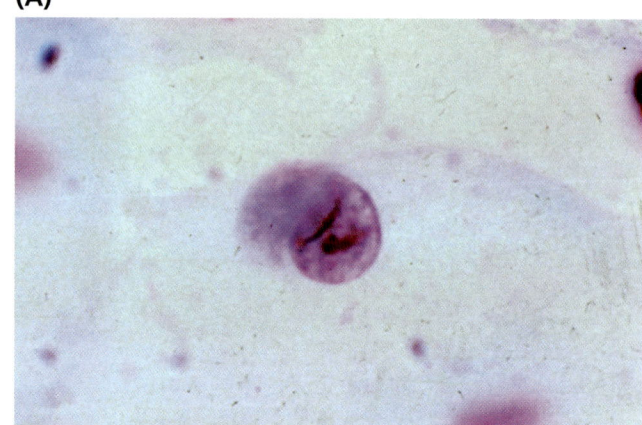

(B)

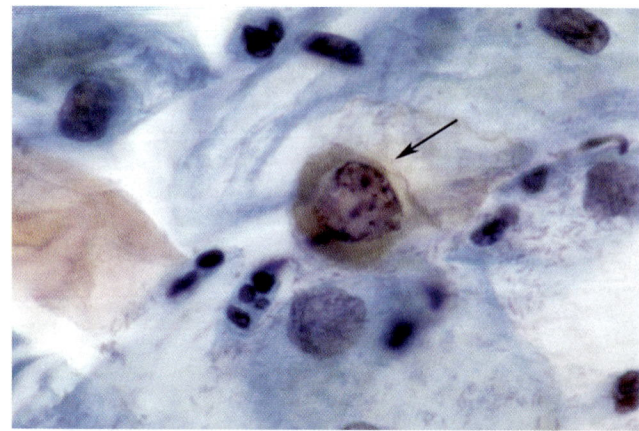

Figure 4.71 Single tumor cells, early endometrial adenocarcinoma. While the cell in (A) has a prominent nucleolus, the cell in (B) reveals chromatin changes (arrow). Vaginocervical smear, Pap stain.

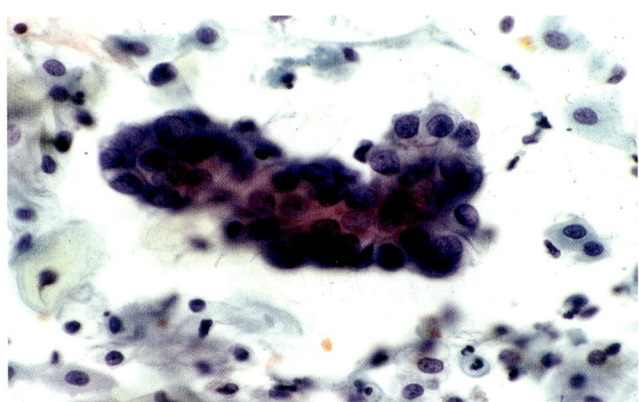

Figure 4.72 Adenocarcinoma ovary. Tumor cells occur as papillary formation. Notice the clean background. Vaginocervical smear. Pap stain.

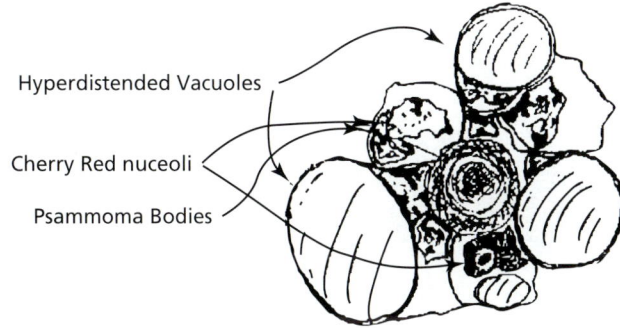

Figure 4.73 Large vacuoles, cherry red nucleoli and laminated psammoma bodies, features commonly associated with ovarian adenocarcinoma.

(A)

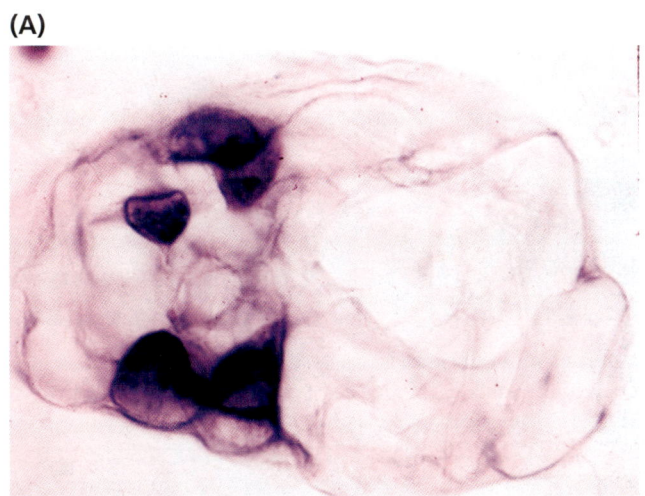

(B)

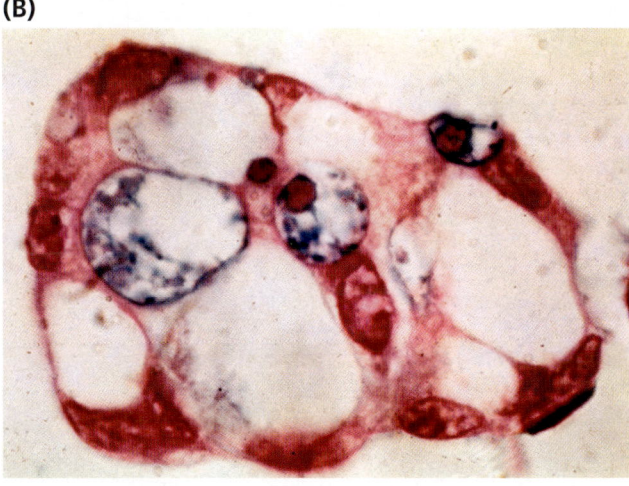

Figure 4.74 Bubblegum cytoplasmic vacuoles ovarian adenocarcinoma (A, B). Abdominal fluid specimen direct smear, Pap stain (A), mucicarmine stain (B).

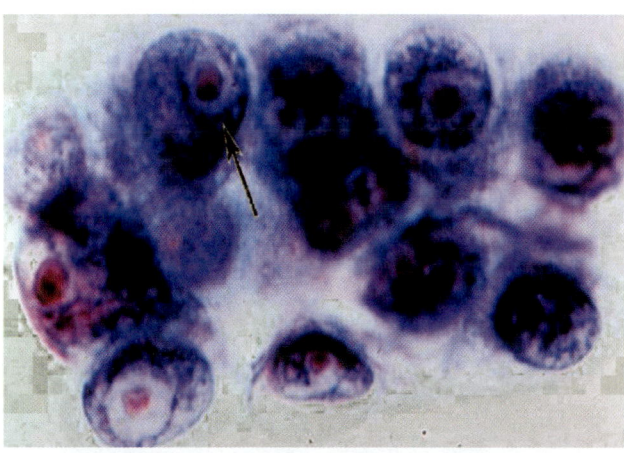

Figure 4.75 Cherry-red nucleoli and perinucleolar halos (arrow), first noticed by William Howdon, MD. They are not specific for ovarian and endometrial adenocarcinoma and may be observed in other adenocarcinoma cells. Vaginocervical smear. Pap stain.

Cells may have variable vacuolation. Vacuoles tend to be large, thin-walled, hyperdistended, and seek the surface, projecting outwards. There may be clear halos around prominent cherry-red nucleoli, psammoma bodies within papillary fragments, "clean" background, MI shift to right (Figures 4.73–4.76).

Bronchoalveolar

These adenocarcinoma cells tend to have hyperdistended single secretory vacuoles (Figures 4.77 and 4.78).

Tumor cells may appear to be very "sticky" (Figure 4.79), and shed together as true tissue fragments or as alveolar casts. The nuclei range from bland (showing few malignant criteria) to obviously malignant. Histiocytes in the specimen usually appear extremely foamy due to abundant phagocytosed material. Nucleoli can be extremely prominent (Figures 4.79–4.83).

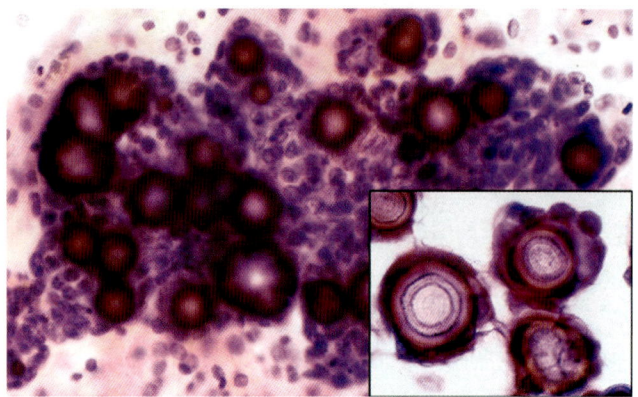

Figure 4.76 Adenocarcinoma ovary with laminated psammoma bodies (insert). Notice the tumor cells spread around the psammoma bodies. Cervicovaginal smear. Vaginal smear, Pap stain.

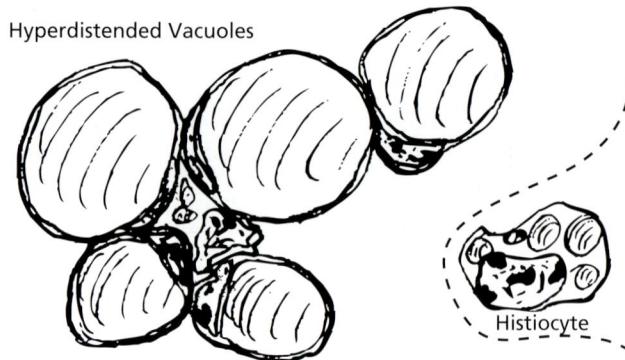

Figure 4.77 Marked cytoplasm vacuolation, often seen in intestinal-type bronchoalveolar carcinoma.

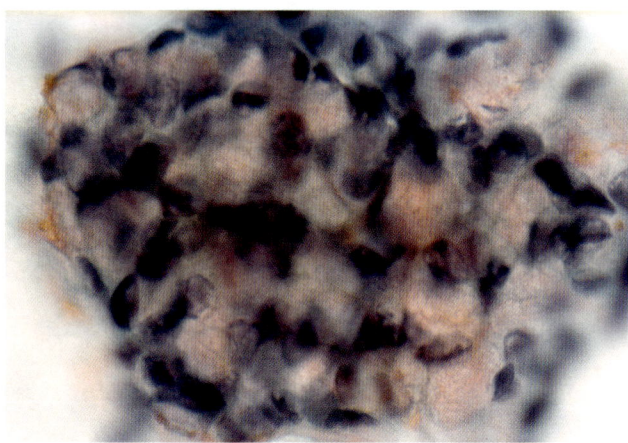

Figure 4.78 Bronchioalveolar carcinoma with tall columnar cells distended with a pale intracytoplasmic mucin. Malignant criteria are not well expressed. FNA lung, Pap stain.

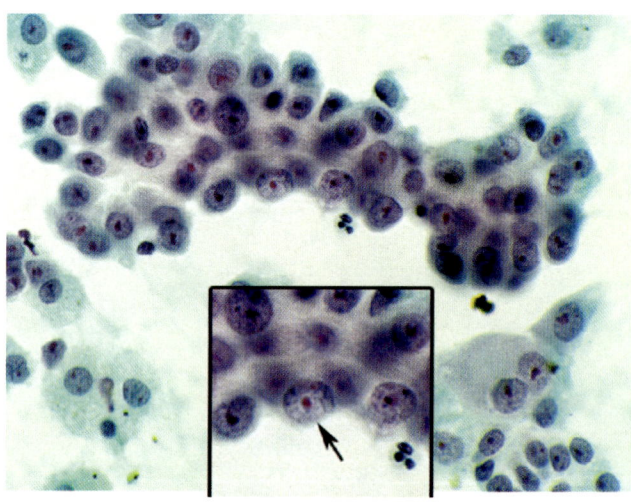

Figure 4.79 Bronchioalveolar carcinoma occurring as an alveolar cast. Bronchoalveolar lavage specimen. Perinuclear halo (arrow, insert), FNA lung, Pap stain.

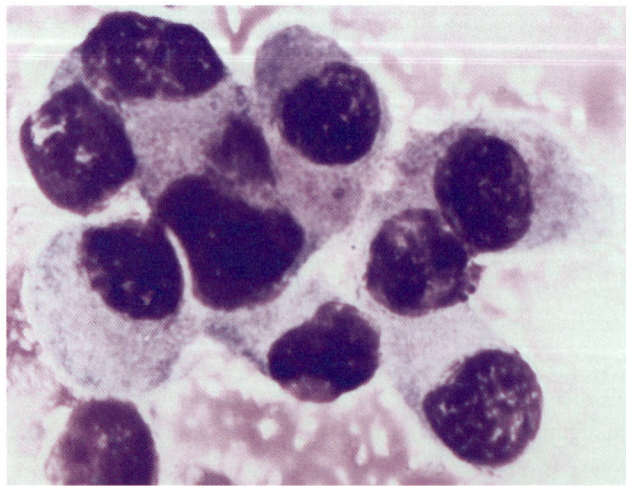

Figure 4.80 Bronchoalveolar carcinoma. Note the columnar appearance of tumor cells. FNA lung. Diff-Quik stain.

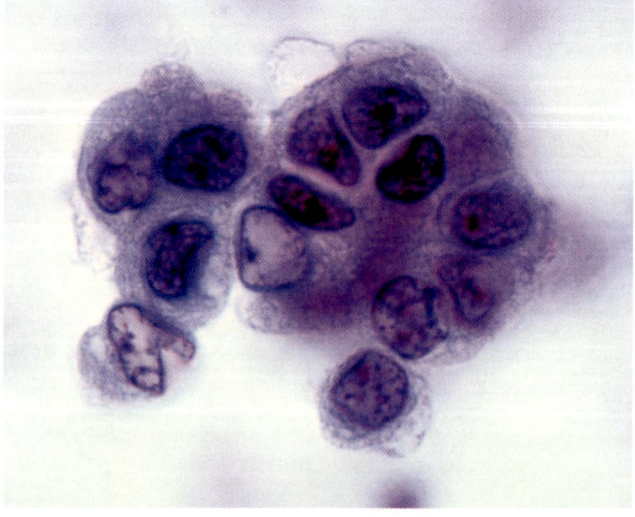

Figure 4.81 Bronchoalveolar carcinoma with distinct malignant features. Tumor cells exhibit alveolar arrangement. BAL specimen, cytospin, Pap stain.

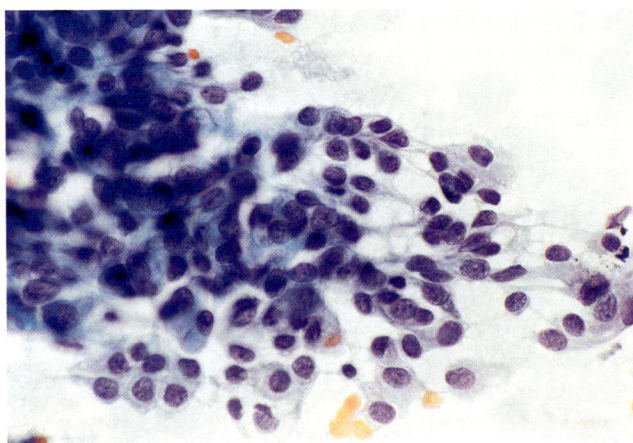

Figure 4.82 Bronchoalveolar carcinoma. The tumor is well-differentiated with minimal malignant criteria among single cells. FNA lung, direct smear, Pap stain.

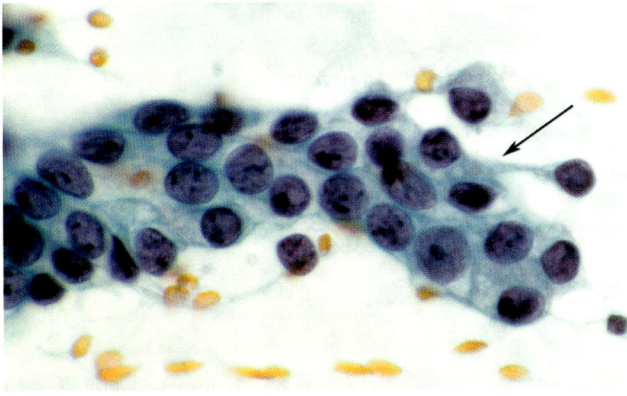

Figure 4.83 Tenacious intracytoplasmic connection (TIC). This thin cytoplasm connection (arrow) is often seen in these tumors. FNA lung, Pap stain. Small cell carcinoma.

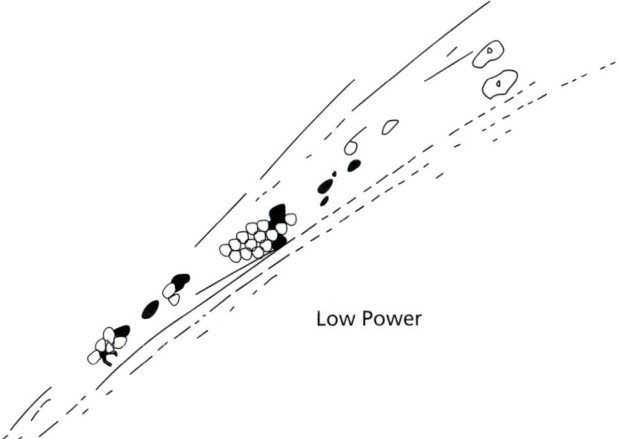

Low Power

Figure 4.84 Characteristic linear exfoliation of small-cell carcinoma cells in sputum specimens. These characteristics are not seen in liquid fixed and prepared slides.

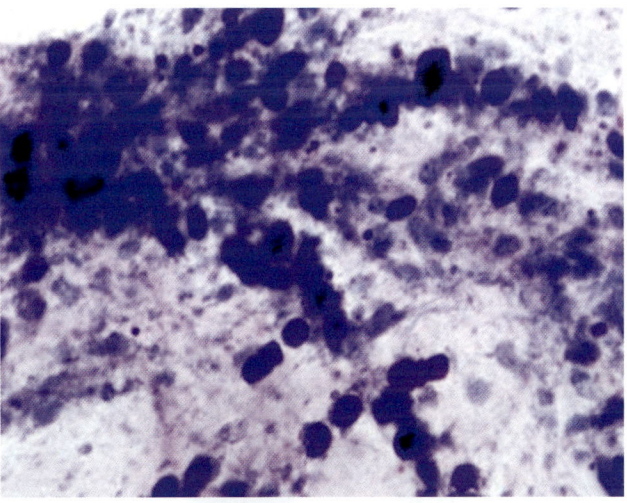

Figure 4.85 Linear distribution of small-cell carcinoma cells along the mucus strands. Sputum specimen, direct smear, Pap stain.

UNDIFFERENTIATED (SMALL CELL) CARCINOMA

These represent undifferentiated carcinoma in most instances, and their prognosis is grave.

In pulmonary material, they characteristically shed as tissue fragments "strung out" along mucus strands (Figures 4.84 and 4.85). They are small cells, but larger than histiocytes. This tumor is rapidly multiplying and tumor necrosis and apoptosis are a common occurrence, appearing as acellular basophilic debris. Sometimes, especially in lymph node aspirates, tumor cells ball up and appear as "blue blobs" or cotton balls (Figure 4.86).

Nucleus

These are generally round or oval, hyperchromatic without prominent chromatin clumps and show molding to the

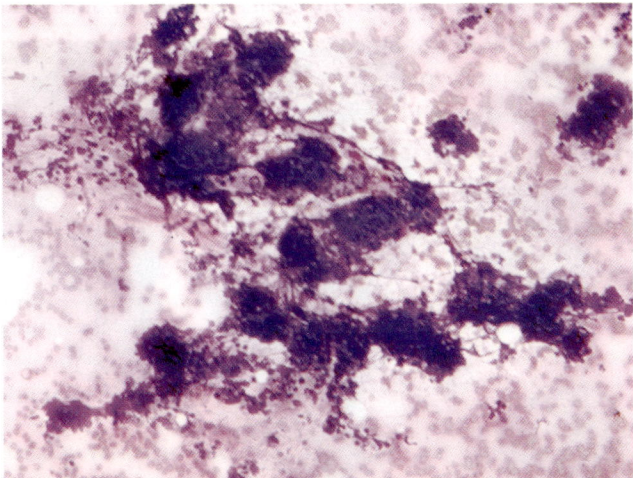

Figure 4.86 "Cotton ball" appearance of small-cell carcinoma aggregates in mediastinal lymph node aspiration. These aggregates need to be distinguished from similar but more tight and irregular structures seen with crushed lymphoid cells. Direct smear, Diff-Quik stain.

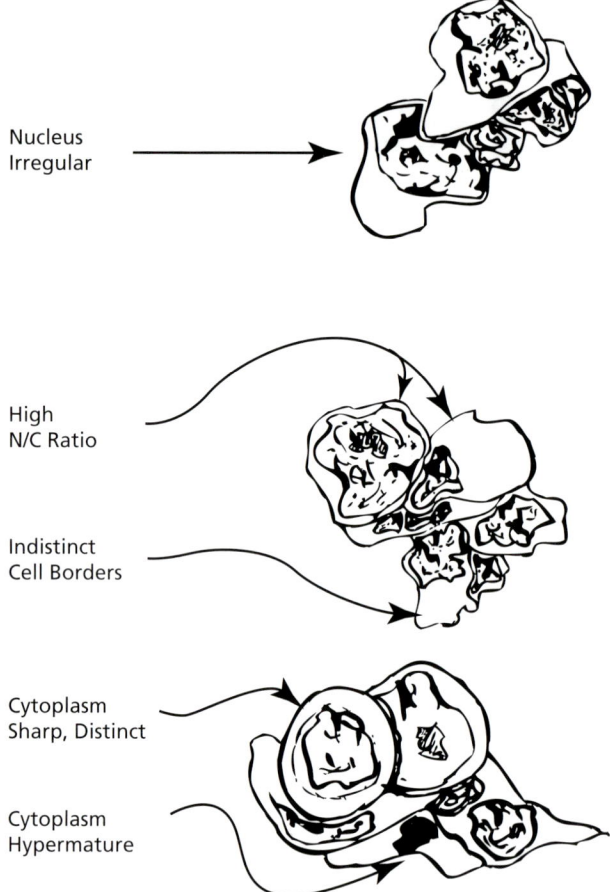

Nucleus
Irregular

High
N/C Ratio

Indistinct
Cell Borders

Cytoplasm
Sharp, Distinct

Cytoplasm
Hypermature

Figure 4.95 Salient features of large cell undifferentiated tumor.

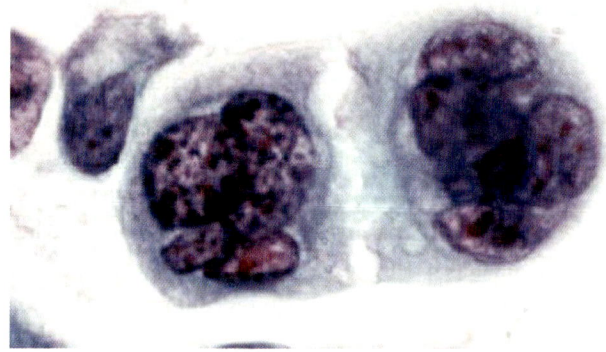

Figure 4.97 Undifferentiated malignant tumor. Notice the nuclear features although the cell size is similar. Bronchial brush. Metastatic sarcoma, Pap stain.

Gastrointestinal stromal tumor (GIST)

GIST is a specific submucosal or wall tumor that is efficiently diagnosed by cytologic examination. These cells occur as well-differentiated smooth muscle tissue with

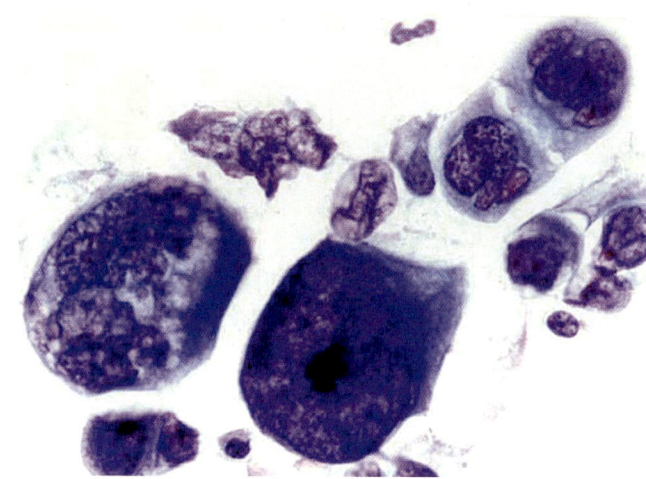

Figure 4.96 Undifferentiated carcinoma lung. Notice the marked variation in the nuclear and cell size. Fine needle aspiration lung, Pap stain.

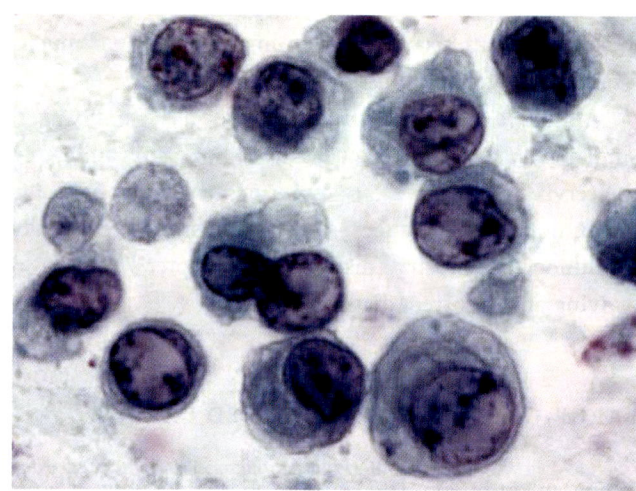

Figure 4.98 Undifferentiated malignant tumor, this represents a high-grade lymphoma. Hilar lymph node fine needle aspiration, direct smear, Pap stain.

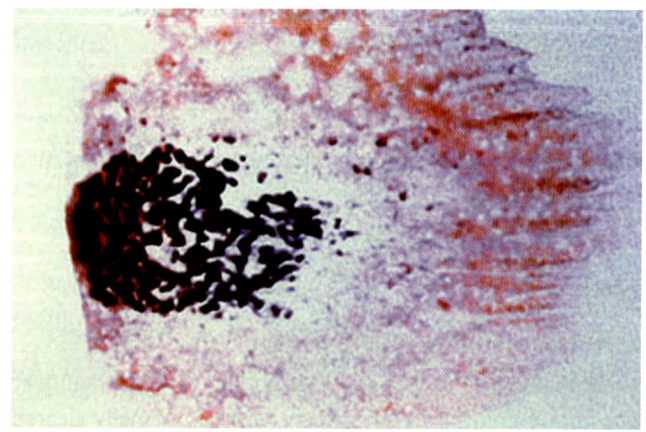

Figure 4.99 Melanoma, metastatic to liver. Notice the melanin pigment in the central concentrate. FNA, unstained slide.

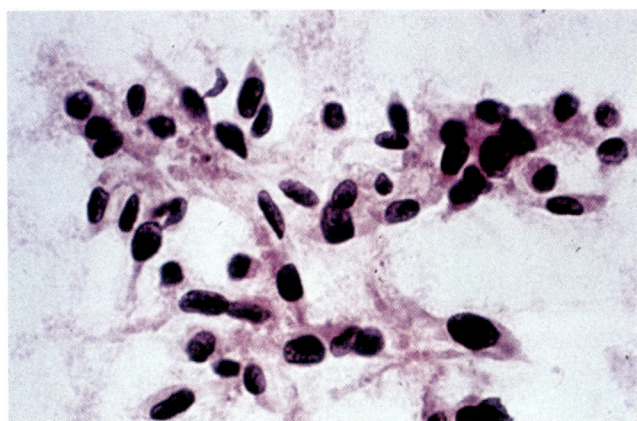

Figure 4.100 Spindle cell sarcoma retroperitoneal area, metastatic to lung. Notice minimal pleomorphism among cells. FNA lung, Pap stain.

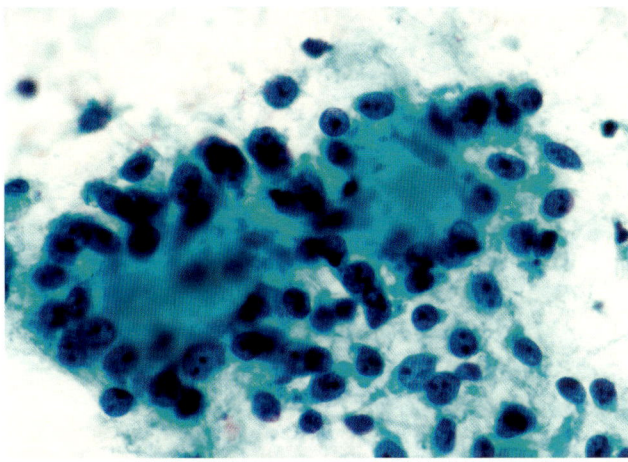

Figure 4.101 Osteosarcoma metastatic, lung. Notice the amorphous osteoid material in the center. FNA lung. Pap stain.

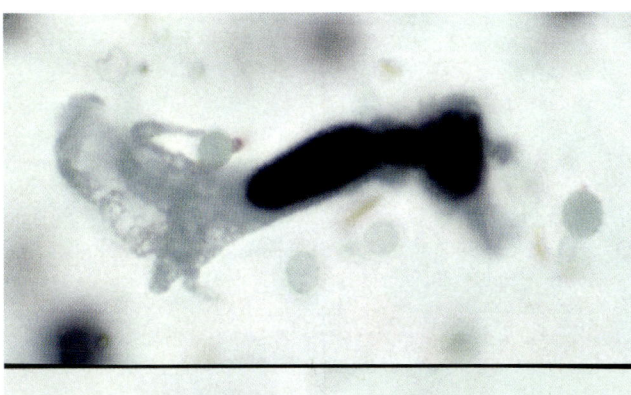

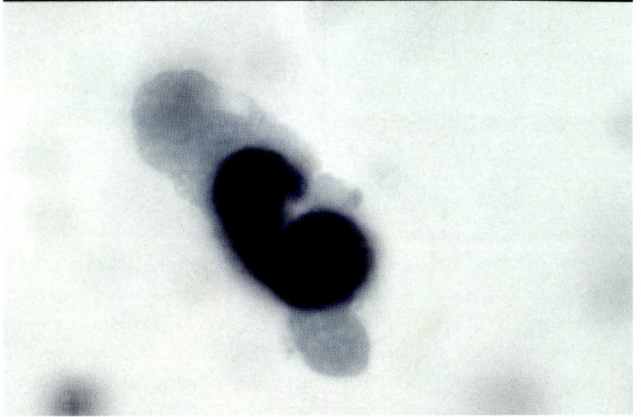

Figure 4.102 Lieomyosarcoma cells, pleural fluid. Tumor cells generally shed singly and may have marked pleomorphism, Pap stain.

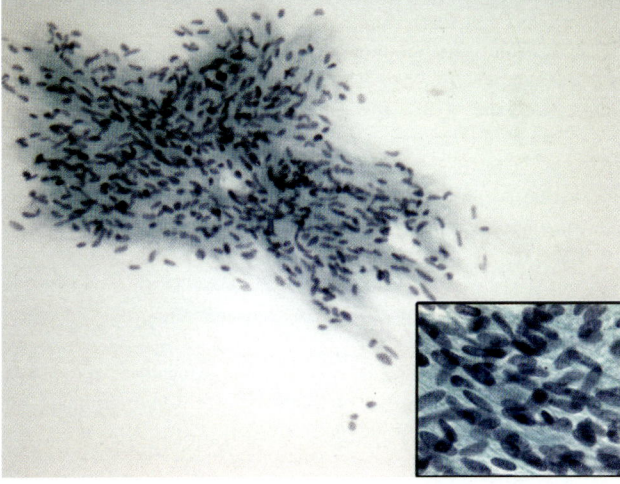

Figure 4.103 Gastrointestinal stromal tumor (GIST). Low power shows a number of mesenchymal spindle cells. The insert reveals higher magnification with some pleomorphism and atypia. Endoscopic-guided gastric FNA, Pap stain.

variable degrees of nuclear atypia. It may be minimal or reveal significant pleomorphism. Occasionally, tumor cells may have an epithelial appearance. Tissue sampling is helpful in the diagnosis which is established by the utilization of specific immunohistochemical antibodies (discussed in Chapter 6). An accurate diagnosis of GIST is critical due to its therapeutic ramifications (Figures 4.103 and 4.104).

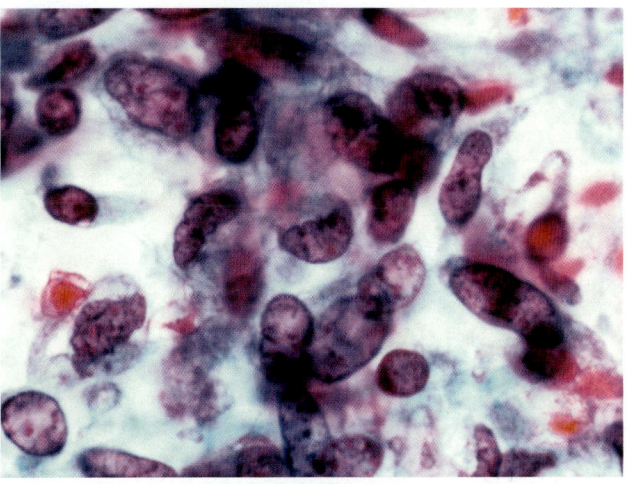

Figure 4.104 GIST with marked nuclear polymorphism and atypia. Endoscopic-guided gastric FNA, direct smear, Pap stain.

FURTHER READING

Arora, V. K., N. Singh, *et al.* (2003). "Significance of cytologic criteria in distinguishing small cell from non-small cell carcinoma of the lung". *Acta Cytol* **47**(2): 216–20.

Baloch, Z. W., M. J. Sack, *et al.* (1999). "Papillary formations in metastatic melanoma". *Diagn Cytopathol* **20**(3): 148–51.

Barros, J. N., M. S. Lowen, *et al.* (2009). "Predictive index to differentiate invasive squamous cell carcinoma from preinvasive ocular surface lesions by impression cytology". *Br J Ophthalmol* **93**(2): 209–14.

Biscotti, C. V., M. A. Gero, *et al.* (1997). "Endocervical adenocarcinoma in situ: an analysis of cellular features". *Diagn Cytopathol* **17**(5): 326–32.

Chang, W. C., J. P. Matisic, *et al.* (1999). "Cytologic features of villoglandular adenocarcinoma of the uterine cervix: comparison with typical endocervical adenocarcinoma with a villoglandular component and papillary serous carcinoma". *Cancer* **87**(1): 5–11.

Chen, K. T. (1990). "Psammoma bodies in fine-needle aspiration cytology of papillary adenocarcinoma of the lung". *Diagn Cytopathol* **6**(4): 271–4.

Chhieng, D. C., D. Jhala, *et al.* (2002). "Endoscopic ultrasound-guided fine-needle aspiration biopsy: a study of 103 cases". *Cancer* **96**(4): 232–9.

Chute, D. J. and E. B. Stelow. (2010). "Cytology of head and neck squamous cell carcinoma variants". *Diagn Cytopathol* **38**(1): 65–80.

Costa, M. J., M. B. Kenny, *et al.* (1991). "Cervicovaginal cytology in uterine adenocarcinoma and adenosquamous carcinoma. Comparison of cytologic and histologic findings". *Acta Cytol* **35**(1): 127–34.

Dallenbach-Hellweg, G. and D. Schmidt. (2002). "Distinction between endometrial and endocervical adenocarcinoma". *Int J Gynecol Pathol* **21**(3): 307–08.

de Brux, J., J. Dupre-Froment, *et al.* (1961). "Exfoliative cytology and experimental cytology of carcinoma in situ. Cytomorphology of carcinoma in situ". *Acta Cytol* **5**: 422–36.

Delgado, P. I., M. Jorda, *et al.* (2000). "Small cell carcinoma versus other lung malignancies: diagnosis by fine-needle aspiration cytology". *Cancer* **90**(5): 279–85.

Domanski, H. A. and M. Akerman. (2005). "Fine-needle aspiration of primary osteosarcoma: a cytological–histological study". *Diagn Cytopathol* **32**(5): 269–75.

Domanski, H. A., M. Akerman, *et al.* (2006). "Fine-needle aspiration of soft tissue leiomyosarcoma: an analysis of the most common cytologic findings and the value of ancillary techniques". *Diagn Cytopathol* **34**(9): 597–604.

Fanning, J., S. N. Markuly, *et al.* (1996). "False positive malignant peritoneal cytology and psammoma bodies in benign gynecologic disease". *J Reprod Med* **41**(7): 504–08.

Frable, W. J. (1994). "Litigation cells: definition and observations on a cell type in cervical vaginal smears not addressed by the Bethesda System". *Diagn Cytopathol* **11**(3): 213–5.

Friedlander, M. A., E. Stier, *et al.* (2004). "Anorectal cytology as a screening tool for anal squamous lesions: cytologic, anoscopic, and histologic correlation". *Cancer* **102**(1): 19–26.

Fu, K., M. A. Eloubeidi, *et al.* (2002). "Diagnosis of gastrointestinal stromal tumor by endoscopic ultrasound-guided fine needle aspiration biopsy – a potential pitfall". *Ann Diagn Pathol* **6**(5): 294–301.

Fushimi, H., M. Kukui, *et al.* (1992). "Detection of large cell component in small cell lung carcinoma by combined cytologic and histologic examinations and its clinical implication". *Cancer* **70**(3): 599–605.

Goldberg, G., G. Learmonth, *et al.* (1985). "Role of cul-de-sac aspiration cytology in the management and follow-up of patients with ovarian carcinoma. A preliminary report". *J Reprod Med* **30**(11): 867–70.

Graham, R. M. (1960). "Cancer detection, including exfoliative cytology". *Acta Unio Int Contra Cancrum* **16**: 377–81.

Graham, R. M., O. T. Messelt, *et al.* (1958). "Panel discussion: radiation changes in carcinoma of the cervix as revealed by cytology and their role in determining prognosis". *Acta Unio Int Contra Cancrum* **14**(4): 364–71.

Gupta, P. K. (1968). "Cytodiagnosis of squamous cell carcinoma. Malignant squamous cell cytology". *Indian J Cancer* **5**(3): 258–68.

Gupta, R. K. (1981). "Value of sputum cytology in the differential diagnosis of alveolar cell carcinoma from bronchogenic adenocarcinoma". *Acta Cytol* **25**(3): 255–8.

Gupta, S. and P. Sodhani. (2004). "Why is high grade squamous intraepithelial neoplasia under-diagnosed on cytology in a quarter of cases? Analysis of smear characteristics in discrepant cases". *Indian J Cancer* **41**(3): 104–08.

Gupta, S. K., D. K. Das, *et al.* (1986). "Cytology of hepatocellular carcinoma". *Diagn Cytopathol* **2**(4): 290–4.

Gupta, S. K., A. K. Rajwanshi, *et al.* (1985). "Fine needle aspiration cytology smear patterns of malignant melanoma". *Acta Cytol* **29**(6): 983–8.

Hernandez, L. V., G. Mishra, *et al.* (2002). "Role of endoscopic ultrasound (EUS) and EUS-guided fine needle aspiration in the diagnosis and treatment of cystic lesions of the pancreas". *Pancreas* **25**(3): 222–8.

Jimenez-Heffernan, J. A., P. Lopez-Ferrer, *et al.* (2008). "Fine-needle aspiration cytology of large cell neuroendocrine carcinoma of the lung: a cytohistologic correlation study of 11 cases". *Cancer* **114**(3): 180–6.

Jobo, T., M. Arai, *et al.* (1999). "Usefulness of endometrial aspiration cytology for the preoperative diagnosis of ovarian carcinoma". *Acta Cytol* **43**(2): 104–09.

Joseph, P., D. N. Rana, *et al.* (2006). "Significance of psammoma bodies in cervical cytology". *Cytopathology* **17**(6): 399–401.

Kalogeraki, A., J. Panayiotides, *et al.* (2000). "Quantitative cytology in ovarian carcinoma ascitic fluids". *Anal Quant Cytol Histol* **22**(2): 139–42.

Kashimura, M., Y. Matsuura, *et al.* (1993). "Cytology of vulvar squamous neoplasia". *Acta Cytol* **37**(6): 871–5.

Kasuganti, D., D. Cimbaluk, *et al.* (2006). "Lymph node metastasis of large-cell carcinoma of the lung in a seventeen-year-old patient: diagnosis by fine-needle aspiration". *Diagn Cytopathol* **34**(12): 852–3.

Klijanienko, J., J. M. Caillaud, *et al.* (2003). "Fine-needle aspiration of leiomyosarcoma: a correlative cytohistopathological study of 96 tumors in 68 patients". *Diagn Cytopathol* **28**(3): 119–25.

Kneafsey, P., M. A. Duggan, *et al.* (2003). "Fine needle aspiration cytology of pulmonary, well-differentiated fetal adenocarcinoma prepared by the ThinPrep method". *Cytopathology* **14**(2): 87–90.

Koss, L. G., M. R. Melamed, *et al.* (2006). *Koss' Diagnostic Cytology and its Histopathologic Bases.* Philadelphia, PA, Lippincott Williams & Wilkins.

Layfield, L. J., M. E. Robert, *et al.* (1992). "Aspiration biopsy smear pattern as a predictor of biologic behavior in adenocarcinoma of the breast". *Acta Cytol* **36**(2): 208–14.

Lee, K. G. and N. H. Cho. (1991). "Fine-needle aspiration cytology of pulmonary adenocarcinoma of fetal type: report of a case with immunohistochemical and ultrastructural studies". *Diagn Cytopathol* **7**(4): 408–14.

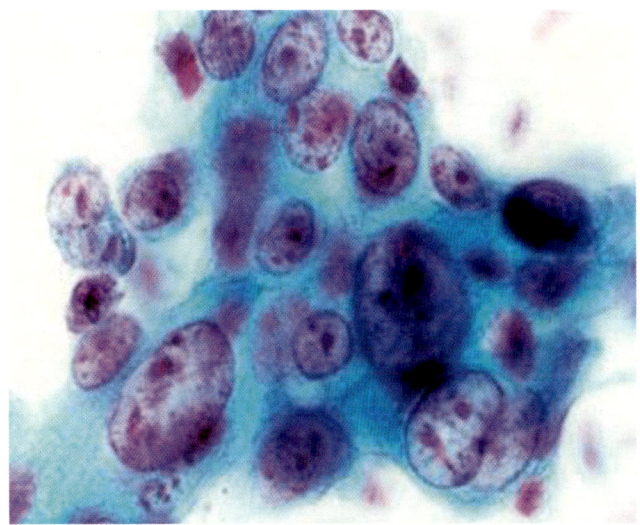

Figure 5.7 Reactive bronchial cells. Notice the marked size variation and nuclear organelle. Bronchial brush specimen. Patient on chemotherapy for leukemia, direct smear, Pap stain.

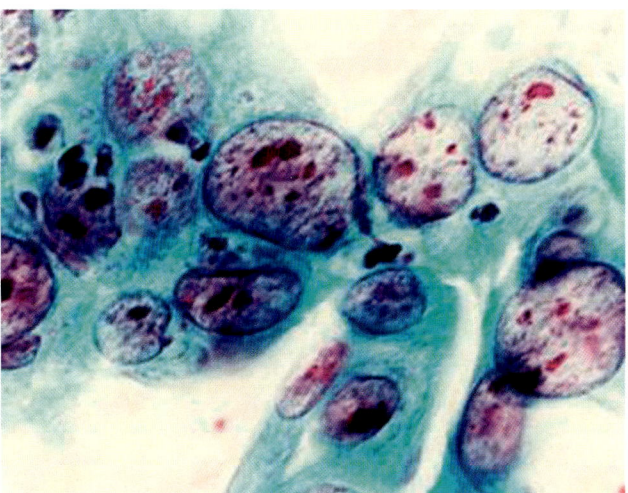

Figure 5.8 Reactive bronchial cells. Notice the size variation and prominent nucleoli which often are misinterpreted to and diagnosed as malignant. Post-radiation, Hilar lymphoma, bronchial brush, direct smear, Pap stain.

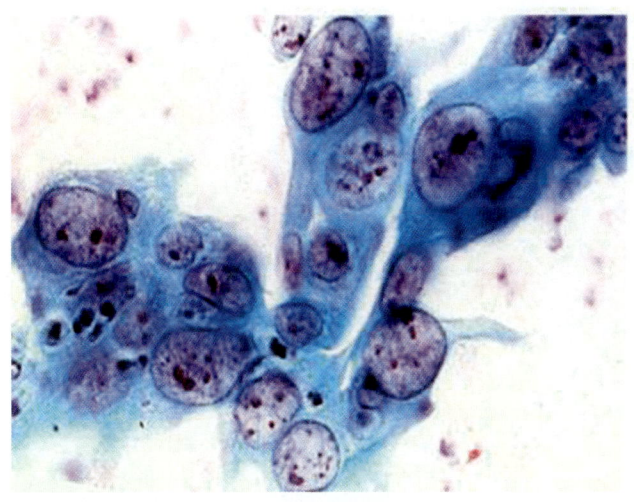

Figure 5.9 Reactive bronchial cells. Notice the uniformly thin and well-stretched nuclear membranes. Reactive bronchial cells (same case as Figure 5.7). Three weeks later, now has pleural effusion also, bronchial brush, direct smear, Pap stain.

NUCLEAR MEMBRANE

Reactive cells and large nuclei have a distinct, sharp, and uniformly thin nuclear membrane. It tends to be well stretched and at times may become irregular and wavy. Nuclear membrane undulation increases with greater cellular activity. However, it does not exhibit the alternate thinning and thickening often observed among neoplastic cells (Figure 5.9).

PARACHROMATIN

Parachromatin and interchromatinic material appears as uniformly pale and generally of cyanophilic hue when examined with Papanicolaou technique. Parachromatin appears "watery" (Figures 5.8–5.10). Similar changes may be observed in certain malignant epithelial tumors.

CHROMATIN

Chromatin in the reactive cells appears as fine and fibrillary or granular. Uniformity of the chromatinic material is the key observation. Size of the chromatin material is proportional to the activity (Figures 5.11–5.13).

NUCLEOLI

Nucleoli do not occur among reactive squamous cells but are commonly seen in the other epithelial (columnar, mesothelium, urothelium) and mesenchymal cells. They are generally small and round. They may be variable in number and size and prominent. Nucleoli tend to stand out and appear distinct against the pale nuclear chromatin. Tinctorial features of nucleoli may be affected by associated chromatinic material (Figures 5.7, 5.8 and 5.13).

Dyskaryotic cells

A constellation of cytoplasmic and nuclear changes are identifiable which can be recognized as representing an epithelial lesion (Figure 5.14).

The slightly atypical lesions shed more of the mature columnar minimally dyskaryotic cells and/or the mature squamous–minimal dyskaryotic cells.

The more disturbed moderately atypical lesions shed more of the moderately mature–moderately dyskaryotic

(A)

(B)

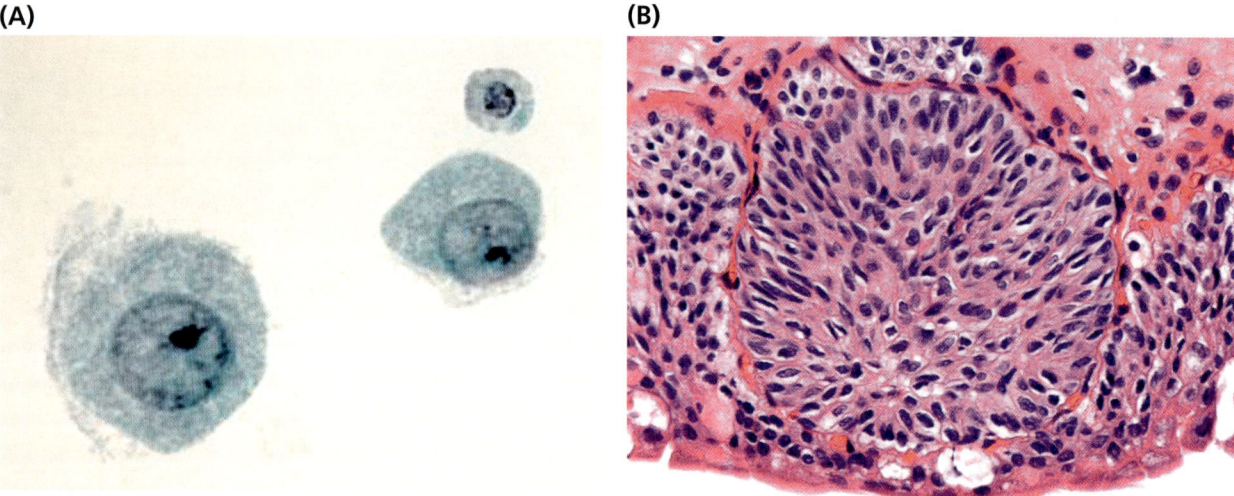

Figure 5.10 Reactive urothelial cells. Notice the pale and uniformly homogenous parachromatin. Urinary bladder wash specimen (A), ThinPrep slide, Pap stain. Corresponding urinary bladder biopsy (B), H/E stain.

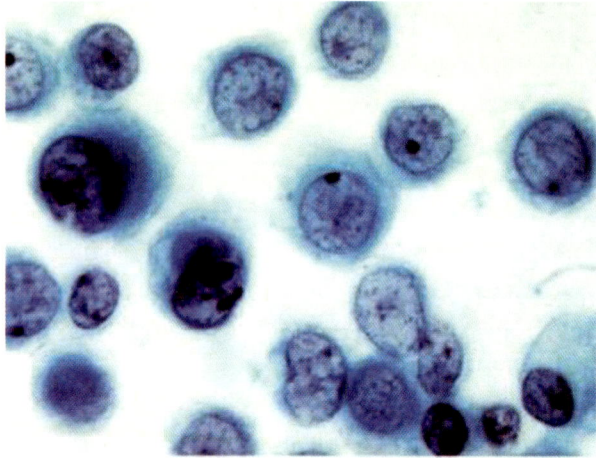

Figure 5.11 Reactive mesothelial cells. Notice the uniformly distributed chromatin despite extremely high N:C ratio. Pulmonary tuberculosis, under treatment developed pleural effusion, Millipore filter, Pap stain. (Same as Figure 2.6.)

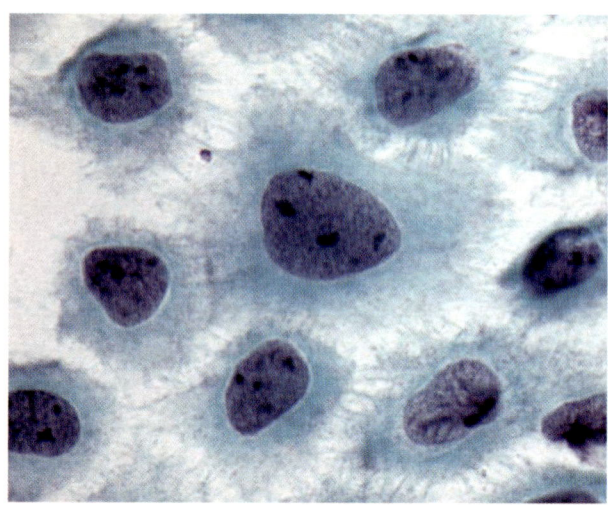

Figure 5.12 Reactive mesothelial cells. Notice the chromatin which is uniform in size and distribution. Abdominal wash, direct smear, Pap stain.

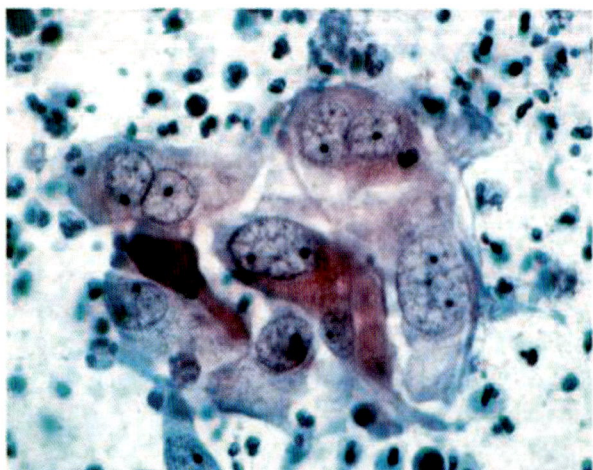

Figure 5.13 Reactive ductal cells. Notice the pale fine chromatin and small nucleoli. Breast cyst, fine needle aspiration, Pap stain.

cells. The grave or "borderline" lesions shed more of the immature markedly dyskaryotic cells.

There is a seamless transition from the markedly dyskaryotic change to cancer cells typical of classical non-keratinizing carcinoma in-situ (CIS); the same dyskaryotic nucleus (usually marked dyskaryotic) acquires an extremely scanty and immature cytoplasm.

These dyskaryotic cells and CIS cells are also present in microinvasive carcinoma; however, there appear also a percentage of cancer cells with clear and cytoplasmic features facilitating invasion.

With the classical invasive squamous cell carcinoma, these nuclear and cytoplasmic features become more prominent and the percentage of cells with these features increases. It must be recognized that there is a substantial

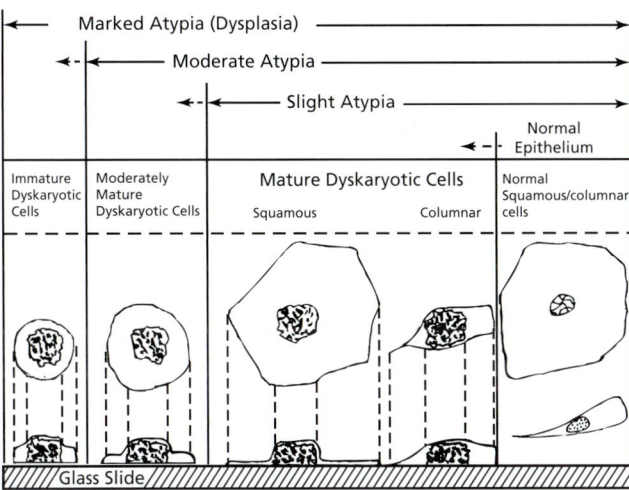

Figure 5.14 Nuclear and cytoplasmic changes that are associated with recognizable epithelial lesions. Depending upon the degree of the above-mentioned changes, among squamous and to a certain degree columnar epithelial cells, "minimal/slight," "moderate," and "marked" dyskaryosis is recognized which correlates with the degree of increased activity. Similar changes can also be observed among other epithelia including urothelial, gastric, esophageal ductal pancreatic, and breast cells.

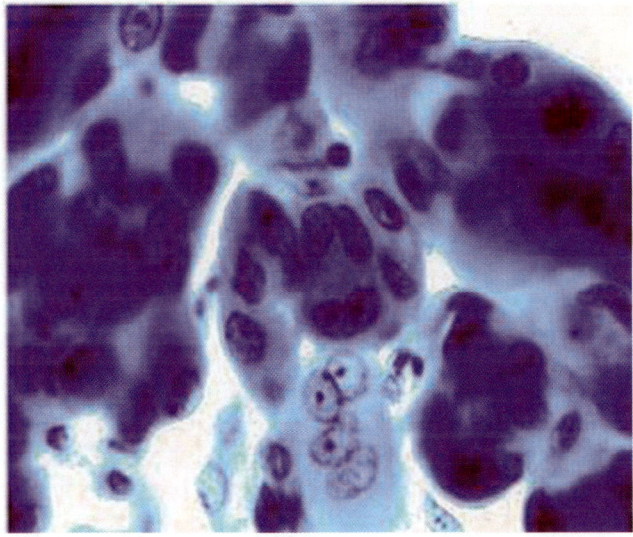

Figure 5.16 Multinucleated mesothelial cells. Reactive changes following intrapleural therapy. Pleural fluid specimen, Millipore filter, Pap stain.

morphological overlap in the appearance and occurrence of the cells and changes. Almost always, in high-grade borderline lesions a galaxy of cells representing a spectrum of proliferative (reactive, proplastic) changes is seen.

Multinucleation

In reactive processes, multinucleation may be seen commonly among various epithelia such as endocervical,

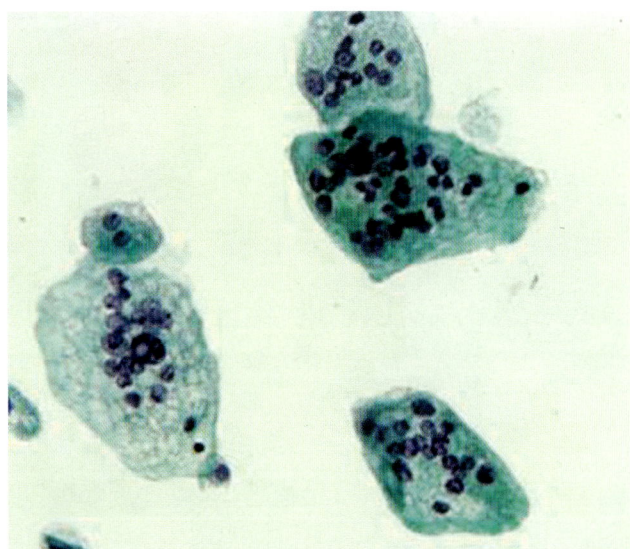

Figure 5.15 Multinucleated reactive urothelial (umbrella) cells. Such cells are commonly seen following instrumentation and in association with bladder stones, voided urine, cytospin, Pap stain.

urothelial and bronchial, and occasionally mesothelial (Figures 5.15 and 5.16).

DECREASED FUNCTIONAL ACTIVITY

Background

In extreme cases, the background changes seen in a smear as well as in modified form in liquid-based preparations may indicate cell death, retroplasia or degenerative changes. Such changes are commonly observed in slides obtained from tumors with extensive cell death from invasive tumors, or resulting from poor cellular preservation and preparation. They may be associated with rapid growth and therapy or ischemia. Care must be exercised in the recognition of degenerative changes; similar cellular alterations may be observed in specimens and cells that are poorly preserved, fixed or infracted to a certain degree. The quantity and quality of injury determines the morphological manifestations of retroplasia and are a common source of such alterations (Figures 5.17 and 5.18).

Cell as a whole

The cell as a whole may exhibit retroplastic or degenerative changes. These depend upon multiple factors including type of cell (soft, low molecular weight epithelial vs. highly keratinized squamous). Protein, lipid, carbohydrate,

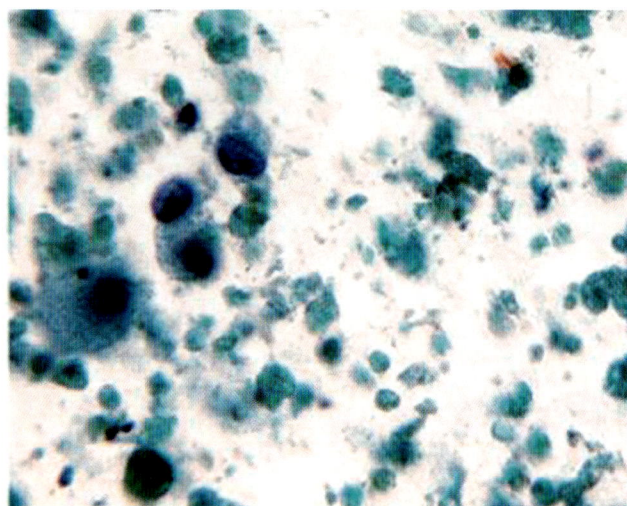

Figure 5.17 Degenerated tumor cells appearing as "ghost structures" following tumor infarction. Neck mass, FNA, direct smear, Pap stain.

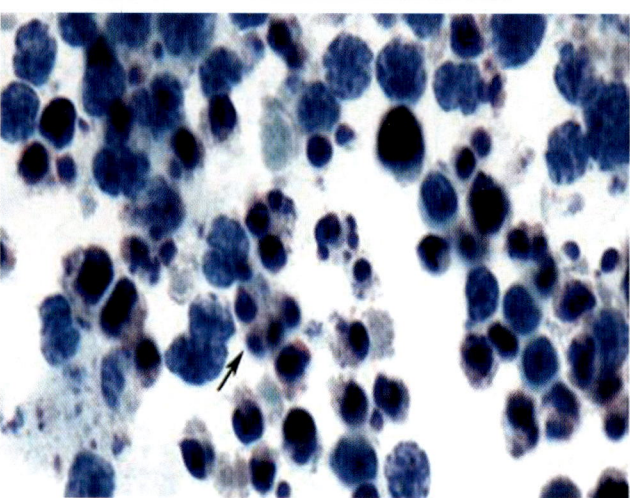

Figure 5.18 Degenerated tumor cells appearing as dense, apoptotic, and dark (arrow). Patient with acute myelogenous leukemia under treatment. Pleural fluid specimen, Millipore filter, Pap stain.

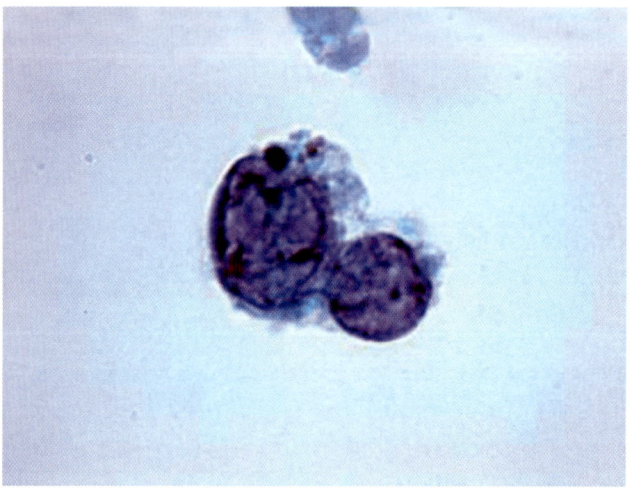

Figure 5.19 Cell-as-a-whole degeneration. Notice the cytoplasmic fraying, nuclear membrane breaks, and pale and blotchy chromatin. Voided urine, ThinPrep, Pap stain.

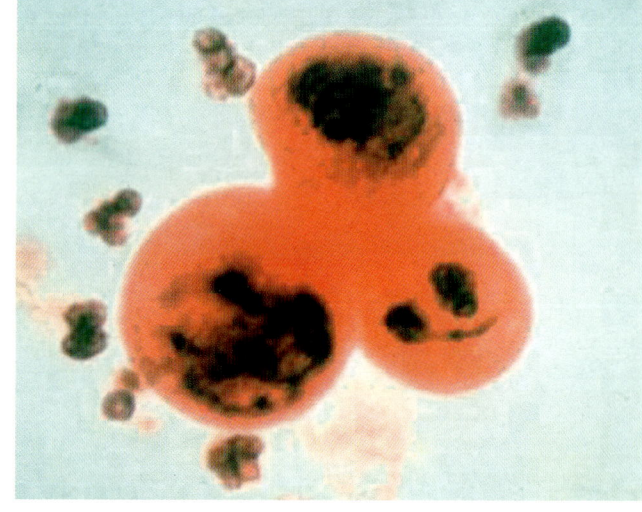

Figure 5.20 Cell-as-a-whole degeneration. Notice the cytoplasmic acidophilia, opacity, nuclear fraying, and chromatin, pleural fluid, cytospin, Pap stain.

and mineral contents of the cells as well as numerous metabolic products such as lipofuscine and calcium determine the degree of observed degenerative changes Factors affecting the degenerative changes seen in cells often include type, nature, and duration of the stimulus leading to degeneration. The introduction of rapid fixation, such as in liquid-based specimens and ethanol, is less likely to cause cellular degeneration when compared to delayed fixations. Similarly, use of methanol and formaldehyde produce different types of cellular degenerative changes. The environmental milieu surrounding the cells, such as mucus, body fluid with low or high protein content (transudate vs. exudates) or pH variations

(urine), affect the preservation and viability of cells and contribute to their degeneration. Cells degenerate by losing fluids, i.e. they become small, dark, and shriveled (Figures 5.19 and 5.20).

Cell fixation

The tinctorial character of cell cytoplasm is altered. Distinct nuclear hematoxynophila is replaced by cytoplasmic acidophilia. Cellular transparency, the hallmark of Papanicolaou-stained cells, is altered; cells become opaque with fuzzy cell margins and migration of nucleo cytoplasmic interphase. These changes often appear as karyo- and

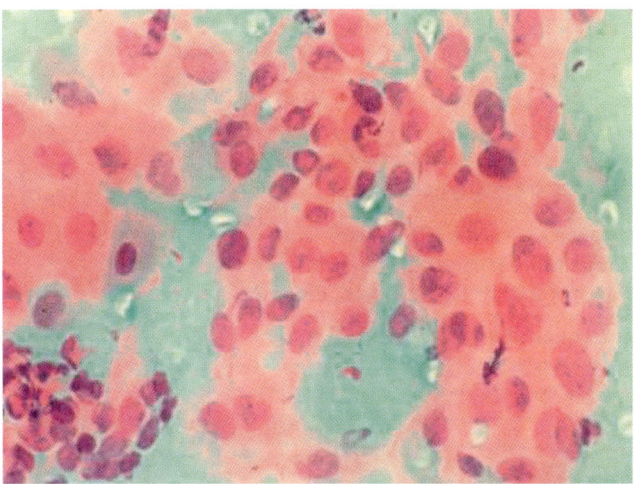

Figure 5.21 Cellular degeneration resulting from air drying of the cells. Notice the lack of nuclear and cytoplasmic differentiation and cellular transparency. Conventional vaginocervical smear, Pap stain.

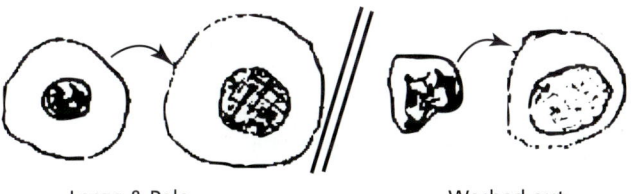

Large & Pale   Washed out

Figure 5.23 These line drawings depict the nuclear degeneration resulting from fluids absorption by the nuclei.

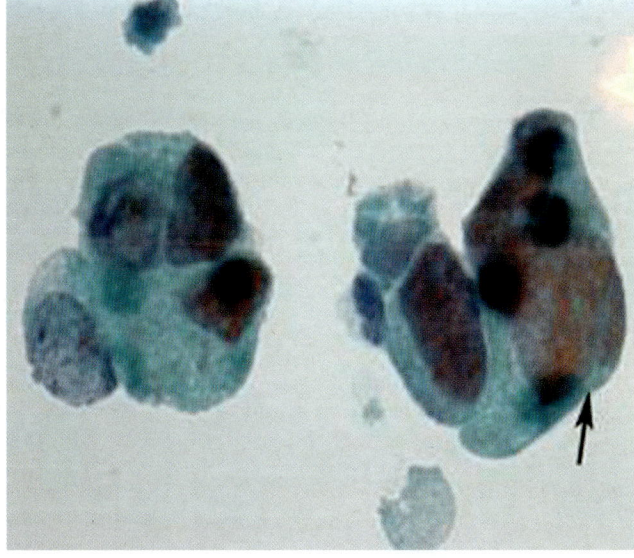

Figure 5.25 Large and washed-out nucleus (arrow) resulting from fluid absorption by the urothelial cells. Bladder wash, ThinPrep slide, Pap stain.

cytomegaly, which can be misinterpreted as "atypical." These air-drying changes, although uncommon among gynecologic liquid-based preparations, are often seen in FNA and many other preparations (Figures 5.21 and 5.22).

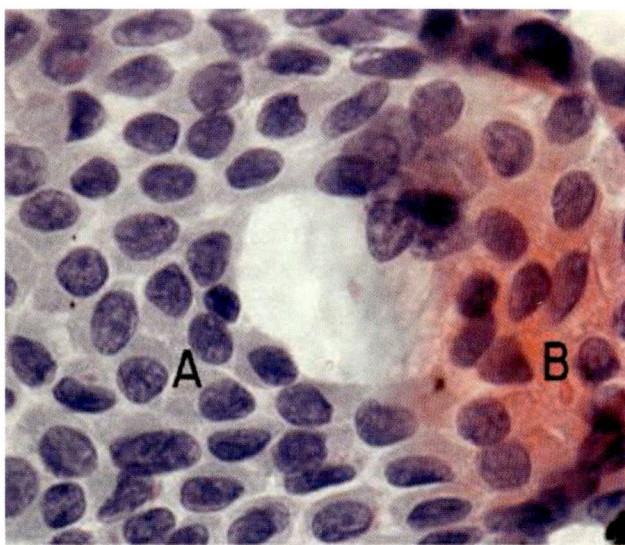

Figure 5.22 Partial air drying. Well-fixed cells (A) reveal diagnostic nuclear details; they are obliterated in air-dried (B) cells. FNA, lung, Pap stain.

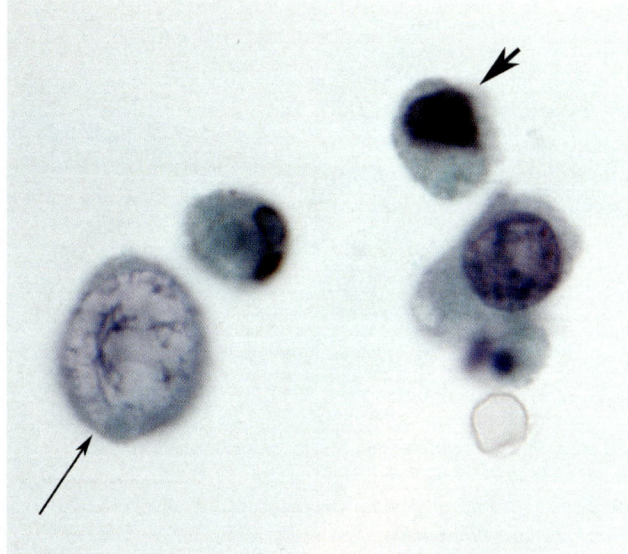

Figure 5.24 Large and pale nucleus (large arrow) resulting from fluid absorption. Note the dark hyperchromatic nuclei (small arrow). Urinary bladder wash, ThinPrep slide, Pap stain.

Nucleus

SIZE

The nucleus most commonly degenerates either by imbibing or losing fluids. This results in swelling and distention of the nucleus that may result in disintegration. Likewise, the nucleus may become condensed, dark, and homogeneous with a loss of organelle details with uniformity of its content. Such changes affect the texture and nuclear chromatin pattern (Figures 5.23–5.26).

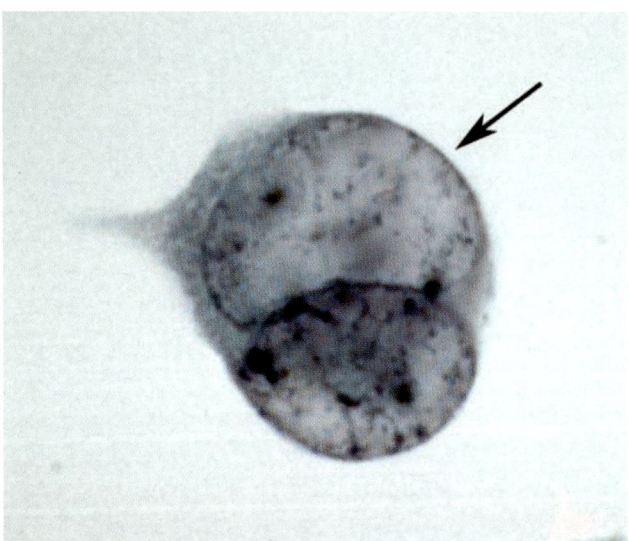

Figure 5.26 Large pale nucleus (arrow) with nuclear membrane changes. Urinary Bladder wash, ThinPrep slide, Pap stain.

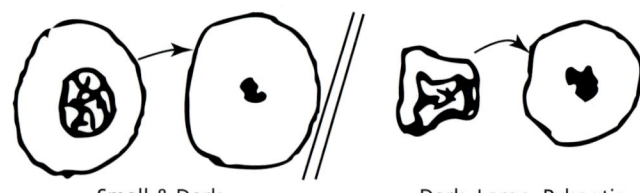

Small & Dark   Dark, Large, Pyknotic

Figure 5.27 Nuclear changes associated with intranuclear fluid loss. Nuclei may become small and dark, or dark, large, and pyknotic; the latter is often associated with neoplastic processes.

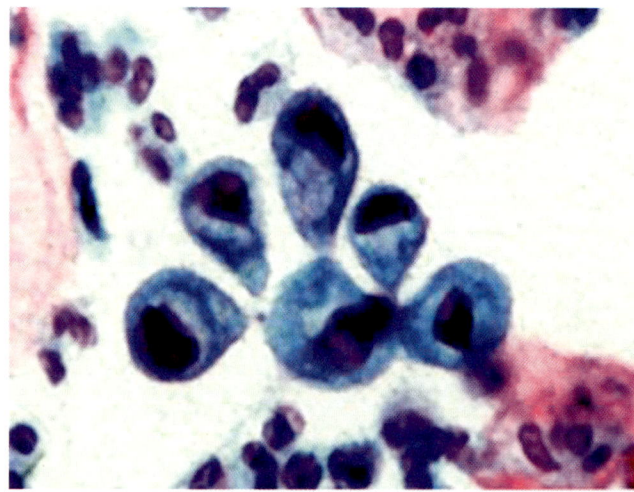

Figure 5.29 Degenerated cells with pyknotic nuclei. These are large cells and hyperchromatic, IUD cells. Vaginocervical smear, Pap stain.

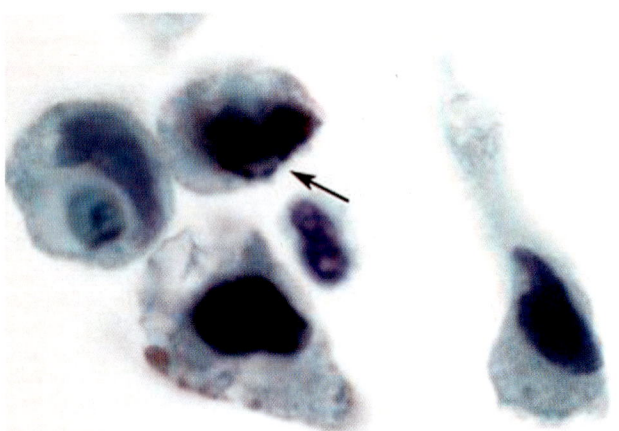

Figure 5.28 Degenerating dark nuclei, urothelial cells showing multinucleation (arrow). Care must be exercised in interpretation as changes can often be misinterpreted as neoplastic. Bladder wash, Cytospin slide, Pap stain.

CHROMASIA

Nuclei tend to become small and dark (pyknotic) when they lose fluids. Sometimes the dark degenerated nucleus is large and pyknotic (at least 4 times in size and intermediate cell nucleus). Such degenerated nuclei may be dyskaryotic or malignant in nature (Figures 5.27–5.30). Dark and large atypical nuclei are more important diagnostically when compared to small and dark cells. It is critical that these changes must not be used as the sole feature for diagnosis of malignancy. They should be recognized and specimens examined carefully for other malignant or dyskaryotic cells (Figure 5.27).

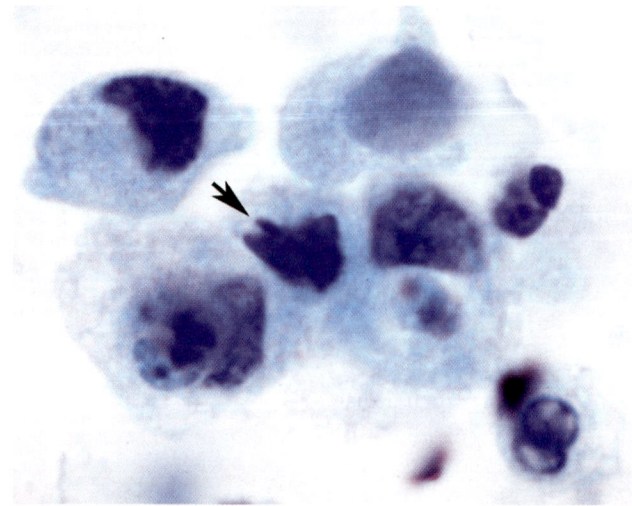

Figure 5.30 Degenerating nuclei with hyperchromasia, pyknosis, and nuclear membrane abnormalities (arrow). These alveolar macrophages represent a case with pulmonary infarct. BAL, ThinPrep slide Pap stain.

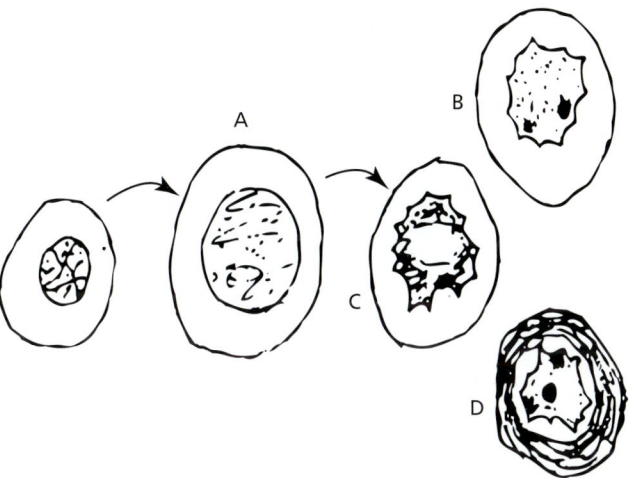

Figure 5.31 Nuclear membrane changes, minimum (A) to marked (D), that occur as a result of cellular degeneration. In some cells, there may also be cytoplasmic changes.

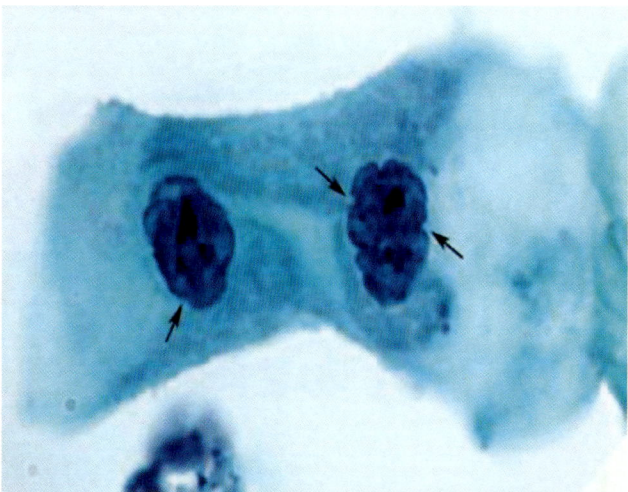

Figure 5.32 Early nuclear membrane degenerative changes (arrow), these bites tend to be at acute angles. These are similar to those depicted in (B) and (C) in Figure 5.31. Voided urine, cytospin, Pap stain.

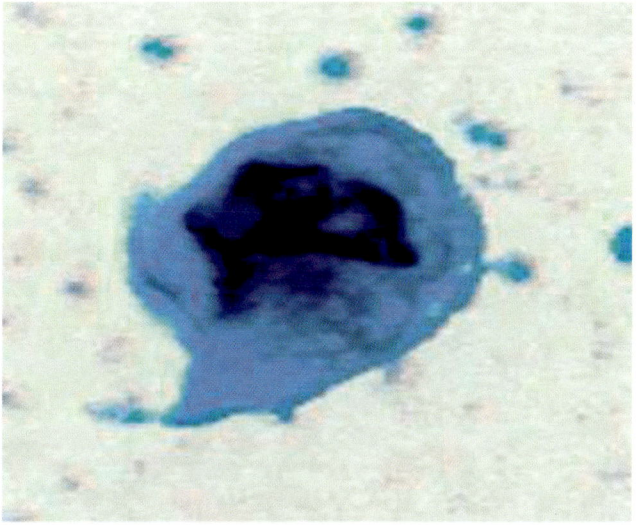

Figure 5.33 Marked nuclear membrane degenerative changes, squamous cell carcinoma sputum specimen, ThinPrep slide, Pap stain.

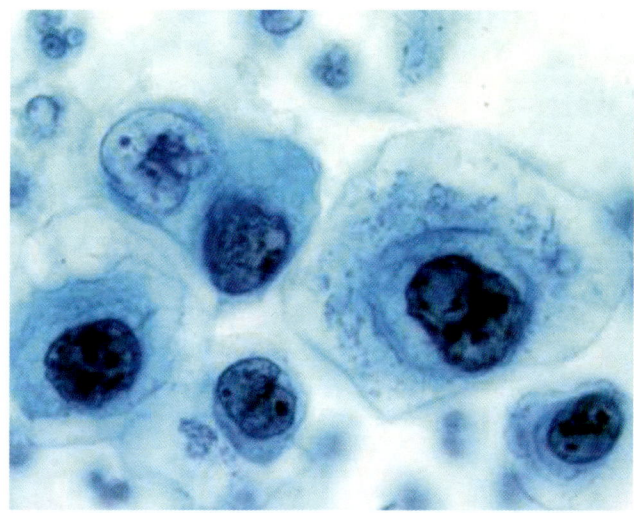

Figure 5.34 Nuclear chromatin degeneration, blurring, clumping, and condensation seen in this pleural fluid specimen from a case with pulmonary infarct, Millipore filter, Pap stain. Chromatin clumping and rounding is a common feature of degeneration and should not be confused with malignant change.

NUCLEAR MEMBRANE

The shape of a degenerated nucleus is often irregular, wrinkled or rasinoid. The nuclear membrane crookedness may be angular with sharp invaginations (Figures 5.30–5.33). Although similar shape changes may occur in malignant cells, they should not be considered diagnostic for cancer, and additional morphologic evidence must be sought before rendering such a diagnosis. Nuclear membrane and chromatinic features are helpful in the diagnostic evaluation of cells with such sharply angled nuclear membranes.

CHROMATIN

There are critical changes that occur in the chromatic material, its distribution and chromatinic blurring. The chromatin parachromatin interface is obliterated and the nuclear chromatin loses its crispness, appearing fuzzy and "cloudy". This is one of the earliest features of a degenerating nucleus. Eventually, the chromatinic material becomes emulsified and blurry, mixing with the parachromatin; it appears as a hematoxylophilic blob (Figures 5.34–5.37).

CHROMATIN CLUMPING

Chromatin acquires irregular shapes and forms. In contrast to chromatin clumping observed in malignant cell nuclei,

135

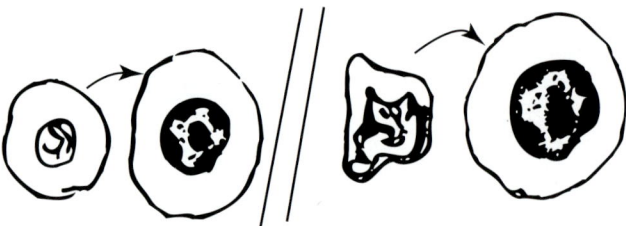

Figure 5.35 Chromatin blurring, rounding, and clumping of the inner membrane layer as compared to the nuclear outer rim. Such changes are a common occurrence in prefixed, such as liquid-prepared, specimens and should be carefully evaluated.

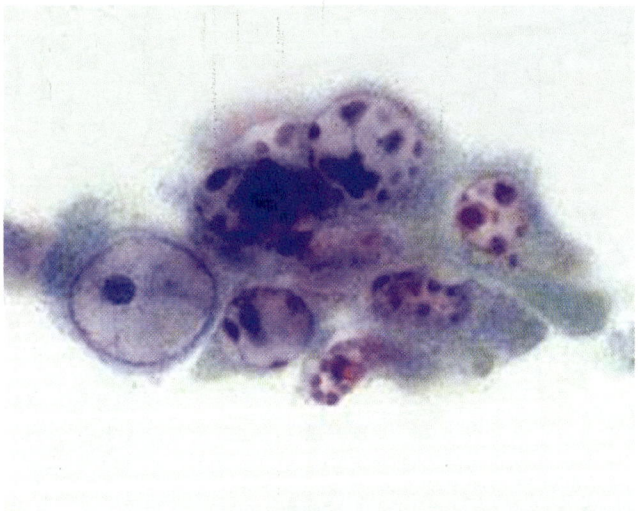

Figure 5.36 Nuclear degeneration with chromatin aggregates and rounding toward the center of the nucleus. Voided urine specimen, ThinPrep slide, Pap stain.

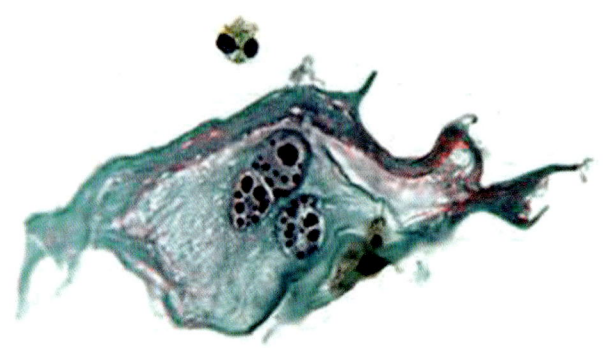

Figure 5.37 Nuclear degeneration with large rounded nuclear clumps in the center of the nucleus. Degenerated epithelial cells. There is an eosinophil for size comparison. Bronchial wash, direct smear, Pap stain.

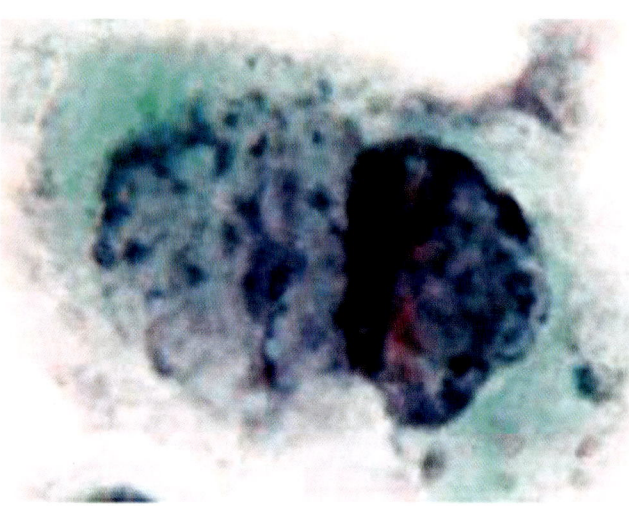

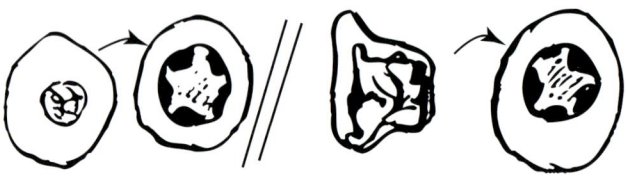

Figure 5.39 Chromatin margination along the nuclear membrane. The appearance can be irregular or beaded.

Figure 5.38 Degenerative nuclear changes with chromatin clumping. Notice the fuzzy edges and beading, mostly along the nuclear membrane. Bronchial wash specimen, adenocarcinoma lung primary. Bronchial brush, ThinPrep slide, Pap stain.

degenerated cell chromatin clumps have poorly defined or indistinct edges (Figure 5.38).

CHROMATIN MARGINATION

The condensed masses of chromatin tend to move toward the periphery of the nucleus. This migration can be uniform and evenly distributed, but more commonly occurs as irregular cobblestones (Figures 5.39 and 5.40). It is important to appreciate that the margin of the chromatin material is poorly delineated and blurred. In some cases such as viral infection, chromatin clumps may be beaded and

uniformly distributed along the nuclear membrane (Figures 5.38 and 5.40). Chromatin may accumulate in the center of the nucleus (Figure 5.36) and is with or without cartwheel-arranged chromatin threads connecting to the nuclear membrane. Some changes occur commonly in the response to viral infection and after radiation and chemotherapy.

CHROMATOLYSIS AND APOPTOSIS

Chromatin may become finely granular and appear as "sand" particles around the cells. These changes are often

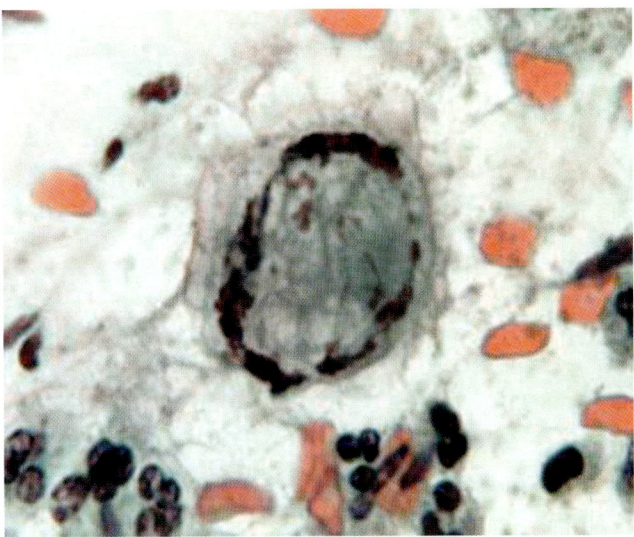

Figure 5.40 Nuclear degeneration with pronounced chromatin change. Notice the margination, sharp edge towards the outside and loss of details. Vaginocervical smear, Pap stain.

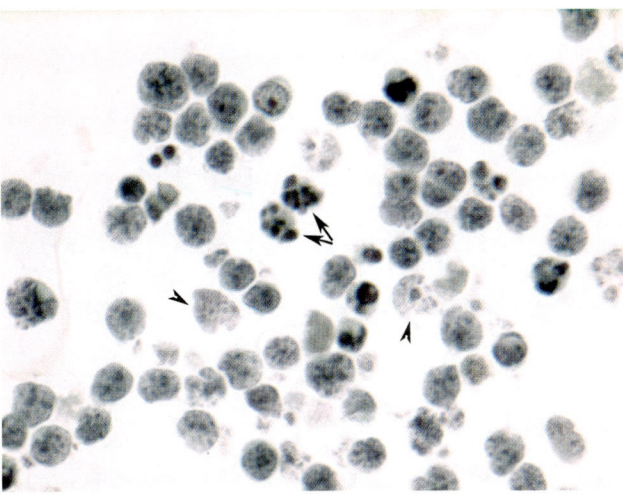

Figure 5.41 Apoptosis and chromatolysis changes in a large cell lymphoma. Notice the nuclear apoptosis (arrows) and chromatolysis (arrowheads). Such changes are commonly observed following chemotherapy. Cerebrospinal fluid specimen, cytospin, Pap stain.

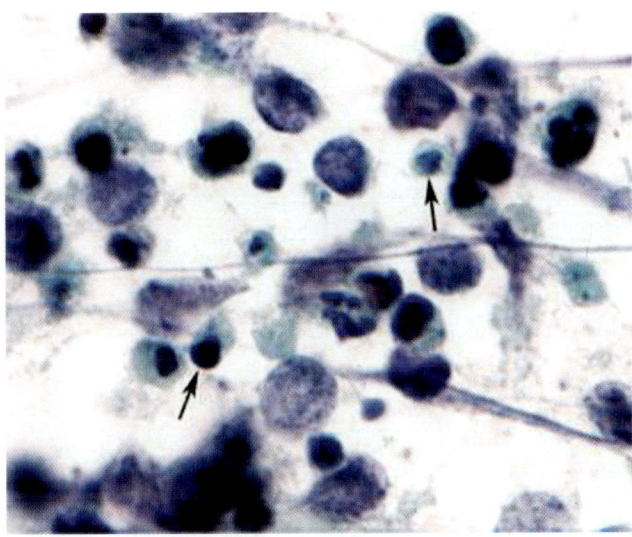

Figure 5.42 Nuclear degeneration and apoptotic change. Notice the small dark nuclear fragments (arrows). Small-cell carcinoma FNA lung, direct smear, Pap stain.

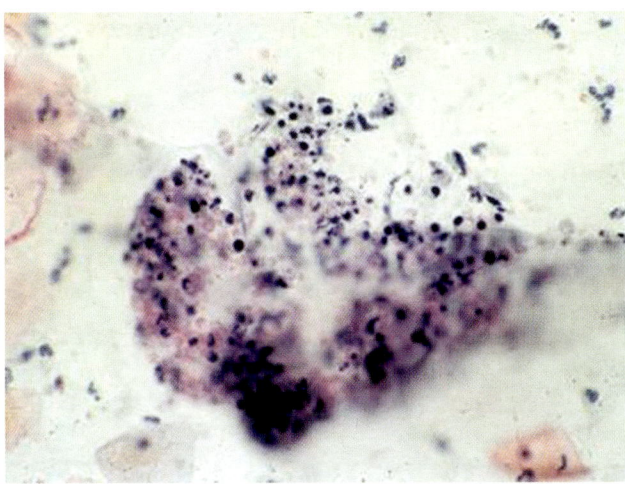

Figure 5.43 Apoptosis, endocervical adenocarcinoma. Vaginocervical smear, Pap stain.

NUCLEOLI

Nucleoli may become pale and inconspicuous. They lose their sharp and crisp appearance. They can also enlarge in size and look prominent and pale (Figures 5.44 and 5.45).

PARACHROMATIN CLEARING

Although parachromatin clearing is often seen in malignant nuclei, its occurrence in degeneration is common and should not be confused as a malignant criterion. Often, blurring of the chromatin along the inner margin of nucleus is common (Figures 5.46 and 5.47).

Cytoplasm

There are a number of common pan-epithelial changes in the cytoplasm that may occur in retroplasia.

seen in rapidly growing tumors and are more common in certain tumors such as small-cell carcinoma of the lung, endocervical adenocarcinoma, and certain forms of lymphomas (Figure 5.41). Apoptosis may occur in reactive and proliferative endocervical cells, especially in the second half of the menstrual cycle and among oral contraceptive users. Chromatolysis and apoptotic changes are frequently seen in body cavity fluid specimens including cerebrospinal fluid obtained from patients under therapy for lymphoreticular malignancies (Figures 5.42 and 5.43).

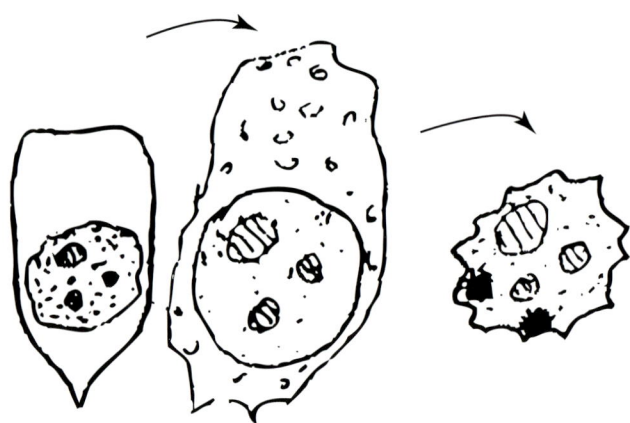

Figure 5.44 Line drawings depicting the nucleolar degeneration. Nucleoli may become pale and faint or dark and prominent.

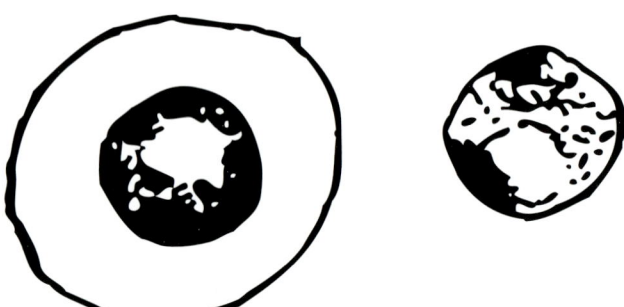

Figure 5.46 Parachromatin clearing in degeneration.

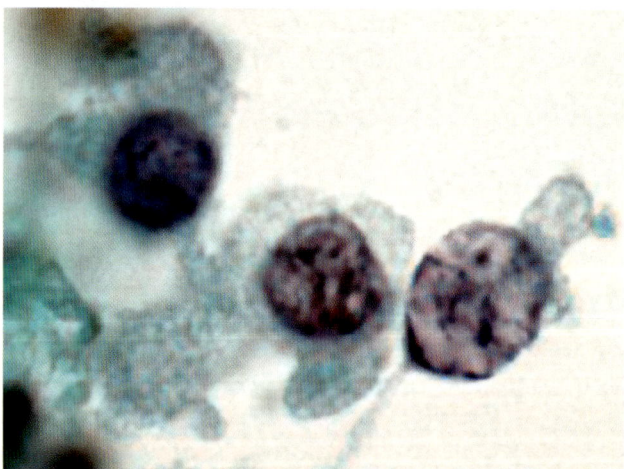

Figure 5.48 Cytoplasmic degeneration; notice the fraying. Urine, bladder wash specimen, ThinPrep slide, Pap stain.

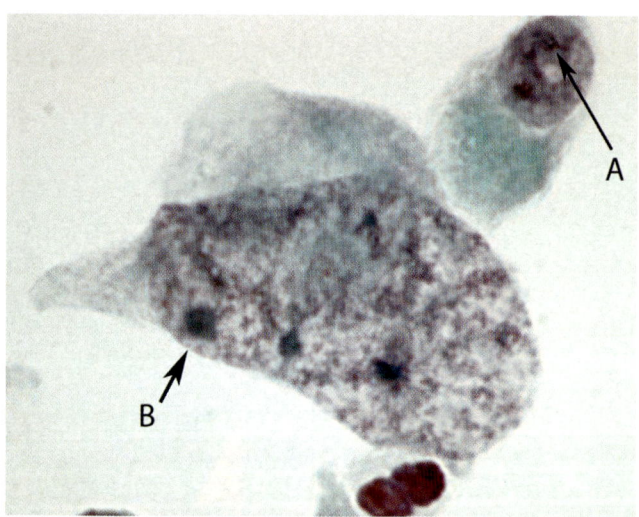

Figure 5.45 Nucleolar degeneration. Notice the faint, poorly defined nucleoli (A) and prominent nucleoli (B). Bladder wash specimen, ThinPrep slide, Pap stain.

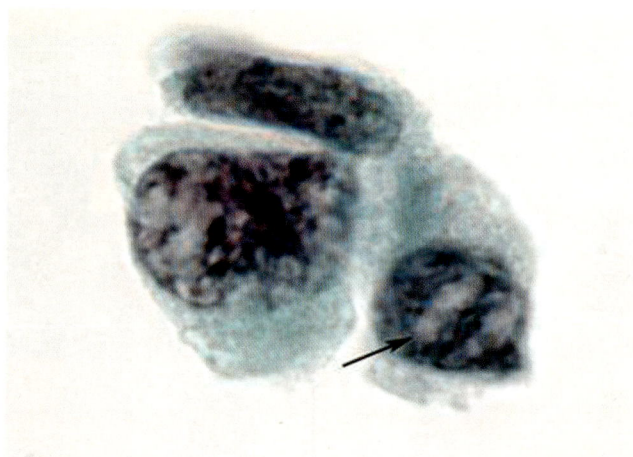

Figure 5.47 Nuclear degeneration. Notice the chromatin blurring (arrow) and clearing. Voided urine specimen, ThinPrep slide, Pap stain.

1. Fraying. The cytoplasm may disintegrate and may appear frayed or torn apart, resulting in ill-defined margins. Care must be exercised in the evaluation and interpretation of the nuclear changes in such situations. These alterations occur commonly in Thin Prep slides obtained from epithelial lesions with low molecular weight cytokeratins such as pancreas, breast, and lung (Figure 5.48).

2. Dissolution. Cytoplasmic edges may dissolve among adjacent epithelial cells. These micro-vacuoles can resemble the intracellular bridges often seen in squamous differentiations (Figure 5.49). Similar degenerative changes can sometimes be observed at the nucleo-cytoplasmic interphase.

3. Vacuolation. Cytoplasmic vacuoles may be continuously seen in degenerating cells. These can occur as multiple, small, or variable size or a large secretory-type vacuole. This secretory-type change is often observed in body cavity fluid and urine specimens with a low protein content and osmolarity. Sometimes the

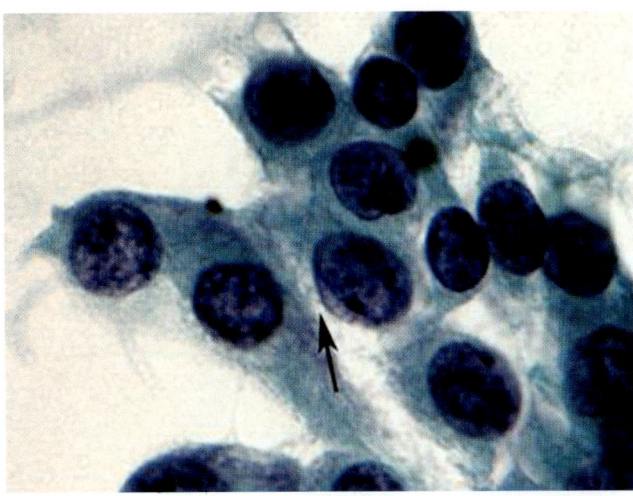

Figure 5.49 Intracytoplasmic degenerative vacuoles (arrow) that resemble intercellular bridges. Bile duct brush specimen, ThinPrep slide, Pap stain.

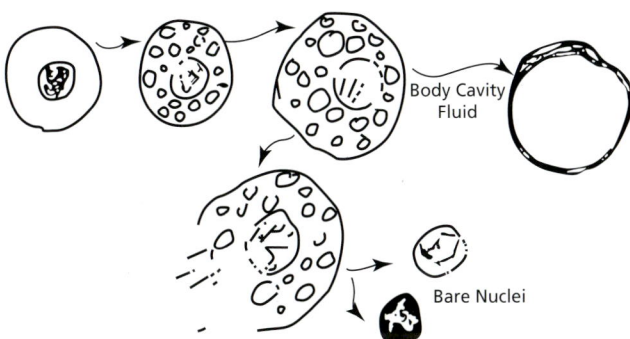

Figure 5.50 Cytoplasmic degeneration and vacuole formation.

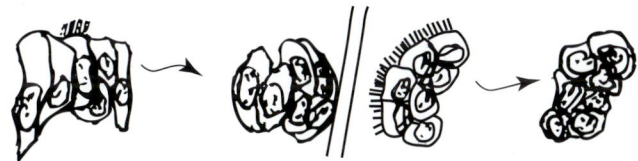

Figure 5.52 Partial and total loss of cilia among bronchial cells.

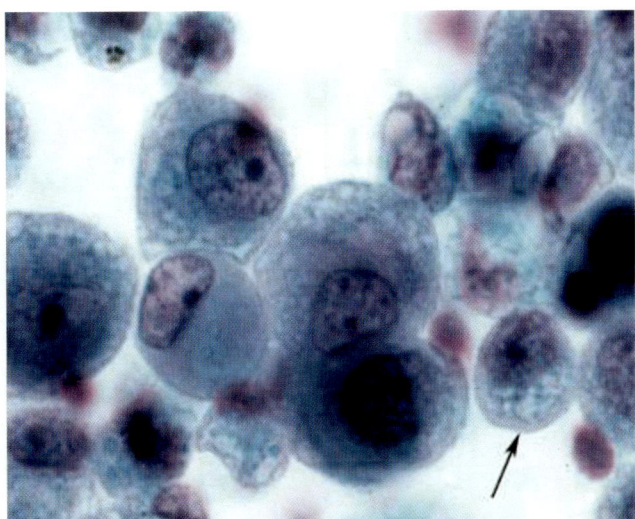

Figure 5.51 Cytoplasmic degeneration with multiple small vacuoles (arrow). Reactive mesothelial cells. Pleural fluid, Millipore filter, Pap stain.

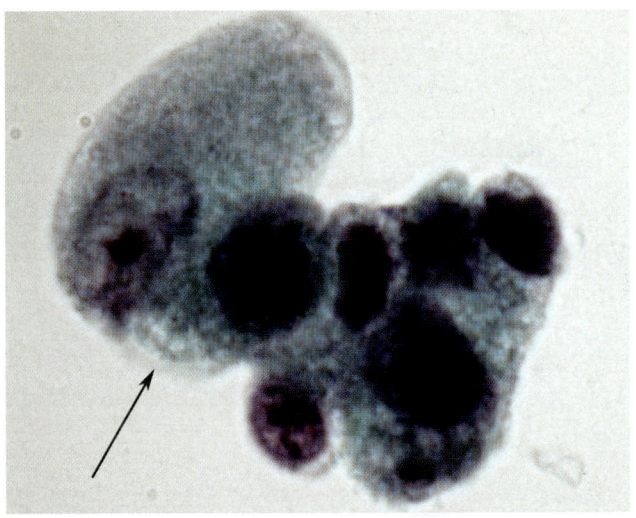

Figure 5.53 Degenerated cilia (arrow). These are often difficult to recognize and a common cause of incorrect diagnosis. Bronchial brush, ThinPrep slide, Pap stain.

vacuoles can become distant and disintegrate, leaving bare nuclei. These degenerative vacuoles may even alter the adjacent nucleus, posing diagnostic problems. Certain cytoplasmic contents such as glycogen may be affected by the microbial environment resulting in bare nuclei (Figures 5.50 and 5.51).

4. Differentiation. Total or partial loss of cilia is one of the earliest manifestations of degenerative changes in ciliated epithelial cells. Often there are associated nuclear changes mimicking a neoplastic process. It is essential that a careful search for cilia, total or partial and a flat terminal plate be made in all suspected cases (Figures 5.52 and 5.53). Detached fragments of ciliary tufts

(discussed in Chapter 2) may be observed as a sign of cytoplasmic degeneration. A similar appearance occurs in ciliocytophthoria, which is often seen in bronchopulmonary cells with viral infections. Similarly, astrocytes may lose their cytoplasmic processes. Care must be exercised as bare nuclei may result from cytopreparation artifacts.

5. Perinuclear halos and acidophilia (pseudokeratinization) commonly develop among degenerated squamous, metaplastic, mesothelial, and columnar cells (Figures 5.54 and 5.55).

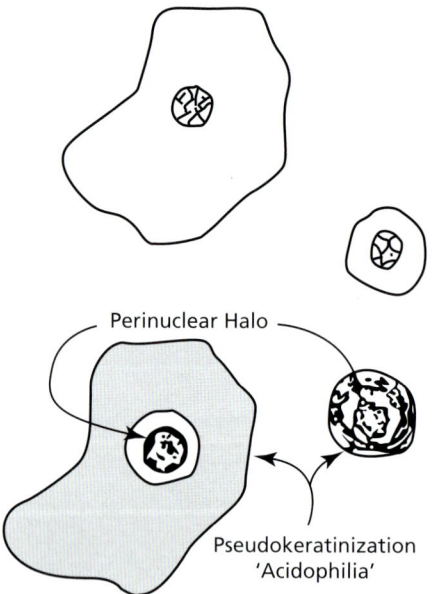

Figure 5.54 Perinuclear halos and pseudokeratinization among degenerating epithelial cells.

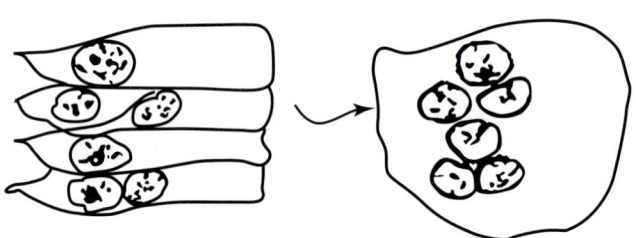

Figure 5.56 Loss of cell borders and a pseudosyncytial formation.

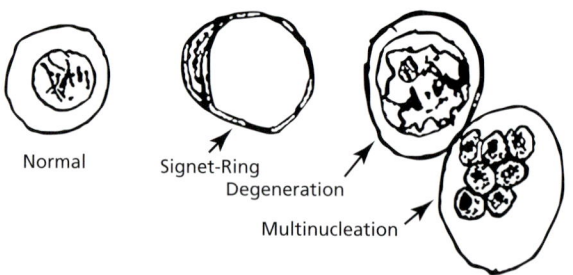

Figure 5.58 Common morphologic changes among mesothelial cells.

Pseudosyncytial formations

Adjacent cells may have total loss of intercellular borders ("pseudo-syncytial"). These often appear multinucleated with poor nuclear preservation and other signs of degenerative changes (Figures 5.56 and 5.57).

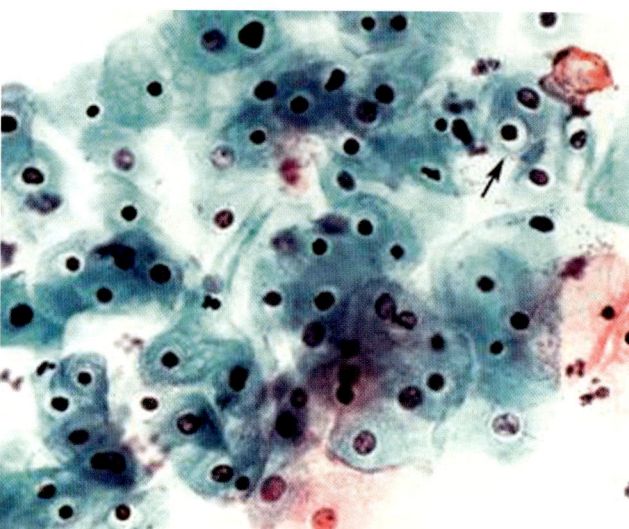

Figure 5.55 Perinuclear halos (arrow) among squamous cells associated with *Trichomonas* infection. Vaginal smear, Pap stain.

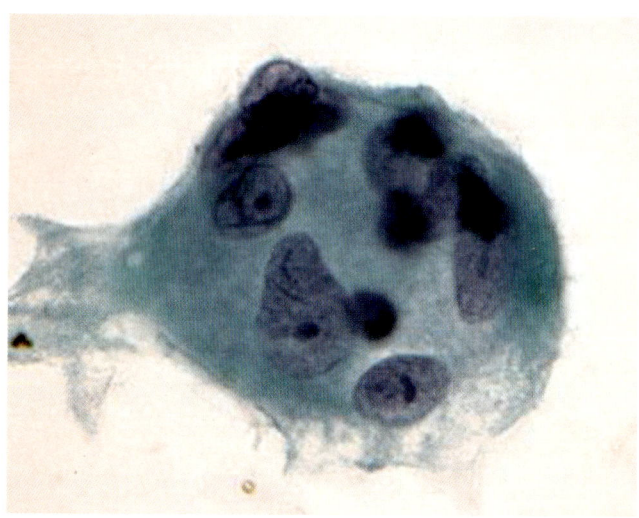

Figure 5.57 Pseudosyncytial formation among degenerated columnar cells. Bronchial wash, direct smear, Pap stain.

SELECTED BODY SITES

Two sites have become noted in the literature for their high percentage of false positive diagnoses and thus lack of dependability. This is unfortunate. They are clinically "diagnostically blind" areas in which accurate cytology can assist. In order to maintain a high diagnostic dependability, the following are routine in our practice for body cavity fluids and urines.

Body cavity fluids

Normal mesothelial cells

Normal mesothelial cells (well-preserved) show the following features (Figures 5.58 and 5.59).

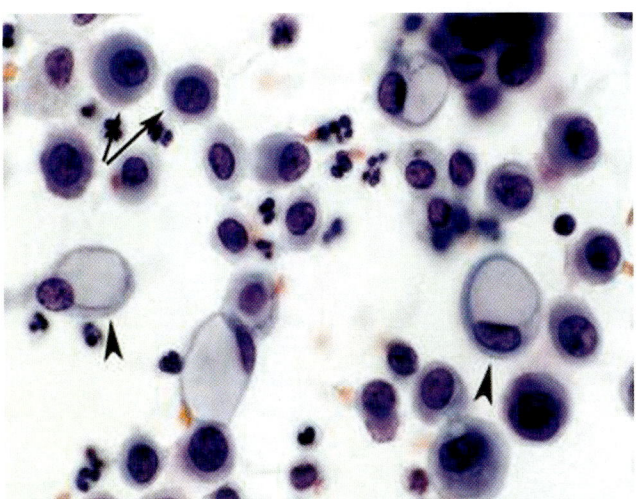

Figure 5.59 "Normal" exfoliated mesothelial cells (long arrows), signet-ring forms (arrowheads). Pleural fluid, Millipore filter, Pap stain.

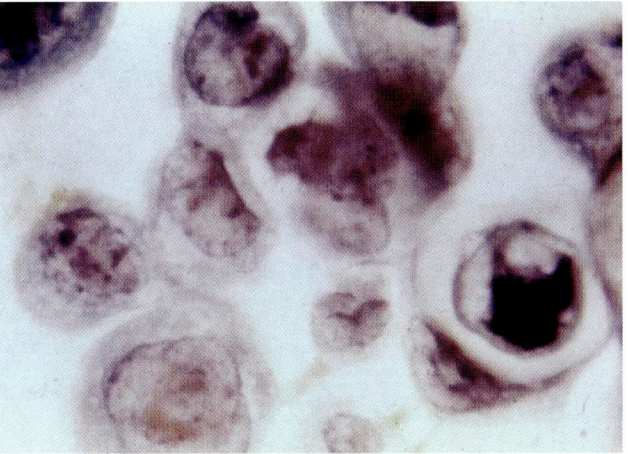

Figure 5.60 Markedly atypical mesothelial cells. Notice the loss of nuclear details. Pulmonary infarct, pleural fluid. Millipore filter, Pap stain.

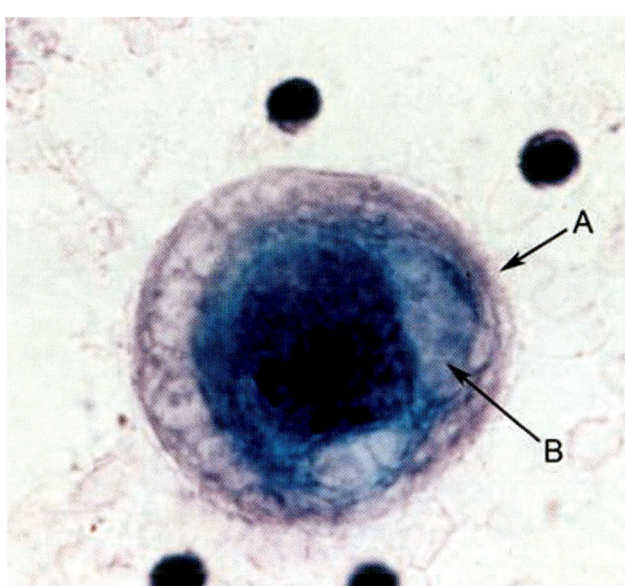

Figure 5.61 Mesothelial cell degeneration, notice the ecto (A) and endoplasmic (B) differentiation (arrows). Patient with chronic lymphocytic leukemia on chemotherapy. Pleural fluid, Millipore filter, Pap stain.

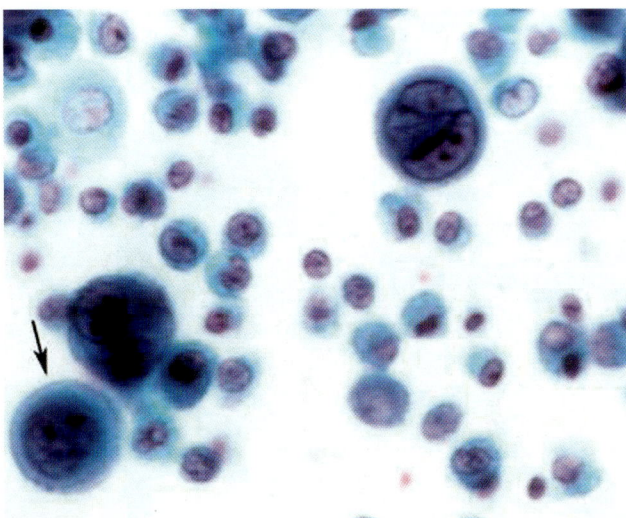

Figure 5.62 Mesothelial cell degeneration. Notice the ecto/ endoplasmic differentiation (arrow). Pulmonary infarct, Millipore filter, Pap stain.

(i) They round up when exfoliated into fluid.

(ii) They may shed singly or as multinucleate cells. Papillary tissue fragments can develop from benign cells obtained from a closed cavity or space, such as the rectovaginal pouch.

(iii) Mesothelial cells may acquire signet-ring appearance resembling malignant cells.

Degenerated mesothelial cells

These show the following features (Figures 5.60–5.62).

(i) Often lose fine nuclear details.

(ii) May acquire ecto-endoplasmic appearance resembling a squamous cell.

(iii) May become orangophilic, resembling a keratinized squamous cell. Such features can occur among mucus-bearing cells. The presence of orangophilic (squamoid) cells in a body cavity fluid specimen per se must not be considered a squamous differentiation and carcinoma

Reactive mesothelial cells

These often occur in various infective processes, pulmonary infarct, following pneumotharax, therapy, and certain

(A)

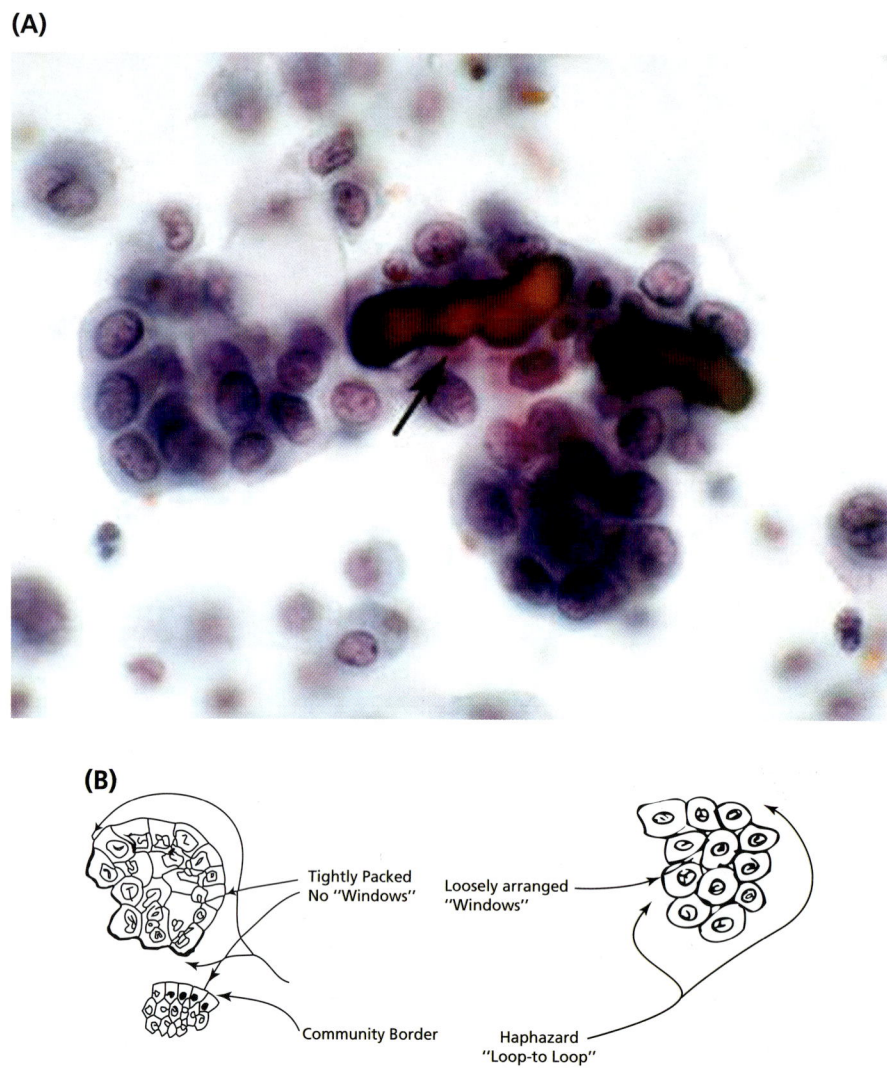

(B)

Tightly Packed No "Windows"

Loosely arranged "Windows"

Community Border

Haphazard "Loop-to Loop"

Figure 5.63 (A, B) Proliferating mesothelial cells with psammoma body formation (arrow). Rectovaginal pouch aspiration, Millipore filter, Pap stain (A). Line drawing depicting salient features of diagnostic tissue fragment/cell groups (B).

autoimmune diseases. These cells often contain intercellular spaces (windows) in contrast to usually the neoplastic proliferation with a community border (Figure 5.63).

(i) Cells acquire extremely atypical and bizarre forms resembling neoplastic processes. Nucleoli may become enlarged associated with abnormal chromatin clearing and clumping.

(ii) Mitosis and rarely abnormal features may appear among reactive mesothelial cells.

(iii) Proliferative tissue fragments may appear as acinic structures with homogeneous luminal secretions rich in mucopolysaccharides. These can be mistaken for evidence of neoplastic processes. Tissue

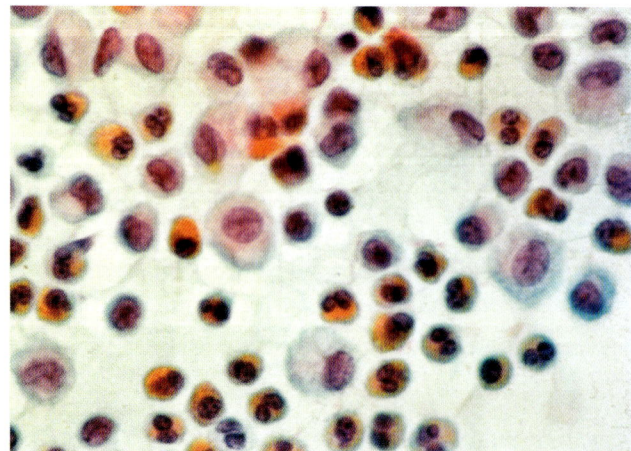

Figure 5.64 Numerous eosinophils, pleural effusion repeat tap, Millipore filter, Pap stain.

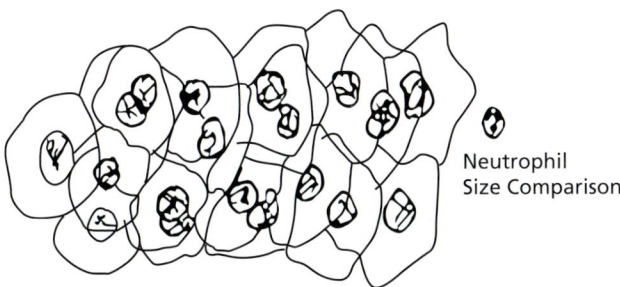

Figure 5.65 Tissue fragment of urothelial cells.

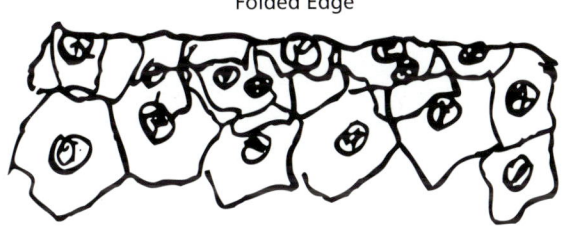

Figure 5.67 Folded edge of urothelial cells, resembling margin of a polyp.

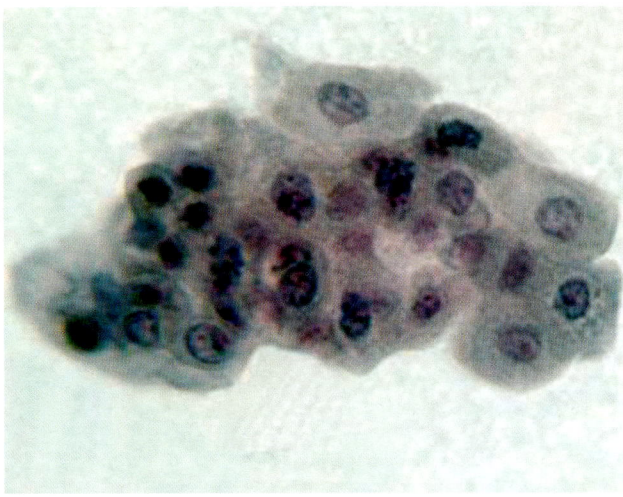

Figure 5.66 Tissue fragment of urothelial cells following instrumentation. These cells can be reactive and extremely bizarre and atypical, Millipore filter, Pap stain.

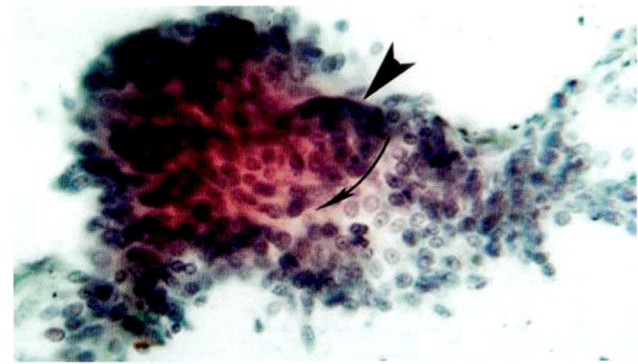

Figure 5.68 Fragment of urothelium, notice the fold (arrowhead) and the free edge (arrow). Ureter brush, direct smear, Pap stain.

fragment formation is considered a hallmark for malignancy diagnosis in the body cavity fluid specimens, and may appear with papillary formations. In proplasia (i.e. reaction, pulmonary infarct), they can become very bizarre with many malignant criteria; however, they retain an "independent" cell appearance, and chromatin is slightly blurred.

Mesothelial cells, when they are reactive and clump, appear not to fit tightly ("windows" between cells), the outside border of the group appears as a "haphazard" cluster of individual cells, and nuclei do not mold.

Malignant cells: unequivocal diagnosis of epithelial malignancy requires true tissue fragments with nuclear malignant criteria, a community border and lack of "windows" among cells. Tumor cells can occur singly in body cavity specimens, but their accurate diagnosis requires caution and experience, especially when occurring in liquid-based slides.

Eosinophilia
This occurs in pleural effusion most commonly in a repeat pleural tap specimen, viral infections, allergic reactions, malignancies after surgical intervention, and parasitic infections (Figure 5.64).

Urine

Normal urothelial cells
These tend to shed singly in a voided specimen. Instrumentation, investigation studies, and therapy may "ream-out" groups of urothelial cells resembling a papillary formation. Such groups have adequate cytoplasm and they stratify (Figures 5.65 and 5.66).

The outside border of the group appears torn off, with the "haphazard" appearance of a conglomeration of individual cell borders. A folded sheet may appear to have a papillary luminal margin (Figures 5.67 and 5.68).

Papillary transitional cell carcinoma
The outside border of a papillary frond has a "community" appearance of an epithelial luminal margin. When the latter is present in a true tissue fragment, it represents a papillary process; however, as this may still be

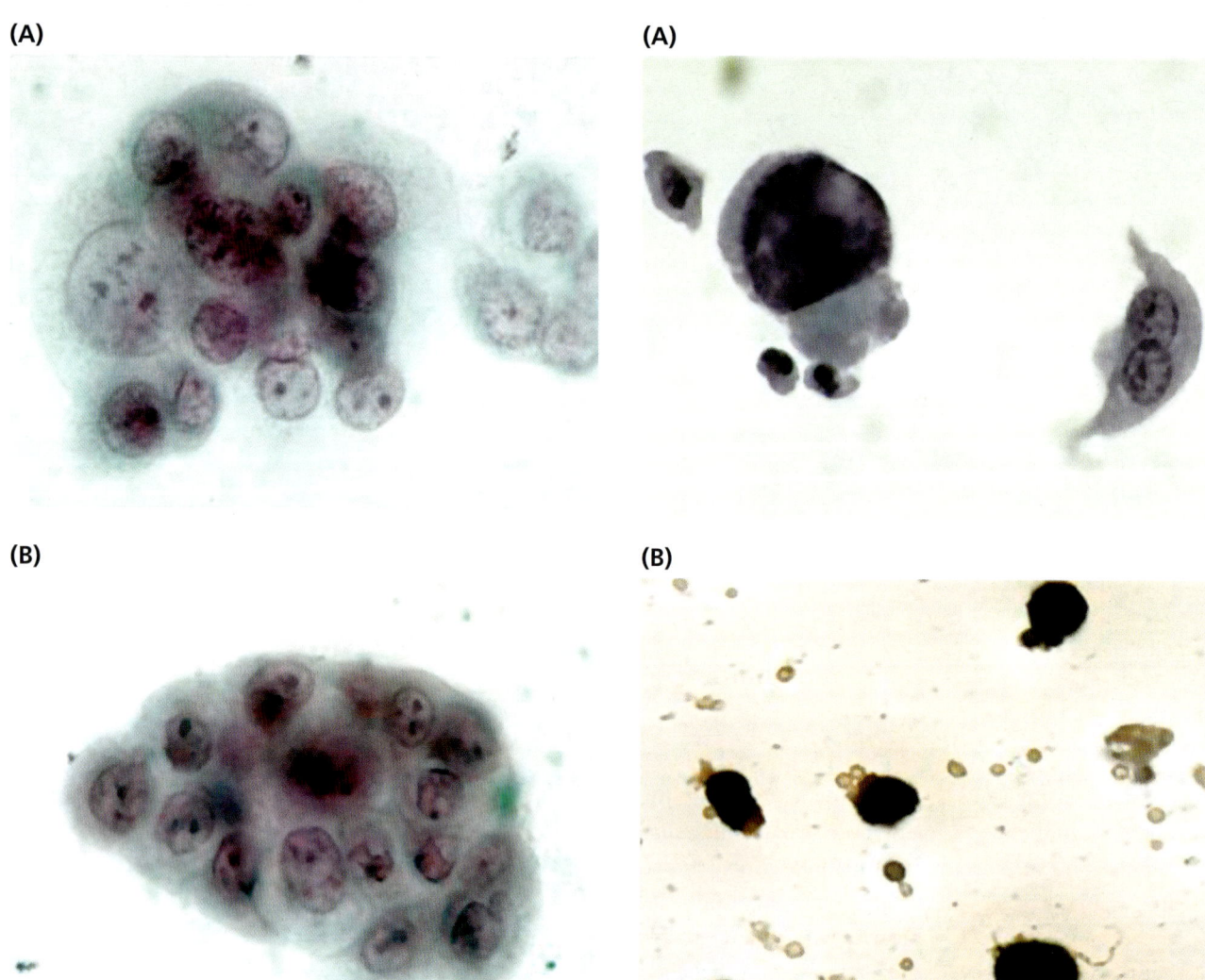

(A)

(B)

Figure 5.69 Reactive urothelial cells (A) and low-grade papillary urothelial carcinoma (B). Notice nuclear features of malignancy. Bladder wash, Millipore filter, Pap stain.

(A)

(B)

Figure 5.70 Intranuclear BK virus infection (A), same specimen stained with Mab 597, specifically staining the viral inclusions (B). Voided urine specimen, cytospin preparation.

inflammatory or irritative, there must also be sufficient criteria in the nucleus to unequivocally indicate malignancy before such a diagnosis may be rendered (Figure 5.69).

Adenocarcinoma
Usually undifferentiated carcinoma cells with abundant cytoplasm shed in tissue fragments. Acini and polyps may be present. They may be degenerated, but strict diagnostic criteria must be practiced.

Viral infections
Although cytomegalovirus and herpes may be observed in the urinary specimen, the most common and clinically significant infection is BK virus. Infected urothelial cells

generally shed singly with large, generally basophilic, intranuclear inclusions that almost totally obliterate the nucleus and cause a peripheral marinating of chromatinic material. At times, a fine lace-like or fish-net appearance of chromatin may appear in the infected cells. These cells resemble CIS urothelial cells and have been called "decoy cells" (Figures 5.70 and 5.71).

CYTOMEGALIC INCLUSION DISEASE
The diagnostic cells are usually the cuboidal columnar cells from renal tubules. They are single and rounded, appearing strikingly darker and larger than the normal transitional cells (Figures 5.72–5.74).

Infected cells reveal both cytoplasmic and intranuclear changes. These include the following:

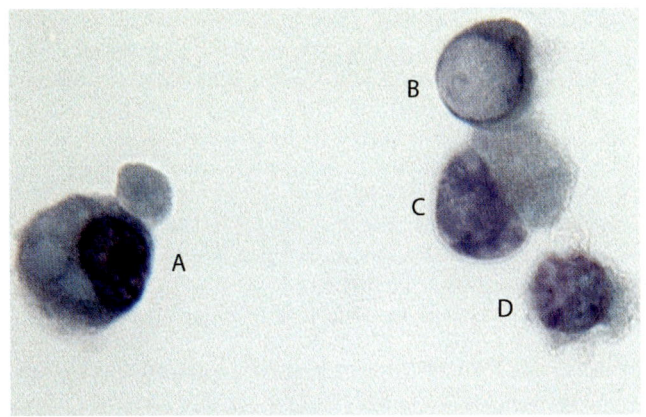

Figure 5.71 This picture depicts the various morphologic appearances of BK-infected urothelial cells. Classic (A), ground glass (B), granular (C, D). Voided urine, ThinPrep slide, Pap stain.

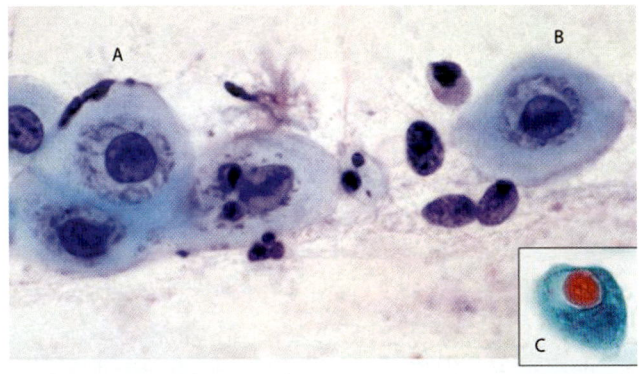

Figure 5.73 Cytomegalovirus infection. Notice the intranuclear and intracytoplasmic basophilic inclusions and an acidophilic inclusion (insert). Picture (A) shows chromatin bridging, chromatin condensation is seen in (B), and an acidophilic intranuclear inclusion is seen in (C). Bronchial brush specimen. Vaginocervical smear (A, B), ThinPrep slide(C), Pap stain.

1. Cytoplasm. Generally, it is abundant as in urothelial cells, but can be scant in other epithelia, such as pneumocytes, bronchial, and gastric epithelia. Various changes may affect: (a) color – darker lavender or redder than normal; (b) consistency – granular or foamy and thick; (c) cell border – sharp, well-preserved; (d) inclusions – intracytoplasmic granular or ropey. Inclusions, generally perinuclear in distribution, may occur. These should not be solely used for diagnostic purposes.

2. Nucleus. This is generally large. It may contain the classic (a) inclusion body, which is eosinophilic with smudgy, degenerated; (b) hematoxylinophilic chromatin around its periphery and mixed in it; (c) peri-inclusion halo with trans-halo bridges of degenerated chromatin strung across it; and (d) nuclear membrane with degenerated chromatin plastered to its inner surface.

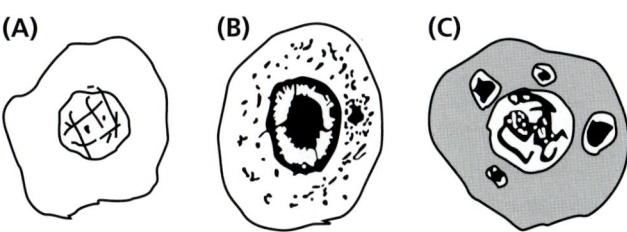

Figure 5.72 Line drawings showing features of cytomegalovirus (CMV) infection. Normal epithelial cell (A), intranuclear inclusion with radiating chromatin filaments (B), intranuclear and intracytoplasmic inclusions (C).

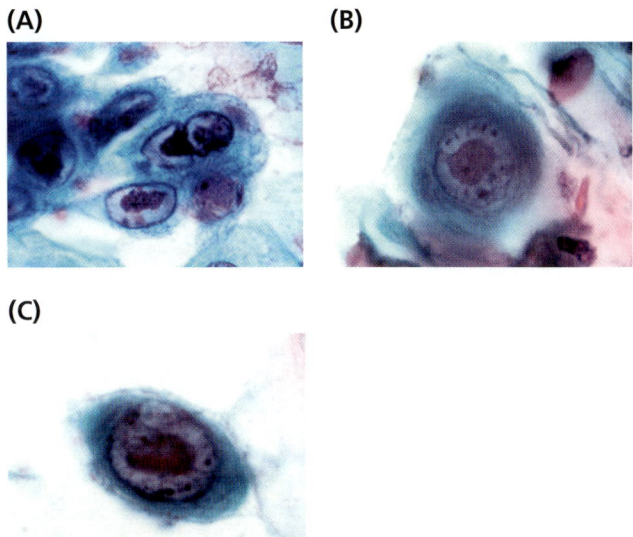

Figure 5.74 CMV-infected cells. Peri-inclusion halo (A), smudge surrounding chromatic (B), peripheral condensation of chromatin (C). Cervicovaginal smears, Pap stain.

FURTHER READING

Agarwal, C. and M. Jain. (2009). "Utility of fibronectin in immuocytochemical differentiation of reactive mesothelial cells from metastatic malignant cells in serous effusions". *Indian J Pathol Microbiol* **52**(1): 25–8.

Ahmed, M. N., A. Lushpihan, *et al.* (1976). "Cytology of transitional cell carcinoma in situ of urinary bladder with extensive prostatic involvement". *Urology* **7**(5): 538–40.

Aron, M., A. Mallik, *et al.* (2006). "Fine needle aspiration cytology of follicular variant of papillary carcinoma of the thyroid: morphologic pointers to its diagnosis". *Acta Cytol* **50**(6): 663–8.

Arora, V. K., N. Singh, *et al.* (2003). "Significance of cytologic criteria in distinguishing small cell from non-small cell carcinoma of the lung". *Acta Cytol* **47**(2): 216–20.

Atkinson, B. F. (2004). *Atlas of Diagnostic Cytopathology*. Philadelphia, PA, Saunders.

Atkinson, B. F. and J. F. Silverman. (1998). *Atlas of Difficult Diagnoses in Cytopathology*. Philadelphia, PA, Saunders.

Baloch, Z. W. and V. A. LiVolsi. (2002). "Etiology and significance of the optically clear nucleus". *Endocr Pathol* **13**(4): 289–99.

Berner, H. S., B. Davidson, *et al.* (2000). "Differential expression of CD44s and CD44v3–10 in adenocarcinoma cells and reactive mesothelial cells in effusions". *Virchows Arch* **436**(4): 330–5.

Bethwaite, P. B., B. Delahunt, *et al.* (1995). "Comparison of silver-staining nucleolar organizer region (AgNOR) counts and proliferating cell nuclear antigen (PCNA) expression in reactive mesothelial hyperplasia and malignant mesothelioma". *Pathology* **27**(1): 1–4.

Boorjian, S., C. Ng, *et al.* (2004). "Abnormal selective cytology results predict recurrence of upper-tract transitional-cell carcinoma treated with ureteroscopic laser ablation". *J Endourol* **18**(9): 912–6.

Bukovsky, A. (1986). "Multinucleation versus 'cell-in-a-cell' pattern". *Acta Cytol* **30**(2): 204–05.

Burja, I. T., S. K. Thompson, *et al.* (1999). "Atypical glandular cells of undetermined significance on cervical smears. A study with cyto-histologic correlation". *Acta Cytol* **43**(3): 351–6.

Cakir, E., F. Demirag, *et al.* (2009). "Cytopathologic differential diagnosis of malignant mesothelioma, adenocarcinoma and reactive mesothelial cells: a logistic regression analysis". *Diagn Cytopathol* **37**(1): 4–10.

Chalon, J., C. K. Tang, *et al.* (1978). "Diagnostic and prognostic significance of tracheobronchial epithelial multinucleation". *Acta Cytol* **22**(5): 316–20.

Chen, G. L., E. A. El-Gabry, *et al.* (2000). "Surveillance of upper urinary tract transitional cell carcinoma: the role of ureteroscopy, retrograde pyelography, cytology and urinalysis". *J Urol* **164**(6): 1901–04.

Chien, C. R., L. L. Ting, *et al.* (2005). "Post-radiation Pap smear for Chinese patients with cervical cancer: a ten-year follow-up". *Eur J Gynaecol Oncol* **26**(6): 619–22.

Cibas, E. S. and B. S. Ducatman. (2009). *Cytology: Diagnostic Principles and Clinical Correlates.* Philadelphia, PA, Saunders Elsevier.

Copeland, J. N., M. B. Amin, *et al.* (2002). "The morphologic spectrum of metastatic prostatic adenocarcinoma to the lung: special emphasis on histologic features overlapping with other pulmonary neoplasms". *Am J Clin Pathol* **117**(4): 552–7.

Crapanzano, J. P. and M. F. Zakowski. (2001). "Diagnostic dilemmas in pulmonary cytology". *Cancer* **93**(6): 364–75.

Demay, R. M. (2000). "Hyperchromatic crowded groups: pitfalls in pap smear diagnosis". *Am J Clin Pathol* **114** (Suppl): S36–43.

DiBonito, L., M. M. Musse, *et al.* (1992). "Cytology of transitional-cell carcinoma of the urinary bladder: diagnostic yield and histologic basis". *Diagn Cytopathol* **8**(2): 124–7.

Domanski, H. A., M. Akerman, *et al.* (2006). "Fine-needle aspiration of soft tissue leiomyosarcoma: an analysis of the most common cytologic findings and the value of ancillary techniques". *Diagn Cytopathol* **34**(9): 597–604.

Ducatman, B. S., H. H. Wang, *et al.* (1993). "Tubal metaplasia: a cytologic study with comparison to other neoplastic and non-neoplastic conditions of the endocervix". *Diagn Cytopathol* **9**(1): 98–103; discussion 103–05.

Elpek, G. O., N. Paksoy, *et al.* (1999). "Value of morphometry in distinguishing atypical reactive mesothelial and adenocarcinoma cells in pleural effusions". *Diagn Cytopathol* **21**(2): 148–50.

Finley, J. L., J. F. Silverman, *et al.* (1988). "Fine-needle aspiration cytology of pulmonary carcinosarcoma with immunocytochemical and ultrastructural observations". *Diagn Cytopathol* **4**(3): 239–43.

Granter, S. R. and E. S. Cibas. (1997). "Cytologic findings in thyroid nodules after 131I treatment of hyperthyroidism". *Am J Clin Pathol* **107**(1): 20–5.

Guarda, L. A., C. E. Peterson, *et al.* (1991). "Anaplastic thyroid carcinoma: cytomorphology and clinical implications of fine-needle aspiration". *Diagn Cytopathol* **7**(1): 63–7.

Hashi, A., T. Yuminamochi, *et al.* (2008). "Intranuclear cytoplasmic inclusion is a significant diagnostic feature for the differentiation of lobular endocervical glandular hyperplasia from minimal deviation adenocarcinoma of the cervix". *Diagn Cytopathol* **36**(8): 535–44.

Hata, S., Y. Mikami, *et al.* (2002). "Diagnostic significance of endocervical glandular cells with 'golden-yellow' mucin on pap smear". *Diagn Cytopathol* **27**(2): 80–4.

Henderson, D. W., K. B. Shilkin, *et al.* (1998). "Reactive mesothelial hyperplasia vs mesothelioma, including mesothelioma in situ: a brief review". *Am J Clin Pathol* **110**(3): 397–404.

Hernandez, E. and B. F. Atkinson. (1996). *Clinical Gynecologic Pathology.* Philadelphia, PA, W.B. Saunders.

Hoda, R. S. and S. A. Hoda. (2007). *Fundamentals of Pap Test Cytology.* Totowa, NJ, Humana Press.

Jhala, N., G. P. Siegal, *et al.* (2008). "Large, clear cytoplasmic vacuolation: an under-recognized cytologic clue to distinguish solid pseudopapillary neoplasms of the pancreas from pancreatic endocrine neoplasms on fine-needle aspiration". *Cancer* **114**(4): 249–54.

Kapila, K., M. R. Nampoory, *et al.* (2007). "Role of urinary cytology in detecting human polyoma bk virus in kidney transplant recipients. A preliminary report". *Med Princ Pract* **16**(3): 237–9.

Karakiewicz, P. I., S. Benayoun, *et al.* (2006). "Institutional variability in the accuracy of urinary cytology for predicting recurrence of transitional cell carcinoma of the bladder". *BJU Int* **97**(5): 997–1001.

Kaur, J. and P. Dey. (2010). "Micronucleus to distinguish adenocarcinoma from reactive mesothelial cell in effusion fluid". *Diagn Cytopathol* **38**(3): 177–9.

Khayyata, S., J. E. Barroeta, *et al.* (2008). "Papillary hyperplastic nodule: pitfall in the cytopathologic diagnosis of papillary thyroid carcinoma". *Endocr Pract* **14**(7): 863–8.

Kim, T. J., H. S. Kim, *et al.* (1999). "Clinical evaluation of follow-up methods and results of atypical glandular cells of undetermined significance (AGUS) detected on cervicovaginal Pap smears". *Gynecol Oncol* **73**(2): 292–8.

Kitazume, H., K. Kitamura, *et al.* (2000). "Cytologic differential diagnosis among reactive mesothelial cells, malignant mesothelioma, and adenocarcinoma: utility of combined E-cadherin and calretinin immunostaining". *Cancer* **90**(1): 55–60.

Koss, L. G. (2005). "Cytological criteria for the diagnosis of intraductal hyperplasia, ductal carcinoma in situ, and invasive carcinoma of the breast". *Diagn Cytopathol* **33**(3): 219.

Koss, L. G. (2007). "Of tissues, cells, and molecules: reminiscences of an old pathologist". *Hum Pathol* **38**(10): 1447–53.

Koss, L. G. (2008). "Atypical urothelial cells". *Anal Quant Cytol Histol* **30**(1): 61–2.

Koss, L. G., M. R. Melamed, *et al.* (2006). *Koss' Diagnostic Cytology and its Histopathologic Bases.* Philadelphia, PA, Lippincott Williams & Wilkins.

Koukoulaki, M., M. O'Donovan, *et al.* (2008). "Prospective study of urine cytology screening for BK polyoma virus replication in renal transplant recipients". *Cytopathology* **19**(6): 385–8.

Lachman, M. F. (1994). "Morphometric comparison of a metastatic transitional cell carcinoma simulating squamous metaplasia in sputum cytology. A case report". *Acta Cytol* **38**(3): 407–09.

Lee, A., Z. W. Baloch, *et al.* (2000). "Mesothelial hyperplasia with reactive atypia: diagnostic pitfalls and role of immunohistochemical studies – a case report". *Diagn Cytopathol* **22**(2): 113–6.

Lee, M. W. and G. K. Nguyen. (2007). "Cytology of papillary low-grade transitional cell carcinoma of the cervix in pap smear". *Diagn Cytopathol* **35**(9): 615–7.

Leslie, K. K., S. A. Walter, *et al.* (2007). "Effect of tamoxifen on endometrial histology, hormone receptors, and cervical cytology: a prospective study with follow-up". *Appl Immunohistochem Mol Morphol* **15**(3): 284–93.

Logani, S., P. K. Gupta, *et al.* (2000). "Thyroid nodules with FNA cytology suspicious for follicular variant of papillary thyroid carcinoma: follow-up and management". *Diagn Cytopathol* **23**(6): 380–5.

Malik, S. N., E. J. Wilkinson, *et al.* (2001). "Benign cellular changes in Pap smears. Causes and significance". *Acta Cytol* **45**(1): 5–8.

Murugan, P., N. Siddaraju, *et al.* (2008). "Significance of intercellular spaces (windows) in effusion fluid cytology: a study of 46 samples". *Diagn Cytopathol* **36**(9): 628–32.

Owens, C. L. and S. Z. Ali. (2005). "Atypical squamous cells in exfoliative urinary cytology: clinicopathologic correlates". *Diagn Cytopathol* **33**(6): 394–8.

Papanicolaou, G. N. (1960). *Atlas of Exfoliative Cytology*. Cambridge, MA, published for the Commonwealth Fund by Harvard University Press.

Pereira, T. C., R. S. Saad, *et al.* (2006). "The diagnosis of malignancy in effusion cytology: a pattern recognition approach". *Adv Anat Pathol* **13**(4): 174–84.

Renshaw, A. A. (2005). *Aspiration Cytology*. Philadelphia, PA, Elsevier Saunders.

Ribotta, M., A. Donna, *et al.* (1992). "Quantitative analysis of nucleoli and nucleolar organizer regions in cultured primary human normal, reactive and malignant mesothelial cells". *Pathol Res Pract* **188**(4–5): 536–40.

Saad, R. S., A. Kanbour-Shakir, *et al.* (2006). "Cytomorphologic analysis and histological correlation of high-grade squamous intraepithelial lesions in postmenopausal women". *Diagn Cytopathol* **34**(7): 467–71.

Sakuma, N., T. Kamei, *et al.* (1999). "Ultrastructure of pleural mesothelioma and pulmonary adenocarcinoma in malignant effusions as compared with reactive mesothelial cells". *Acta Cytol* **43**(5): 777–85.

Saleh, H. A., M. El-Fakharany, *et al.* (2009). "Differentiating reactive mesothelial cells from metastatic adenocarcinoma in serous effusions: the utility of immunocytochemical panel in the differential diagnosis". *Diagn Cytopathol* **37**(5): 324–32.

Saleh, H. A., J. Haapaniemi, *et al.* (1998). "Bronchioloalveolar carcinoma: diagnostic pitfalls and immunocytochemical contribution." *Diagn Cytopathol* **18**(4): 301–06.

Sandhyamani, S., C. C. Kartha, *et al.* (1984). "Reactive mesothelial nodule of the pericardium". *Indian Heart J* **36**(3): 169–72.

Schaefer, F. V., R. P. Custer, *et al.* (1983). "Induction of squamous metaplasia: requirement for cell multiplication, and competition with lobuloalveolar development in cultured mammary glands". *Differentiation* **25**(2): 185–92.

Schulte, E. (1986). "Air drying as a preparatory factor in cytology: investigation of its influence on dye uptake and dye binding". *Diagn Cytopathol* **2**(2): 160–7.

Selvaggi, S. M. and H. K. Haefner. (1997). "Microglandular endocervical hyperplasia and tubal metaplasia: pitfalls in the diagnosis of adenocarcinoma on cervical smears". *Diagn Cytopathol* **16**(2): 168–73.

Silverberg, S. G. and R. A. DeLellis. (2006). *Silverberg's Principles and Practice of Surgical Pathology and Cytopathology*. Edinburgh, Churchill Livingstone/Elsevier.

Soosay, G. N., M. Griffiths, *et al.* (1991). "The differential diagnosis of epithelial-type mesothelioma from adenocarcinoma and reactive mesothelial proliferation". *J Pathol* **163**(4): 299–305.

Stanley, M. W., M. J. Henry-Stanley, *et al.* (1992). "Hyperplasia of type II pneumocytes in acute lung injury. Cytologic findings of sequential bronchoalveolar lavage". *Am J Clin Pathol* **97**(5): 669–77.

Ueda, J., T. Iwata, *et al.* (2006). "Comparison of three cytologic preparation methods and immunocytochemistries to distinguish adenocarcinoma cells from reactive mesothelial cells in serous effusion". *Diagn Cytopathol* **34**(1): 6–10.

Vrtacnik Bokal, E., S. Rakar, *et al.* (2005). "Human papillomavirus infection in relation to mild dyskaryosis in conventional cervical cytology". *Eur J Gynaecol Oncol* **26**(1): 39–42.

Wang, N., S. N. Emancipator, *et al.* (2002). "Histologic follow-up of atypical endocervical cells. Liquid-based, thin-layer preparation vs. conventional Pap smear". *Acta Cytol* **46**(3): 453–7.

Wiatrowska, B. A., J. Krol, *et al.* (2001). "Large-cell neuroendocrine carcinoma of the lung: proposed criteria for cytologic diagnosis". *Diagn Cytopathol* **24**(1): 58–64.

Willen, R., T. Bruce, *et al.* (1976). "Squamous epithelial cancer in metaplastic pleura following extrapleural pneumothorax for pulmonary tuberculosis". *Virchows Arch A Pathol Anat Histol* **370**(3): 225–31.

Williams, S. K., K. J. Denton, *et al.* (2008). "Correlation of upper-tract cytology, retrograde pyelography, ureteroscopic appearance, and ureteroscopic biopsy with histologic examination of upper-tract transitional cell carcinoma". *J Endourol* **22**(1): 71–6.

Ylagan, L. R., S. Edmundowicz, *et al.* (2002). "Endoscopic ultrasound guided fine-needle aspiration cytology of pancreatic carcinoma: a 3-year experience and review of the literature". *Cancer* **96**(6): 362–9.

Zusman-Harach, S. B., H. R. Harach, *et al.* (1991). "Cytological features of non-small cell carcinomas of the lung in fine needle aspirates". *J Clin Pathol* **44**(12): 997–1002.

Fixation in the context of diagnostic cytopathology today traces its roots to Dr. Papanicolaou's use of equal parts of diethyl ether and 95% ethyl alcohol. He first described this fixative in a 1917 paper about the existence of a typical estrous cycle in the guinea pig – although there is no mention of that fixative in that paper. Thus, Papanicolaou published no rationale for his choice of alcohol and ether. This fixative became the standard in diagnostic cytopathology after Dr. Papanicolaou recorded its use in the 1942 monograph that he co-authored with Dr. Herbert Traut.

Papanicolaou did not publish his rationale for including ether in alcohol. Ether has no fixative properties. Since it is an effective fat solvent, ether may serve as an adjuvant, which speeds alcohol's penetration into cells. In blinded comparisons with cells fixed only in 95% alcohol, no discernible difference is evident.

Ether, of course, is highly volatile and explosive. More than a few non-explosion proof refrigerators have exploded when storing ether that was ignited by a spark. Consequently, its use was generally discontinued by the late 1950s, leaving 95% ethanol alone as the standard fixative for Pap smears (Figure 6.1). Indeed, the very first issue of *Acta Cytologica* published in 1957 included a write-in symposium that addressed "experiences with various methods of fixation of smears."

In practice, a fresh cellular sample is spread onto a glass slide and immediately fixed by plunging it into alcohol (i.e. wet-fixation). Air-drying should not be allowed to occur either before, during, or after fixation. "Fresh" means the cell sample had just been collected and had not been suspended in preservative prior to being applied to the slide surface.

As Papanicolaou's cytological method became more widely used, it was applied in more settings and to non-gynecologic cytologic specimens. The standard method of immediate wet-fixation of fresh cells could not be readily adapted, which led to many variations of fixatives and fixation methods, not all of which produced cytomorphologically equivalent results.

Cytologic specimens that can be spread on slides at the collection site can be fixed by several methods. Cell suspensions that cannot be spread on slides until first processed in a laboratory require either refrigeration or preservation in dilute alcohol when lengthy time delays are anticipated (e.g. non-hospital based sites). Nowadays, most (80–90%) gynecologic cytologic specimens are

(A) **(B)**

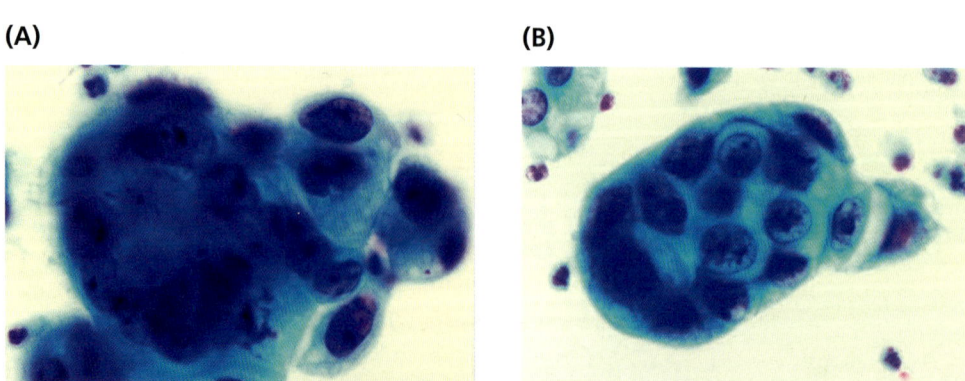

Figure 6.1 (A) Ether-alcohol vs. (B) 95% ethanol fixation.

Cytohistology: Essential and Basic Concepts, Prabodh Gupta and Zubair Baloch. Published by Cambridge University Press. © Cambridge University Press 2011.

collected in proprietary or patented preservatives. As a result of the availability of various denatured alcohols and collection circumstances, there are many possible preservation and fixation combinations – some produce results indistinguishable from those produced by the standard fixation method, most produce useful but different results, and a few are unsatisfactory.

The Papanicolaou stain used for all photomicrographs in this chapter is a modified Pap stain that incorporates Gill Hematoxylin – No. 1 (2 min), and Gill modified OG (15 s) and EA (10 min).

There are four basic alternatives to immediate wet-fixation in 95% ethanol:

- substitute alcohols,
- air-drying of protected fixed cells,
- air-drying and rehydration of unprotected cells, and
- preservation.

Parenthetically, alcohol used alone by convention means ethanol.

SUBSTITUTE ALCOHOLS

The goal of fixation is to make every cell reveal its health or disease status by its cytomorphology. The goal is not to preserve the life-like appearance of cells, unless one seeks to study the life-like appearance of cells per se (Figure 6.2(A) and 6.2(B)).

Substitute alcohols are those that can be used in the same manner as 95% ethanol without noticeable morphological differences. "Same manner" means immediate wet-fixation of fresh specimens. These substitute alcohols include: (1) absolute methanol, (2) reagent alcohol, (3) 80% isopropanol, and (4) 90% acetone (Figure 6.3).

Acetone is not an alcohol, but it is included in this category for convenience.

Absolute methanol

Methanol is the first of three possible substitute alcohols. Methanol shrinks cells less relative to the shrinkage observed with 95% ethanol. For this reason, methanol can be used at absolute (i.e. 100%) strength.

Reagent alcohol

Reagent alcohol is comprised of 9 parts ethanol, and 0.5 part each of methanol and isopropanol. The latter

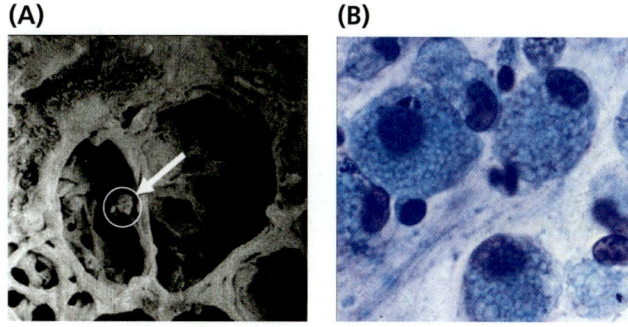

(A)   **(B)**

Figure 6.2 Macrophages (arrow): (A) life-like appearance vs. (B) artifactual.

two alcohols denature the ethanol. According to the US federal law, "reagent alcohol shall be packaged by the manufacturer in containers not exceeding four liters."

It is not necessary to dilute reagent alcohol to 95% concentration, as it makes no visibly discernible difference in cytomorphology when used full-strength. Indeed, ethanol can be used full-strength as well.

Reagent alcohol is 1 of 50 specially denatured alcohol formulations approved by the federal government for manufacture for assorted applications. Some of the formulations are not denatured by denaturants likely to impact cytomorphology, and also are not restricted to sale in containers not to exceed 4 liters capacity. Special denatured alcohol Formula No. 3-C, for example, is 100 gallons of alcohol and 5 gallons of isopropyl alcohol.

80% isopropanol

Absolute isopropanol shrinks cells excessively. Diluting isopropanol to 80% concentration diminishes the shrinkage to that comparable to ethanol.

90% acetone

Historically, acetone has been used full-strength, but it hardens cells and tissues unacceptably. Diluting acetone to 90% concentration produces acceptable results. Its odor, however, makes it unattractive for routine use.

AIR-DRYING OF PROTECTED FIXED CELLS

Air-drying of protected fixed cells is a process by which cells on a slide are fixed in alcohol with polyethylene glycol (PEG) and subsequently air-dried. At least two obvious approaches are possible.

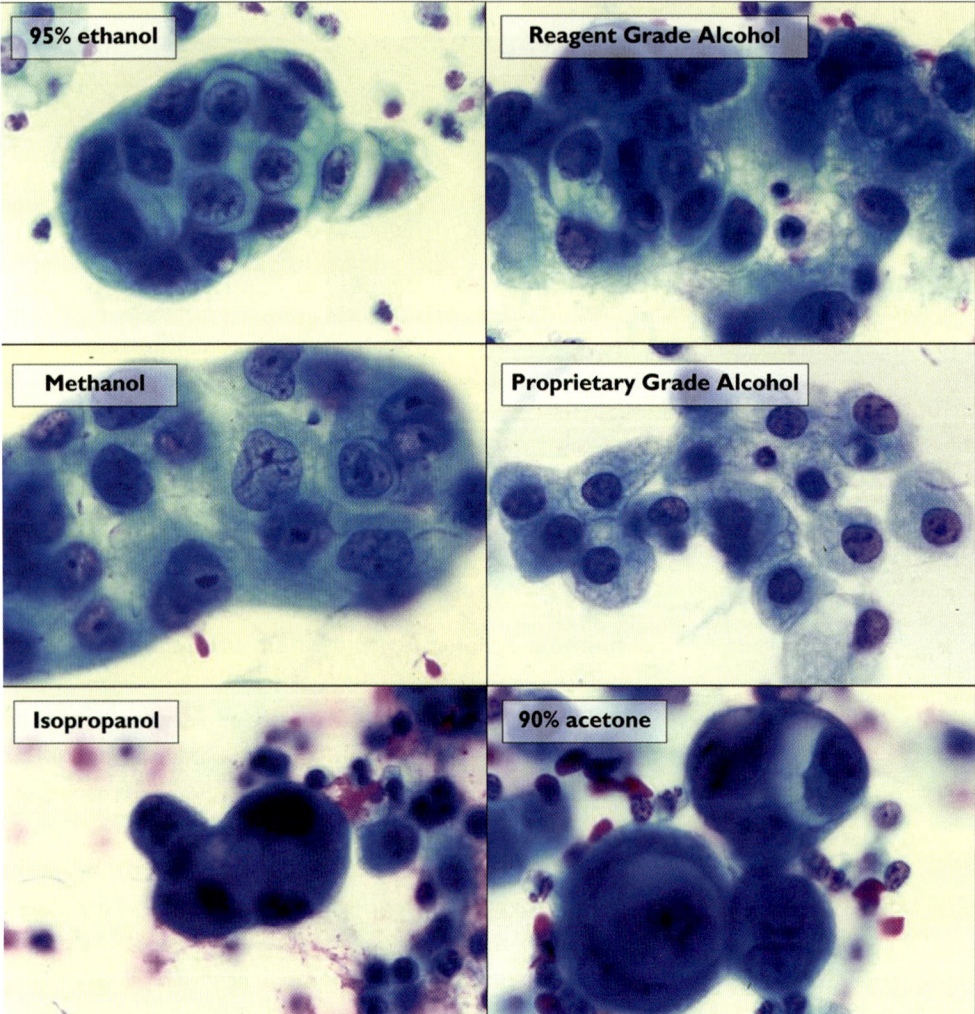

Figure 6.3 Array of mesothelial cells fixed by six different fixatives.

■ Fresh cells can be spread onto a slide and immediately immersed in alcohol (i.e. wet-fixed) with PEG, removed after several minutes, and allowed to air-dry.

■ Fresh cells can be spread onto a slide – avoiding air-drying – and covered with alcohol with PEG, which may be dropped on the slide or delivered as a spray (i.e. spray fixation), and then allowed to air-dry.

The optimal range of distance from which most fluorocarbon propellant powered spray fixative should be delivered to a cell spread is 25–30 cm (10–12 inches). Nearer distances result in nuclear shrinkage, while farther distances result in air-drying. Although the causes of these limitations was not suggested, it is possible that at near distances the propellant-driven blast of spray fixative tears cells from their moorings and shrinks them as they float in the pool of fixative. Additionally, at farther distances, it is possible that the inverse square law diminishes the density of spray

particles and so retards the rate of deposition on the cells, thus allowing sufficient time for partial air-drying. Therefore, the optimal distance may vary with the force of delivery and the density of spray droplets of a given aerosol fixative. Short-distance sensitivity has not been reported for pump spray fixatives.

AIR-DRYING AND REHYDRATION OF UNPROTECTED CELLS

Cells that are spread on a slide and simply air-dried are unsuitable for interpretation cytomorphologically. Indeed, air-drying is one of the major causes of unsatisfactory conventional Pap tests; it has helped spur the development of liquid-based cytology.

Air-drying alters cells physically in at least three observable ways: it *irreversibly* (1) degrades chromatin structure

(A)   **(B)**

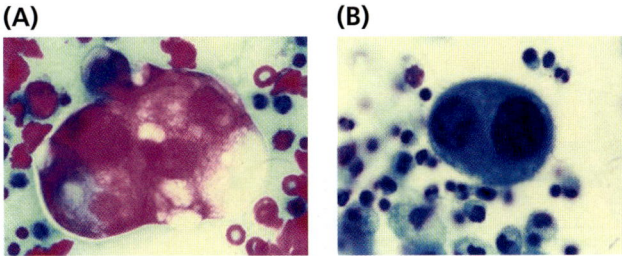

Figure 6.4 (A) Air-dried vs. (B) rehydrated tissue fragments.

and detail, and (2) enlarges or shrinks cells; and it *reversibly* (3) slows dye uptake.

Changes in chromatin display and cell diameter are *irreversible* by all rehydration methods. The effects of the more tightly woven protein texture that selectively blocks stain uptake, however, are *reversible* upon immersion in glycerin (Figure 6.4).

A trihydric alcohol (i.e. it has three OH groups instead of one like isopropanol, which is the same carbon chain length), glycerin penetrates and "wets" protein molecules, thereby allowing all dyes of the Pap stain to penetrate and color the cells normochromatically. The quality of the restoration is dependent on the quality of the Pap stain in use at the time in any given laboratory.

While morphologically more interpretable than if not rehydrated and diagnostic outcomes may be comparable to those of wet-fixed cohorts, rehydrated air-dried cells are not identical with alcohol wet-fixed cells in diameter or chromatin patterns. Given the choice between examining alcohol wet-fixed cells and rehydrated air-dried cells, cyto-professionals usually choose the standard presentation – probably on the basis of subjective familiarity rather than on objective utility. Wet-fixation in alcohol is an empirical method used in no other comparable biomedical application. Alcohol precipitates chromatin in normal and abnormal cells in visibly distinctive and visually distinguishable ways, and that such patterns constitute the foundation of our collective memory banks of cytopathological images. It also permits improved dye permeation as the Papanicolaou stains are alcohol-based. This is in sharp contrast to the classic H/E water-based staining protocol.

PRESERVATION

Preservation was sometimes referred to as prefixation; is collecting cells in preservative, either gynecologic cytologic samples for liquid-based cytology, or non-gynecologic

cytologic cell suspensions such as sputum, urine, and body cavity fluids. Preservatives and fixatives are alike but different: all fixatives are preservatives, but not all preservatives are fixatives. Briefly, a preservative is dilute fixative (e.g. 95% alcohol fixes; 50% alcohol preserves). Fixatives and preservatives kill cells and microorganisms, stop autolysis, alter chemical constituents, and harden protein. Alcohol as a fixative hardens protein by coagulation, which shrinks cells, while alcohol as a preservative partially hardens protein and swells cells (e.g. 50% ethanol swells cells, as evidenced by hemolysis of suspended erythrocytes). For alcohol, therefore, the difference between its acting as a preservative or as a fixative is primarily one of concentration, for which there is no bright line cut-off.

In general, collecting cell suspensions in an equal volume of 50% ethanol, or comparable substitute alcohol, is recommended. If cells will be air-dried after being spread on a slide, include PEG (Carbowax 1450) at a 2% (w/v) concentration. Otherwise, do not include Carbowax, as Carbowax does not preserve or fix cells. It's acceptable to use Carbowax-based preservatives.

MAKING SENSE OF IT ALL

In diagnostic cytopathology visually interpretable chromatin detail is everything. Such detail is exhibited best when every material and method in the cytopreparatory chain is selected for its contribution to the final result (Figure 6.5).

Sound biological, chemical, physical, and optical principles underpin the foundation of the practice. When the links in the chain are strong, useful cytomorphology results; when weak, cytomorphology is compromised (Figure 6.6).

From the standpoint of cytopreparation, regardless of the originating body site, cells are more alike than different. The goal is to transfer the cells from suspension onto a surface for fixing, staining, mounting, and microscopy. Albeit with technique and preparation artifacts, it matters little whether the cells are prepared as a cell spread, a cytocentrifuged preparation, a cellulosic or polycarbonate filter preparation, a liquid-based preparation, or cell blocks. It is true, however; that the morphologic features are preparation-dependent and the observer's familiarity with them is critical for accurate diagnosis.

Based upon our number of years of observations, it can be confidently stated that "depending upon personal preferences, training and experience, high-quality cytologic

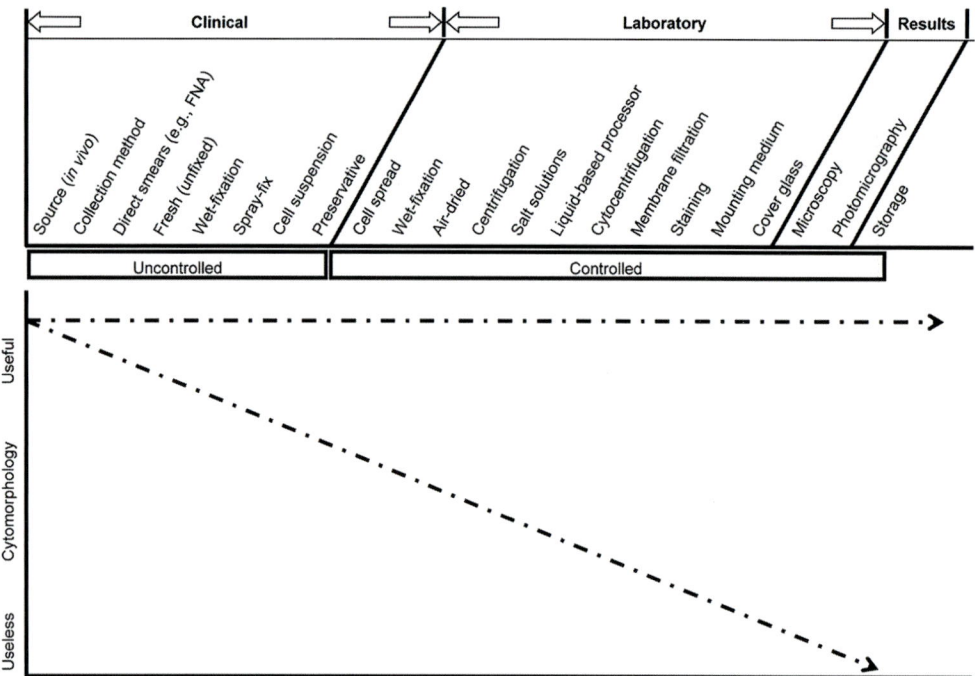

Figure 6.5 Links in the cytopreparatory chain.

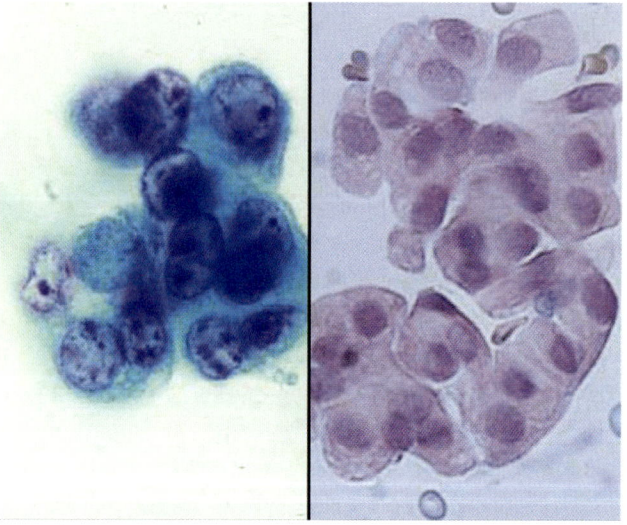

Figure 6.6 Satisfactory and unsatisfactory object/image quality.

preparations can be either a help or a hindrance to the interpretation." These reactions underscore the artifactual nature of cytomorphology and the need to control it tightly.

A cytologic preparation has two basic components when viewed microscopically: the object itself and the image derived from the object. Thus, there are four possible combinations of satisfactory and unsatisfactory quality (Figure 6.7).

One skilled in the art and science of cytopreparation should be able to discern microscopically the reasons for deviations from optimal results and implement stable corrections as needed.

Fixation is a forward-looking process that anticipates the intended use of cells and tissue: microscopic examination for diagnostic applications. Fixatives of different chemical constitutions cannot be used interchangeably for the same application without producing dissimilar morphological results (e.g. 10% formalin is good for tissue but bad for cells). The choice of fixative is coupled with the staining method. For example, methyl alcohol fixes air-dried blood films that will be Romanovsky-stained and ethyl alcohol fixes non-air-dried cells that will be Pap-stained. In the latter examples, differences in the degree of flattening *and* the fixative account for the differences in stain uptake and morphological display. Cell flattening is good (Figure 6.8); cell shrinkage is bad.

Extremes are undesirable. Standard fixation methods strike a balance in specified applications. It is nearly impossible to foresee every conceivable fixation scheme readers may employ or encounter; only the general chemical and physical mechanisms that influence fixation outcomes are discussed here.

The degree to which shrinkage does or does not occur depends on: (1) cellular water content, (2) cell location when preserved or fixed (i.e. in suspension or on a surface), (3) alcohol chain length (i.e. methyl, ethyl, isopropyl [1, 2, 3 carbons, respectively]), (4) alcohol

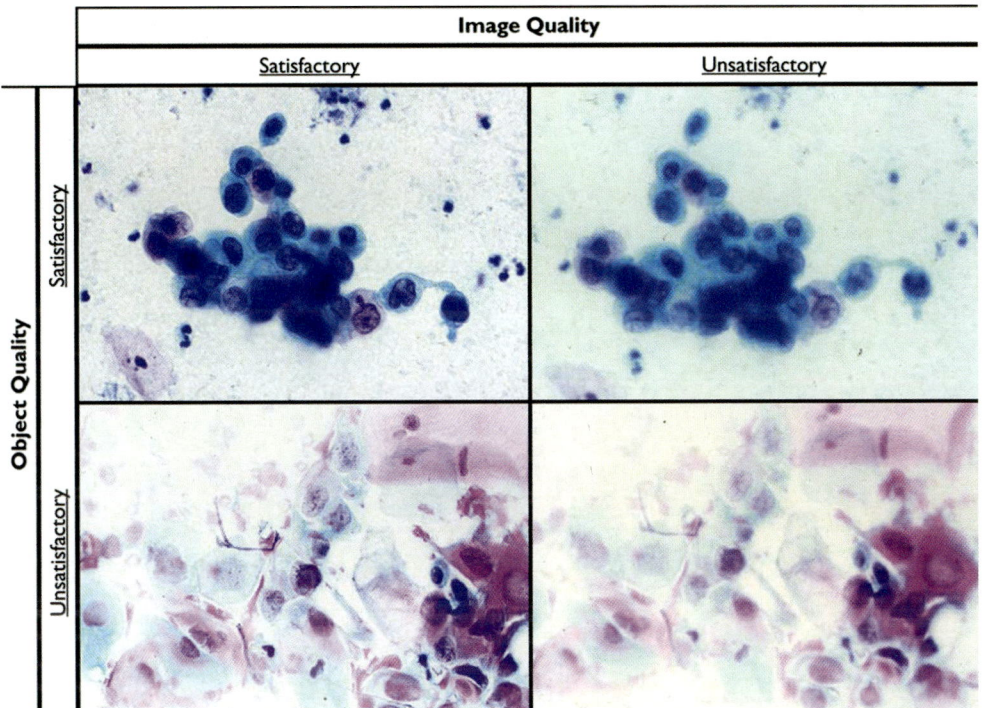

Figure 6.7 Combinations of object and image quality.

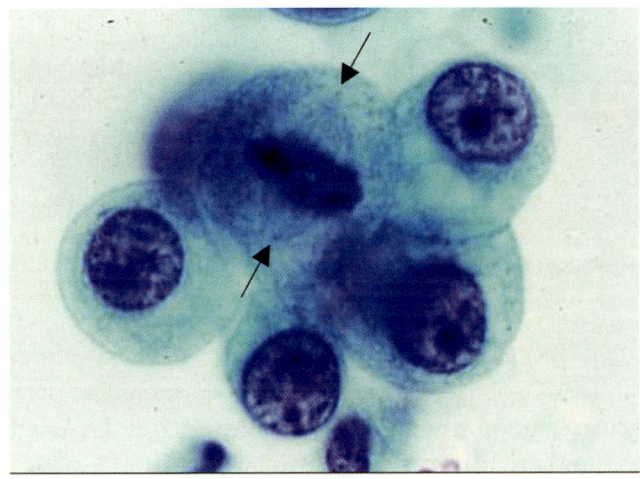

Figure 6.8 Gold standard flattening: cytospin BCF with metaphase plate, spindle apparatus, and centrioles intact (arrows).

concentration, (5) whether maintained wet or allowed to air-dry, (6) location if and when air-dried (i.e. separate from, or in contact with, the slide surface), and (7) whether Carbowax is present in the preservative or fixative when air-drying takes place.

Cellular water content

The water content of materials in the human body ranges from practically nothing in tooth enamel up to

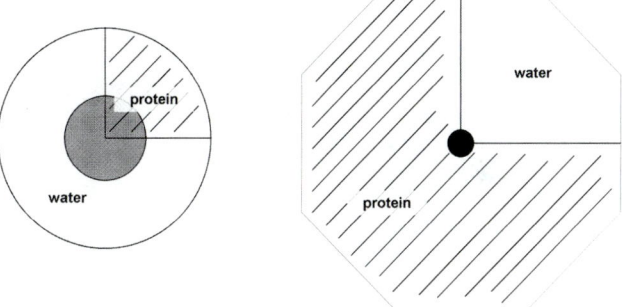

Figure 6.9 Cellular water content.

approximately 85% in neurons of the brain's gray matter. This leads to the notion of cells with low and high water content in considerations of cellular responses to alternative fixatives and fixation methods used in diagnostic cytopathology (Figure 6.9).

Low water content cells include normal and abnormal intermediate and superficial squamous cells, while high water content cells are everything else. Water content is important because alcohol and air-drying independently extract water and will change cell diameters – with associated changes in nuclear area, thickness, and chromatin display – to different degrees.

As shown in Figure 6.10, low water content cells collected in preservative are essentially unchanged in diameter

153

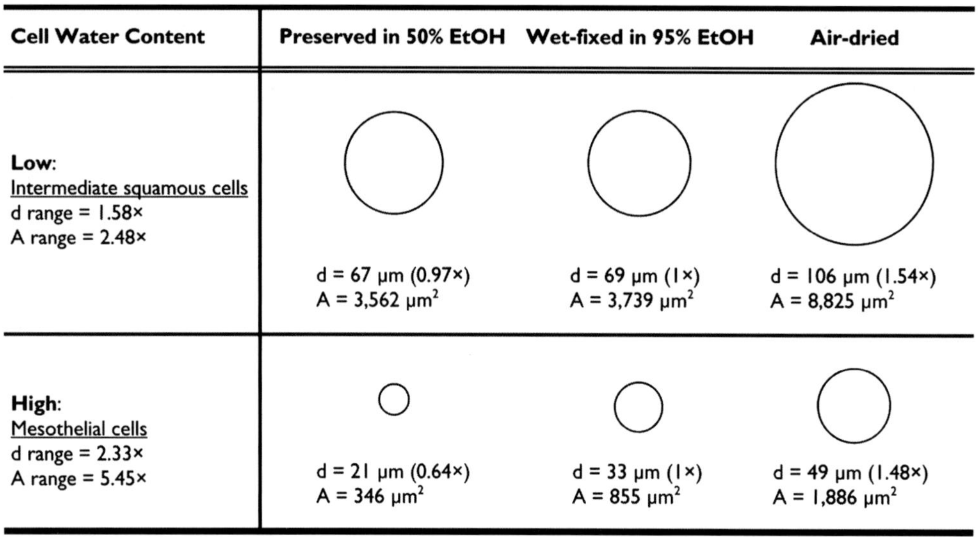

Cell Water Content	Preserved in 50% EtOH	Wet-fixed in 95% EtOH	Air-dried
Low: Intermediate squamous cells d range = 1.58× A range = 2.48×	d = 67 μm (0.97×) A = 3,562 μm²	d = 69 μm (1×) A = 3,739 μm²	d = 106 μm (1.54×) A = 8,825 μm²
High: Mesothelial cells d range = 2.33× A range = 5.45×	d = 21 μm (0.64×) A = 346 μm²	d = 33 μm (1×) A = 855 μm²	d = 49 μm (1.48×) A = 1,886 μm²

Figure 6.10 Alternative materials and methods effects on cells of low and high water content.

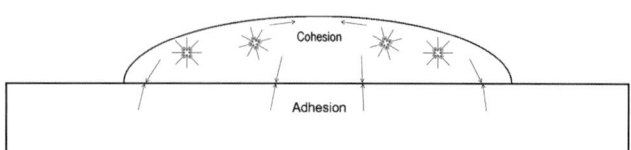

Figure 6.11 Cell flattening.

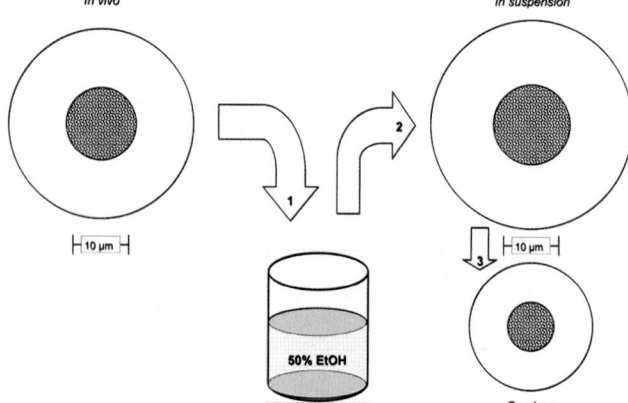

Figure 6.12 Consequences of preserving cells in suspension.

relative to alcohol wet-fixed controls. When air-dried on glass, however, such cells increase in diameter nearly 1.5 times. High water content cells collected in preservative shrink to two-thirds the diameter of control cells, becoming thicker and more optically dense when stained. Preservatives swell cells in suspension initially [e.g. erythrocytes leak hemoglobin] and increase cohesive forces, promoting subsequent shrinkage after the cells are spread on a slide and wet-fixed. When air-dried on glass, high water content cells display diameters enlarged also by nearly 1.5 times – approximately the same amount as by air-dried low water content cells. Air-dried high water content cells are up to 5.5-times greater in area than their preserved counterparts. Such enlargement is a plus – indeed essential – for Romanovsky-stained preparations (Figures 6.10 and 6.14).

Cell location when preserved or fixed

In the standard fixation method – whether for gynecologic or non-gynecologic specimens – fresh cells are in contact with the slide surface when fixed. Such contact is essential to flattening cells, as the contact favors the adhesive forces between the cells and the glass, which are generally stronger than the cohesive forces within fresh cells that resist flattening (Figure 6.11).

Adhesion may be defined as a property that causes unlike substances to stick together; cohesion, like substances to cling together. Collecting cells as preserved suspensions, however, has the opposite effect and increases the cohesive forces within cells. While cells in preservatives first swell, they ultimately shrink when immersed in fixative because the increased cohesive forces are greater than the adhesive forces. Thus, preserved cells resist flattening and become smaller and thicker. Such cells are more optically dense when stained, which masks nuclear details (Figure 6.12).

Alcohol chain length

All alcohols are organic derivatives of water. The chemical formula for water, H_2O, can be written as H-OH, which shows a single hydrogen atom and a hydroxyl group OH, which is the basis for alcohols. Methanol, ethanol, and isopropanol consist of 1, 2, and 3 carbon atoms and a single hydroxyl group: CH_3OH, C_2H_5OH, and C_3H_7OH. As the carbon chain length increases, changes in fixative properties occur: the longer the chain length, the greater the cellular shrinkage that results.

The relationship between alcohol chain length and cellular shrinkage may be due to several factors: (1) greater solubilities of lipids in the higher alcohols, (2) the polarity of the alcohol, the greater the polarity the faster the penetration of the cell and the faster the solvation of cellular structure, and (3) cellular water leaves the cell by diffusion and the cellular contents become progressively more dehydrated. It is believed that the dehydration is the result of the coagulation of the proteins, which brings the molecules closer together, thereby in effect squeezing the water out of the cells.

Solvation, commonly called dissolution, is the process of attraction and association of molecules of a solvent with molecules or ions of a solute. As ions dissolve in a solvent they spread out and become surrounded by solvent molecules. The bigger the ion, the more solvent molecules are able to surround it and the more it becomes solvated.

Alcohol concentration

Alcohols are coagulating, non-additive fixatives. "Coagulating" means transforming protoplasm into a microscopical spongework. "Non-additive" means there is no obvious permanent addition of atoms to some part of the protein. As might be expected, the degree of coagulation, or hardening, is greatest for each alcohol at its maximum concentration. At lower concentrations, alcohols lose their fixative properties – those making cells and tissues capable of resisting subsequent treatments – and gain preservative properties. Collecting a small volume of cells in a large volume of concentrated alcohol, for example, coagulates dissolved protein and shrinks cells unacceptably, which complicate subsequent cytopreparation.

An alternative expression of shrinkage in alcohol can be seen in Figure 6.13.

Whether maintained wet or allowed to air-dry

As a cell air-dries, the air–water interface that passes through the cell exerts tremendous surface tension forces that denature and disrupt proteins, forever altering chromatin display relative to its alcohol wet-fixed appearance.

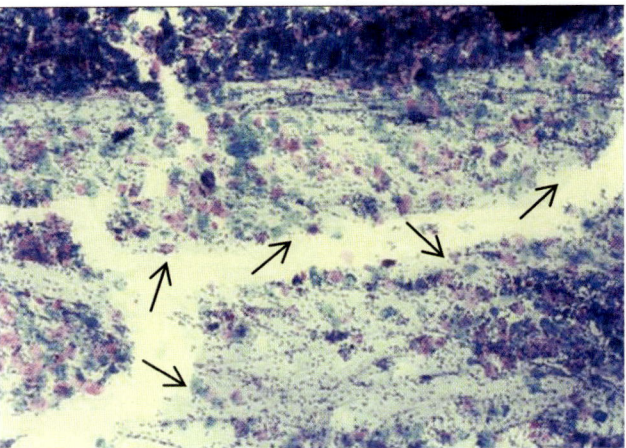

Figure 6.13 Shrinkage fissures (arrows) in conventional Pap smear.

This force has been calculated to be 320 tons/in^2, which – less dramatically – equals 450 mg/μm^2.

Location if and when air-dried

When in contact with a clean glass surface during air-drying, cells increase in diameter as the forces of extracellular adhesion exceed those of intracellular cohesion. The opposite electrostatic charges of cell and glass surfaces are attractive, as are the inward cohesive forces. In other words, the balance of forces favors cells flattening like sunny-side up cooked eggs instead of rounding-up like hard-cooked eggs.

On the other hand, a cell suspended above the glass surface (e.g. on an albumin adhesive film or frosted slide surface, in a mucus stream or tissue fragment) becomes smaller in diameter as the intracellular cohesive forces are now relatively greater (Figure 6.14).

So air-drying may enlarge or shrink cells diametrically, depending on which force is stronger under the circumstances – with the cells becoming thinner or thicker in the process, respectively (Figure 6.15). Cells that are air-dried and then fixed flatten/shrink more than if fixed first and then air-dried.

Air-drying compresses protein and reduces the intermolecular spaces through which dyes must subsequently pass to reach bonding sites. Of the Papanicolaou stain dyes, eosin is most effective at penetrating small spaces. Consequently, air-dried cells appear eosinophilic throughout. Diffuse eosinophilia eliminates color and optical density differences among cellular components, makes cells visually impenetrable, blurs particle boundaries, and exaggerates the apparent visible effects of air-drying.

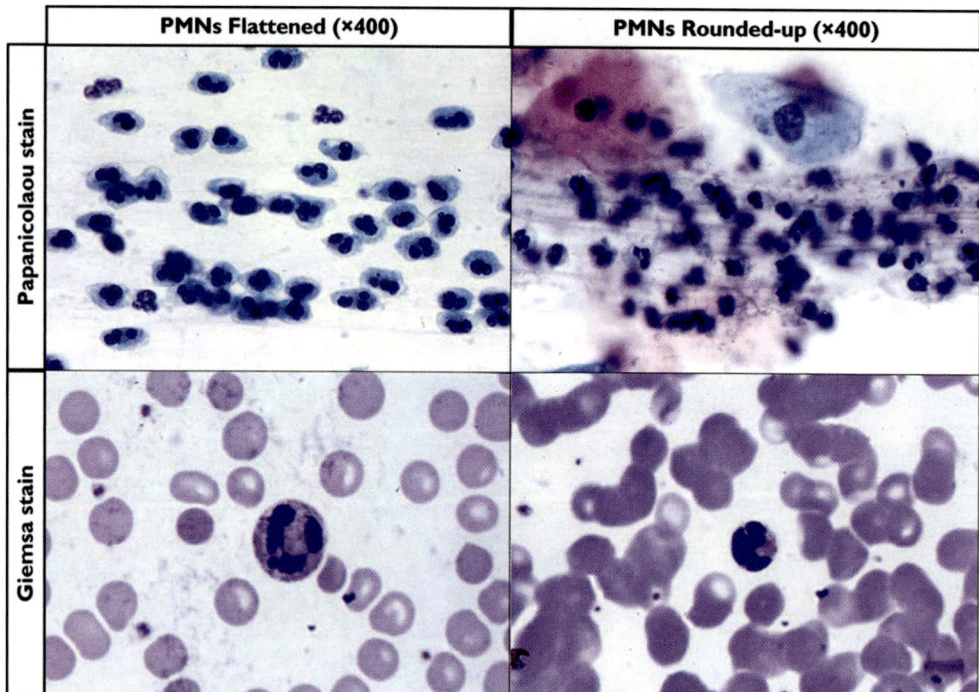

| PMNs Flattened (×400) | PMNs Rounded-up (×400) |

Papanicolaou stain

Giemsa stain

Figure 6.14 2×2 array of well-flattened vs. air-dried cells.

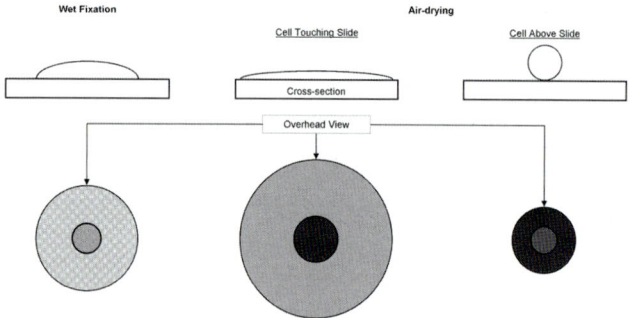

Figure 6.15 Wet-fixation vs. air-drying.

A potential practical consequence is that normal squamous cells with nuclei as small as 8 μm may be misinterpreted as ASC-US because air-drying artifactually enlarges them to 12 μm, while reducing their thickness to 3.4 μm. Rehydrated air-dried cells in groups may appear more optically dense. Some automated coverslippers allow xylene to evaporate from slides before applying the cover glasses. Direct microscopic examination of cells in groups reveals that they shrink suddenly as the xylene evaporates completely – although not in single cells anchored to the slide surface. Such an observation raises the question of whether such coverslippers should be used at all, and underscores the basis for coverslipping slides one at a time. Once fixed, cells should always be kept wet until mounted. Overall, air-drying may make it difficult to compare quantitative cellular features with those of wet-fixed cells. Any quantitative study of cellular features should control the materials and methods of fixation and so specify the details of fixation in reporting findings. Since rehydration is not considered to be standard practice, it might be considered unfavorably in any false-negative Pap smear litigation. If using any alternative fixative and fixation method, evaluate high water content cells as they are more sensitive quality indicators.

Whether Carbowax is present when air-drying takes place

In no instance should cells be allowed to air-dry before being fixed unless intended (e.g. FNA, blood films). After being applied to the cells, the alcohol evaporates. As it does, an air–alcohol interface recedes – or advances, depending on one's perspective – through the cells. Ordinarily, if PEG were not present, substantial denaturation forces would be exerted between the protein molecules and the air–liquid interface, twisting and distorting molecules. When part of the fixative, PEG precipitates as the alcohol evaporates and preempts the forces of distortion, in effect embedding and protecting the fixed cells in situ.

Carbowax is The Dow Chemical Company's trademarked name for its line of polyethylene glycols of varying molecular weights, of which there are approximately 11 – depending on the application – that range from 300 to 8000. Numbers below 600 are liquids; above 900, solids.

Table 6.1 Materials and methods used before, during and after cells come into contact with a glass surface, and promote either cohesion that favors rounding-up, or or adhesion that favors cell flattening

Contact timing	Promote cohesion (shrink)	Promote "balance" (standard)	Promote adhesion (enlarge)
Pre-	High water content cells	Low or high water content cells	Low or high water content cells
	Preserved cells in suspension	Fresh cells	Fresh cells
	Higher alcohol concentrations		
During	Dirty slide surface	Clean slide surface	Clean slide surface
	Above slide	On slide	On slide
	Glycerin–albumin coating	Force: centrifugal, negative pressure	Force: centrifugal, negative pressure
	Slow immersion	Immediate immersion	Immediate immersion
	Isopropanol	95% ethanol, methanol, reagent alcohol, 80% isopropanol, 90% acetone	Methanol
Post-	Air-drying	Keep wet	Keep wet
		Use Carbowax ad hoc	Use Carbowax ad hoc

The melting points of the solids become progressively higher with increasing number. Carbowax 1450 is a water-soluble solid wax with a melting temperature range of 43–46°C, which makes it suitable for cytological applications. Carbowax 1450 was known as Carbowax 1540 at one time (e.g. in 1963, when Saccomanno included it in 50% ethanol as part of his preservative for sputum). The inclusion of Carbowax in a fixative in cytology can be traced back to 1946.

SUMMARY

Table 6.1 summarizes the factors that contribute to cell flattening before, during, or after cells are put in contact with a glass surface.

After the standard fixation method (i.e. immediate wet-fixation of fresh cells spread thinly on a clean slide) in conjunction with the Papanicolaou stain, the hierarchy of potential alternatives, best first, is as follows.

Gynecologic and fine needle aspirations

1. Immediate wet fixation in absolute reagent alcohol, absolute methanol, 80% isopropanol, or 90% acetone.
2. Immediate wet fixation in any of the 4 reagents above with 2% Carbowax 1450 (w/v), followed by air-drying.
3. Spray fixation with ethanol-based fixative that contains Carbowax (polyethylene glycol, PEG).
4. Air-drying followed by rehydration in 50% glycerin x 3 minutes, followed by immersion in 95% alcohol.

Non-gynecologic specimens

1. Collection in equal parts of 50% alcohol with Carbowax, followed by concentration, spreading, air-drying.
2. Collection in commercial preservatives per manufacturer's instructions (e.g. CytoLyt®, CytoRich Red™).

Avoid unprotected air-drying, unless it is an essential step in the SOP (e.g. preparations that will be stained with Diff-Quik or a Romanovsky stain).

TECHNICAL NOTES AND TIPS

- In applications of cytomorphology, cell and nuclear size, N:C ratios, chromatin patterns are relative to the materials and methods of fixation employed. There are no absolute, immutable features. Thus, the materials and methods of cytopreparation must be controlled to produce consistently and reliably useful cytomorphology.
- High water content cells should be used to assess the effects of alternative fixatives and fixation methods. Low water content cells (i.e. superficial and intermediate squamous cells) are practically indestructible, and therefore, are not sensitive indicators of possible deleterious effects.
- Collecting fresh effusions in heparinized containers prevents clotting that can interfere with efficient cytopreparation. At many institutions, Department of

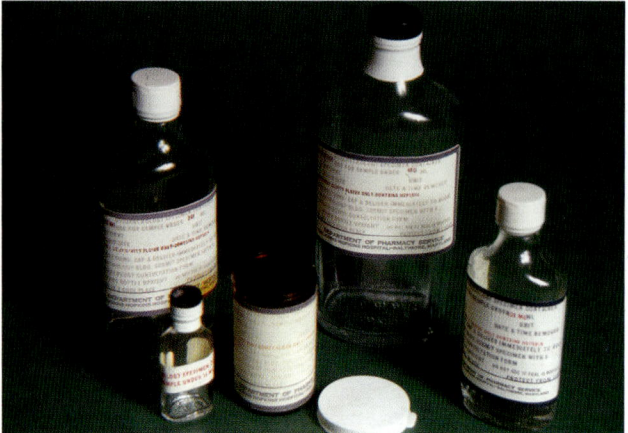

Figure 6.16 Heparinized bottles in four sizes.

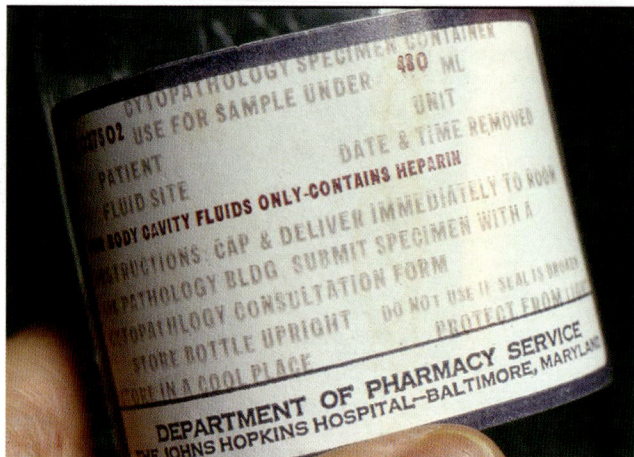

Figure 6.17 Close-up of label on heparinized bottle.

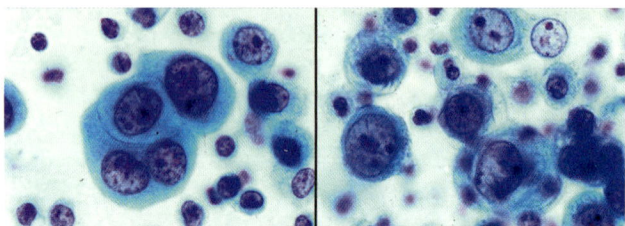

Figure 6.18 Fresh vs. 5-day-old body cavity fluid.

Pharmacy Service prepares specimen containers in different capacities with three units of heparin per cc capacity (Figure 6.16).

- A close-up of the label is shown in Figure 6.17. Details have been published.
- Suspensions of fresh non-gynecologic cytologic specimens can tolerate delays of at least 4 h from collection to cytopreparation and fixation. If longer delays are anticipated, the specimens can be safely refrigerated for up to several days (Figure 6.18).
- The absolute best way to learn what's happening to specimens during cytopreparation is to concentrate them by conventional centrifugation, re-suspend them in BES (balanced electrolyte solution) if fresh or in same preservative if preserved, and examine an unstained drop microscopically. Examine drops at subsequent steps as needed. Partially closing the substage condenser iris diaphragm will create a poor man's phase contrast microscope that will let you see all you need to see.
- Bloody non-gynecologic cell suspensions may result in a laboratory cytopreparatory technique-based false-negative result *unless* the red blood cells are removed prior to collecting the specimen on a slide. If, upon

microscopically examining a drop of specimen as described above, one sees a disproportionate imbalance of erythrocytes to nucleated cells, the erythrocytes will crowd out the nucleated cells and prevent their appearing in the preparation. In such cases, hemolyze the erythrocytes first. Saponin or glacial acetic acid can be used with fresh specimens, or commercial preservatives with hemolytic properties can be used for non-gynecological specimens (e.g. B-D TriPath's CytoRich™ Red Preservative or Cytyc Corporation's CytoLyt®).

If fresh non-gynecologic specimens are to be exposed to a salt solution (e.g. bronchial lavage, re-suspending a cell concentrate), do not use normal saline. Contrary to popular belief, normal saline is not physiologic. It destroys cells within seconds upon exposure (Figure 6.19). Instead, use a balanced electrolyte solution (BES) for in-vivo and in-vitro applications, or use a balance salt solution (BSS) such as Hanks for in-vitro applications only. Be aware that BES costs approximately twice as much as normal saline, and BSS approximately four times as much. Tables 6.2 and 6.3 summarize the properties of these solutions and the composition.

- At the author's first laboratory of employment, glass slides were coated with a thin film of albumin–glycerin to promote cell adhesion. Unfortunately, the cells adhered to the albumin and not the slide, and therefore rounded-up. The cells were stained impenetrably optically dense. Quantitative recovery was achieved at the expense of qualitative display excellence. Direct microscopic observation of cells as they were spread between two slides (i.e. the two-slide pull technique) revealed

Table 6.2 Properties of normal saline, balanced electrolyte solutions, and balanced salt solutions commonly used to collect, wash, or resuspend cells. Normal saline is sometimes referred to as physiological saline or isotonic saline, although neither alternative term is strictly accurate

Solutions	Properties				
	pH	Buffered?	Iso-osmotic?	Inorganic ion complement	Energy source
Normal saline	6.0	No	Yes	Unbalanced	None
Balanced electrolyte solution	6.0	No	Yes	Balanced	None
Balanced salt solution	7.4	Yes	Yes	Balanced	Glucose

Table 6.3 Properties of normal saline, balanced electrolyte solutions and balanced salt solutions commonly used to collect, wash, or resuspend cells. Balanced electrolyte solutions are sterile and pyrogen-free, which means the solution can be used in vivo and/or in vitro. Balanced salt solutions are sterile only, which means the solution can only be used in vitro. BSS were originally intended as a transfer medium for cells grown in culture. If injected into a human, BSS may induce fever in response to the pyrogenic particles that are present

No.	Ingredients (g/l)	Normal saline	Balanced electrolyte solution	Hanks' BSS
1	Sodium chloride	9.0	4.96	8.0
2	Sodium acetate		7.48	NA
3	Potassium chloride		0.746	0.4
4	Calcium chloride		0.368	0.14
5	Magnesium chloride • 6H$_2$O		0.305	0.1
6	Magnesium sulfate • 7H$_2$O			0.1
7	Disodium phosphate • 2H$_2$O			0.06
8	Monopotassium phosphate			0.06
9	Sodium bicarbonate			0.35
10	Dextrose			1.0

that round cells rolled along, squamous cells rolled-up like crepes, and neither configuration was able to make contact with the glass slide surface, adhere to it, and flatten. Those observations led to the following

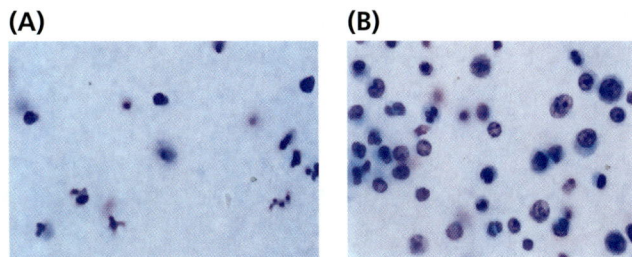

Figure 6.19 (A) Normal saline vs. (B) balanced salt solution.

modifications of the two-slide pull technique: (1) eliminate glycerin–albumin coatings, (2) use squeaky-clean slides (see next bullet), (3) apply a few drops of cell suspension so that the specimen does not spread spontaneously to the edges of the slides, (4) pull the two slides apart along their facing surfaces (in other words, do not lift them apart), one can feel resistance to pulling when done correctly, and (5) immediately immerse in fixative.

- When making cell spreads, first clean the slides by simply dipping in alcohol and wiping with cheesecloth to make them squeaky clean. It is convenient to keep a slide rack full of slides immersed in a covered staining dish of alcohol on the work bench, and clean the slides as needed. Simply wipe the slides dry with cheesecloth. Apply the cells to the slide as a very thin layer to promote contact with the glass surface, adhesion, and flattening. Using slides cleaned this way, the author never had to resort to using slides coated with poly-L-lysine or silane. Poly-L-lysine-coated slides are commercially available and routinely used for specimens submitted for special staining procedures.

- Negative pressure when applied in cell collection using membrane filtration is rarely used nowadays – although none the less valuable in the right hands – and centrifugal force applied during cytocentrifugation promotes constructive cell flattening.

- Immerse cell spreads into fixative rapidly, not slowly. Slow immersion creates alternating bands of cellular and acellular areas that Naylor characterized as a "ribbing effect" (Figure 6.20).

- Although seldom used today, Carnoy's fixative will hemolyze erythrocytes in bloody cell spreads. Such spreads should remain immersed in Carnoy's for no longer than approximately 30 min. Longer exposure shrinks cells excessively, causing them to round-up and become smaller in diameter and thicker. See Table 6.4.

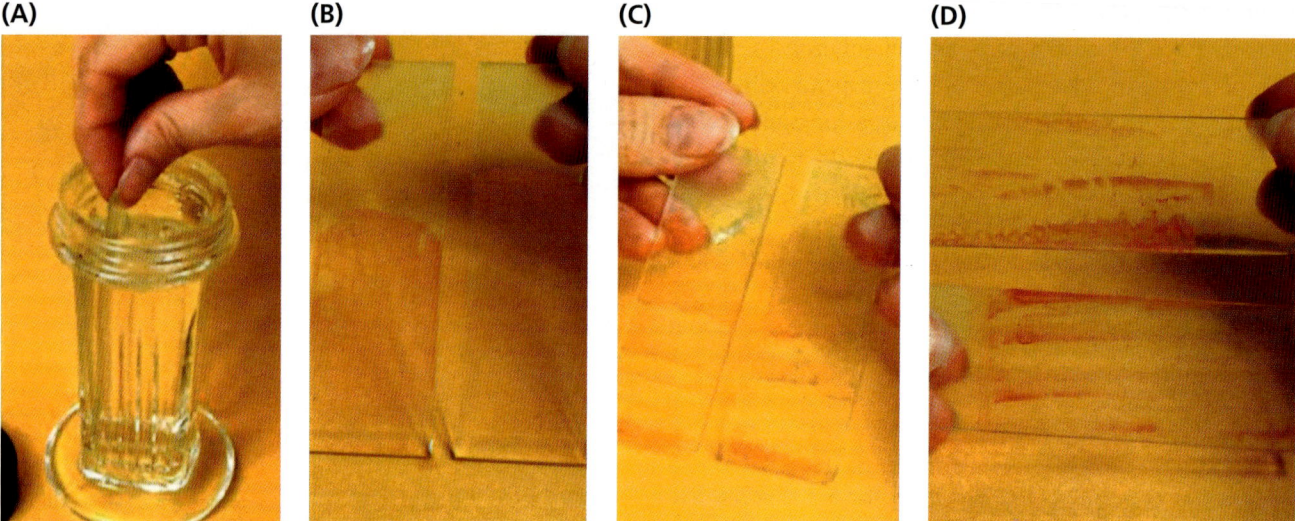

(A) **(B)** **(C)** **(D)**

Figure 6.20 Ribbing effect.

Table 6.4 There are three variants of Carnoy's fixative: (1) Clarke's, (2) Carnoy's, and (3) modified Carnoy's. Decreasing concentrations of glacial acetic acid mean increasing concentrations of alcohol, which chrink cells more. Thus, fixation should be limited to 30 min or less

Formulation	Parts by volume			
	95% Alcohol	Absolute alcohol	Chloroform	Glacial acetic acid
Clarke's fixative	–	3	–	1
Carnoy's fixative	–	6	3	1
Modified Carnoy's fixative	7	–	2.5	0.5

CONCLUSIONS

It is unknown why Papanicolaou chose ether:alcohol as a fixative. Alcohol is not widely used as a fixative in any applications other than diagnostic cytopathology. None the less, Papanicolaou established immediate wet-fixation of fresh cells in ether: alcohol – and later 95% ethanol alone – as the standard material and method of fixation, and the differences produced in nuclear morphology between benign and malignant cells, and all shades-of-gray in between are what we rely on visually to assess the differences. Alternative materials and methods of fixation that vary from the standard produce discernible differences. Those differences are acceptable as long as they do not contribute to misinterpretation of the biological significance relative to the health or disease status of the cells and their potential impact on patient care.

It is also unknown why fixation in alcohol elicits the microscopically visible differences in nuclear morphology among benign and malignant cells at a submicroscopic, molecular level. According to Baker, alcohol does not fix nucleoprotein, it precipitates it. If that is indeed the case, then differences in chromatin appearance may be due to larger pieces of stained nucleoprotein in abnormal cells being distributed in nuclear space more or less usefully and serendipitously in response to the details of the fixation method.

The criteria of cellular health and disease are nothing more than descriptions of cytomorphology that has been artifactually modified by fixation. As a result, fixation's materials, methods, and results are mutually dependent and consistent: the results we expect determine our materials and methods, and the materials and methods we use determine our results. Although such a relationship is obvious and inevitable, so stating it emphasizes the fact that the cytomorphologic changes on which we rely to signal cellular health and disease are not fundamental immutable features of cells in vivo.

Understanding the relationship among the various biological, chemical, mechanical, and physical factors that contribute to cytomorphology equips cytologists to better control the quality of their work, advise clinicians in the collection and handling of specimens, and troubleshoot the causes of unsatisfactory results. The uniformly high quality of cellular display that will result should promote interpretive accuracy and precision. Nature provides the starting materials, and man provides the finishing touches.

FURTHER READING

21 CFR Chapter 1 (4–1–08 Edition), PART 21 – FORMULAS FOR DENATURED ALCOHOL AND RUM, pp. 530–60. Available at: http://frwebgate1.access.gpo.gov/cgi-bin/PDFgate.cgi?WAISdocID= 397749409919±1±1±0&WAISaction=retrieve. Accessed July 18, 2008.

Anderson, T. F. (1955). "Electron microscopy of microorganisms". In: Oster, G. and Pollister, A. W., eds. *Cells and Tissues, Vol. III of Physical Techniques in Biological Research*. New York, NY: Academic Press, pp. 177–240.

Ayre, J. E. and E. Dakin. (1946). "Cervical cytology tests in cancer diagnosis: glycerine technique for mailing". *Canad Med Assoc* 54: 489–91.

Baker, J. R. (1966). *Cytological Technique – The Principles Underlying Routine Methods*, 5th edition. London, Methuen & Co. Ltd.

Baker, J. R. (1968). *Principles of Biological Technique – A Study of Fixation and Dyeing*. London, Methuen & Co. Ltd, reprint.

Beyer-Boon, M. E., M. J. van der Voorn-Den Hollander, et al. (1979). "Effect of various routine cytopreparatory techniques on normal urothelial cells and their nuclei". *Acta Pathol Microbiol Scand Section A* 87(1): 63–9.

Bonime, R. G. (1966). "Air-dried smear for cytologic studies". *Obstet Gynecol* 27(6): 783–90.

Carnoy, J. B. (1886). "Conférence donnée à la Société belge de Microscopie" *Cellule* 3: 1.

Clarke, J. L. (1851). "Researches into the structure of the spinal cord". *Phil Trans R Soc Lond* 141: 607–21.

DeWitt, S. H., R. R. DelVecchio, et al. (1957). "A method for preparing wound washings and bloody fluids for cytologic evaluation". *J Natl Cancer Inst* 19(1): 115–21.

Dey, P. (2005). "Chromatin pattern alteration in malignant cells: an enigma". *Diagn Cytopathol* 32(1): 25–30.

Freeman, J. A. (1969). "Hair spray: an inexpensive aerosol fixative for cytodiagnosis". *Acta Cytol* 13(7): 416–9.

Gill, G. W., K. A. Miller, J. K. Frost, et al. (1973). "Cytomorphological consequences of fixation methods other than ethanolic wet fixation". American Society of Cytology 21st Annual Scientific Meeting, Salt Lake City, UT, November 8, 1973 (platform presentation).

Gill, G. W. (1998). "Air-dried and rehydrated cervicovaginal smears are different". *Diagn Cytopathol* 18(5): 381–2.

Gupta, S., S. Pushpa, et al. (2003). "Rehydration of air-dried cervical smears: a feasible alternative to conventional wet fixation". *Obstet Gynecol* 102(4): 761–4.

Hajdu, S. I. (1983). "A note on the history of Carbowax in cytology". *Acta Cytol* 27(2): 204–06.

Hanks, J. H. and R. E. Wallace. (1949). "Relation of oxygen and temperature in the preservation of tissues by refrigeration". *Proc Soc Exp Biol Med* 71(2): 196–200.

Holmquist, M. D. (1978). "The effect of distance in aerosol fixation of cytologic specimens". *Cytotechnol Bull* 15(2): 25–7.

Kirby, J. P. (1976). "The effects of different fixatives and fixation methods on cell areas". The Johns Hopkins Hospital School of Cytotechnology, Baltimore, MD, June 29, 1976 (student thesis, Gill, G. W. and Erozan, Y. S., advisors).

Manosca, F., M. Schinstine, et al. (2006). "Diagnostic effects of prolonged storage on fresh effusion samples". *Diagn Cytopathol* 35(1): 6–11.

Mikat, K. W. and D. M. Mikat. (1972). "Tissue flattening – a method of enhancing histologic detail". *Lab Med* 7(3): 41–2.

Nasuti, J. F., S. R. Fleisher, et al. (2000). "Semiquantitative analysis of the cellular preservation quality of Normosol® and Carbowax® solutions for thyroid fine-needle aspiration specimens". *Diagn Cytopathol* 22(5): 319–22.

Naylor, B. (1958). "The elimination of a 'ribbing' effect observed in cytologic smears". *Am J Clin Pathol* 30(2): 143–4.

Overman, R. R. and C. M. Pomerat. (1956). "Electrolytes and plasma expanders. I. Reaction of human cells in perfusion chambers with phase contrast, time-lapse cine records". *Z Zellforsch Mikrosk Anat* 45(1): 2–17.

Pundel, J. P., C. D. A. Ferreira, et al. (1957). "Experiences with various methods of fixation of smears". *Acta Cytol* 1: 62–9.

Randall, B. and L. van Amerongen. (1997). "Commercial laboratory practice evaluation of air-dried and rehydrated cervicovaginal smears vs. traditionally-fixed smears". *Diagn Cytopathol* 16(2): 174–6.

Roffe, B. D., F. H. Wagner, et al. (1979). "Heparinized bottles for the collection of body cavity fluids in cytopathology". *Am J Hosp Pharm* 36(2): 211–4.

Saccomanno, G., R. P. Saunders, et al. (1963). "Concentration of carcinoma or atypical cells in sputum". *Acta Cytol* 7: 305–10.

Sagi, E. S. and L. L. Mackenzie. (1957). "The use of acetone in exfoliative cytological studies". *Am J Obstet Gynecol* 73(2): 437–9.

Stockard, C. R. and G. N. Papanicolaou. (1917). "The existence of a typical oestrous cycle in the guinea-pig – with a study of its histological and physiological changes". *Am J Anat* 22: 225–83.

Umlas, J. (1972). "Preparation of bloody specimens for cytologic examination using saponin". *Acta Cytol* 16(2): 186–8.

Watson, P. (1966). "A slide centrifuge: an apparatus or concentrating cells in suspension onto a microscope slide". *J Lab Clin Med* 68(3): 494–501.

Waymouth, C. (1970). "Osmolality of mammalian blood and media for culture of mammalian cells". *In Vitro* 6(2): 109–27.

Wolman, M. (1955). "Problems of fixation in cytology, histology, and histochemistry". *Int Rev Cytol* 4: 79–102.

Yang, G. C. H. (1994). "The mathematical basis for the increased sensitivity in cancer detection in air-dried cytopreparations". *Mod Pathol* 7: 681–4.

7 ANCILLARY TECHNIQUES APPLICABLE TO CYTOPATHOLOGY

Classical pathomorphology (as presented in the preceding chapters) relies on a basic principle: the nucleus reveals whether a cell is benign or malignant, whereas the cytoplasm and the cells architectural arrangements hold the clues to the cell's origin and the direction of its differentiation. However, even the combined power of pattern recognition and individual cell morphology may fall short of achieving these goals. Nuclear changes indicative of malignancy may be obvious in one case, but missing in another. Some malignant cells, for example those of mesothelioma, have deceptively bland nuclei and are best recognized by a combination of their associated clinical data, morphological phenotype, and immunoprofile. Poorly differentiated neoplasms may offer no phenotypical clue as to the cell type involved.

Ancillary studies may assist further in elevating the precise nature of the lesion in such cases. These have evolved over the past 50 years and now include molecular analyses. The exact identification of cell populations in cytological specimens can be accomplished through: (1) special stains, with various reagents used in histochemical methods; and (2) immunological reactions, with a variety of antibodies that detect diagnostically helpful antigens either by immunofluorescence (IF) or immunohistochemistry (IHC). By far, IHC is the most widely used ancillary technique in the practice of pathology. Its main advantage derives from the limitation of IF, since IF does not permit the simultaneous visualization of a positive reaction and the morphological features of the sample under study. With IF, the reaction may fade over time, requiring image documentation.

MULTIMODAL APPROACH

One should follow a systematic diagnostic approach when selecting and utilizing ancillary techniques to interpret the various types of samples. *Clinical* data and the *cytomorphology* play a crucial role. The main utility of ancillary techniques resides in their ability to *confirm* and *establish* a specific diagnosis; to identify cell types correctly; to determine the site of origin of the neoplasm; to assist in therapeutic and prognostic decisions; or, at a minimum, to recognize the correct lineage of a given cell population. These must not be used for the primary diagnosis of a cancer. The logical approach to such diagnostic modalities is depicted in Table 7.1.

This chapter's purpose is to provide an overview of various ancillary methods in the study of small tissue and

Table 7.1 Systematic approach to cytological examination

(1) Clinical interaction	(4) Cytomorphological transliteration
History and physical	Cell group architecture
Laboratory results	Cohesive vs. isolated cells
Clinical impression	Intercellular relationships
Radiologic appearance	Extracellular matrix
Previous material	Criteria of malignancy
(2) Site and sample verification:	(5) Individual cell morphology
Knowledge of terrain	Cellular borders
Location of sampling device	N:C ratio
Adequacy determination	Cytoplasmic texture
Collection medium	Nuclear features
Triage of specimen	Nucleolar region
(3) Cell populations	(6) Multimodal techniques:
Character of background	Liquid-base preparations
Rich vs. poorly cellular	Electron microsocpy
Single vs. mixed	Special stains
Alien vs. native	Immunocytochemistry
Normal vs. abnormal	Flow cytometry
	Image analysis
	Molecular biology

Cytohistology: Essential and Basic Concepts, Prabodh Gupta and Zubair Baloch. Published by Cambridge University Press. © Cambridge University Press 2011.

cytologic samples. It is important to stress that the use of IHC to examine small samples has to be adapted with proper quality controls. The reported efficacy of IHC markers is usually based upon formalin-fixed and paraffin-processed tissue sections. As sophisticated as these methods have become, their use remains ancillary; they are no substitutes for classical morphology using impeccable methods for the collection, preparation, and routine staining of specimens. In essence, immunological techniques are used for the detection and localization of specific antigens within the cell. It is crucial to have a basic concept of the cell and its compartments at the ultrastructural level, even though electron microscopy is seldom used today.

ULTRASTRUCTURAL EXAMINATION

The degree of resolution of light microscopy is insufficient to evaluate the subcellular architecture of individual cells and their relationships to one another. Electron microscopy (EM) covers this gap and has a role in selected cases. The pathologist versed on ultrastructural architecture has a great advantage when interpreting cellular alterations with the light microscope. This knowledge is also crucial for the appreciation of immunocytochemical patterns of reactivity, an ironic development since IHC is the very technique that debunked EM from the daily practice of pathology.

Connected to the cell membrane, the cytoskeleton is responsible for the cell's shape. It supports the secretory apparatus represented by the endoplasmic reticulum and the various organelles involved in vital functions. Certain ultrastructural features are far superior to IHC in the recognition of cell types, as no "false-positive reaction" occurs at the ultrastructural level. The differential diagnosis between benign and malignant mesothelial cells and metastatic adenocarcinoma can be accomplished by both transmission (TEM) and scanning EM (SEM) with a great degree of accuracy. The observation of profuse, slender, and bushy microvilli with a length to diameter ratio greater than 15:1 is virtually pathognomonic for malignant mesothelioma. In contrast, the surface of adenocarcinoma cells contains only short and stubby microvilli (Figure 7.1).

The perinuclear distribution of keratin AE1/AE3 is clearly demonstrated by the presence of profuse intermediate filaments encircling the nucleus of neoplastic

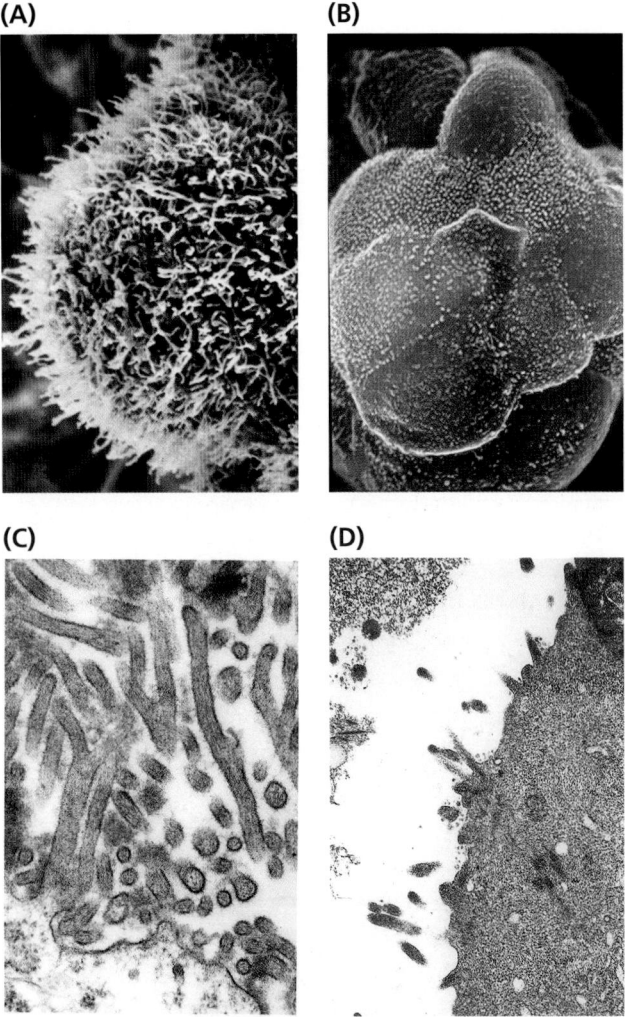

Figure 7.1 Contrast between cell surfaces of malignant mesothelioma (MM) and adenocarcinoma. (A) Florid and bushy microvilli in MM (SEM). (B) Flat surface (Frost's "community border") of breast carcinoma (SEM). (C) Long and slender microvilli in malignant mesothelioma (TEM). (D) Short and stubby microvilli in colon cancer (TEM).

mesothelial cells. The thick membrane pattern of epithelial membrane antigen (EMA) and other successor antigens is understandable by the trapping of antigen and antibody in the profuse, intertwined microvilli on the surface of mesothelial cells. The periphery of mesothelial cells also contains prominent, glycogen-rich submembranous vacuoles, which explain the peripheral PAS-positive vacuolization of mesothelial cells, removed by diastase reaction, indicative of glycogen accumulation. Positivity with the Alcian Blue stain can also be removed by hyaluronidase, attesting to the secretion of hyaluronic acid by neoplastic mesothelial cells. Cytoplasmic globs of hyaluronic acid can be visualized with EM and elucidate the presence of vacuoles in mesothelial cells. Giant desmosomes of tumor cells

(A) **(B)**

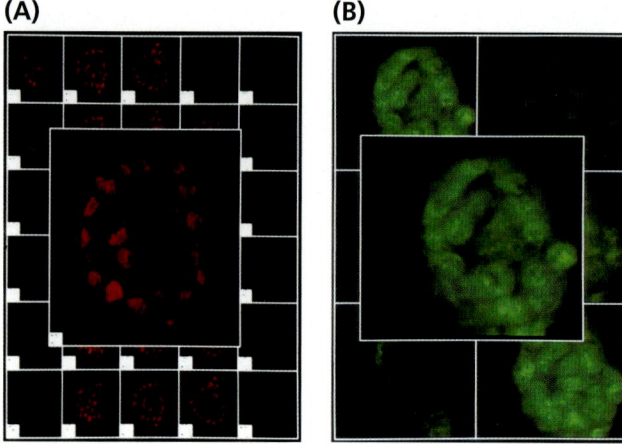

Figure 7.2 Confocal microscopy. (A) Malignant mesothelioma (MM) with wide intercellular spaces. (B) Adenocarcinoma with closely adherent tumor cells.

Table 7.2 Special stains applicable to the study of cell blocks or smears from the sediment of effusions

Stain	Substance demonstrated	Applications
PAS	Glycogen particles	Mesothelioma vs. adenocarcinoma
PAS-D	Muco-substances	Identification of adenocarcinoma
Alcian Blue	Acid muco-substances	Mesothelioma vs. adenocarcinoma
Alcian Blue-H	Hyaluronic acid	Identification of mesothelioma
Mucicarmine	Neutral muco-substances	Identification of adenocarcinoma
Grocott's	Capsule of various fungi	South American and North American blastomycosis
GMS	Wall of certain fungi	*Pneumocystis carinii*
Churukian's	Neuroendocrine granules	Identification of neuroendocrine differentiation

PAS-D: PAS with diastase digestion; Alcian Blue-H: Alcian Blue with hyaluronidase digestion

are additional ultrastructural features which support the diagnosis of mesothelioma in small specimens. The advantage of SEM resides in its ability to highlight the tridimensional architecture of cell groups. This can also be accomplished with confocal microscopy (Figure 7.2).

In neuroendocrine tumors, the typical double membrane of small, electron-dense secretory granules is a more reliable marker of these tumors than immunohistochemical reactions. Other reliable organelles that allow rather specific diagnoses include: pre-melanosomes in melanomas; racket-shaped Birbeck granules in Langerhans histiocytosis; lamellar bodies and Clara cell granules in so-called bronchioloalveolar carcinoma; excessive intracytoplasmic phospholipids in amiodarone toxicity; and florid extracellular phospholipidosis in pulmonary alveolar proteinosis. Add to these the characterization of the various storage diseases, the recognition of intranuclear viral particles, the demonstration of excessive organelles (e.g. mitochondria in oncocytoma and lysosomes in granular cell tumors) and one has a better appreciation of the role that EM may still play in the study of small tissue and cell samples.

HISTOCHEMICAL "SPECIAL" STAINS

The exact identification of various cell types in minute specimens can benefit from the use of: (1) special stains, mainly histochemical methods; and (2) immunochemical reactions, primarily by IHC and IF. By far, IHC has replaced histochemistry for the examination of small samples. IHC is the most popular ancillary technique in the practice of slide-based pathology. The decision to use IHC should be based on routinely stained preparations. Plus, IHC may not always demonstrate cellular components with diagnostic significance. Histochemical techniques tend to be helpful in selected situations. They have a role in diagnostic pathology, particularly in the recognition of infectious agents, lipids, glycogen, mucopolysaccharides, collagen, elastin, and glycoproteins (Table 7.2).

IMMUNOFLUORESCENT TECHNIQUES

Various antigens can be conjugated with a number of fluorescent molecules and used to detect their presence and localization in various tissues. Commonly utilized fluorochromes include fluorescein (green) and rhodamine (red). Owing to its small size and hydrophilic properties, fluorescein isothiocyanate (FITC) can demonstrate cytomorphological characteristics not detectable by other fluorescent molecules. Fluorochomes can be used for direct labeling of primary antibodies or to tag secondary antibodies which may increase signal detectability. For best results, the sample must be properly fixed using an agent that permeabilizes the cell membrane while still preserving the morphological integrity of the cell's cytoplasm. Organic solvents such as cold acetone and methanol fall into this

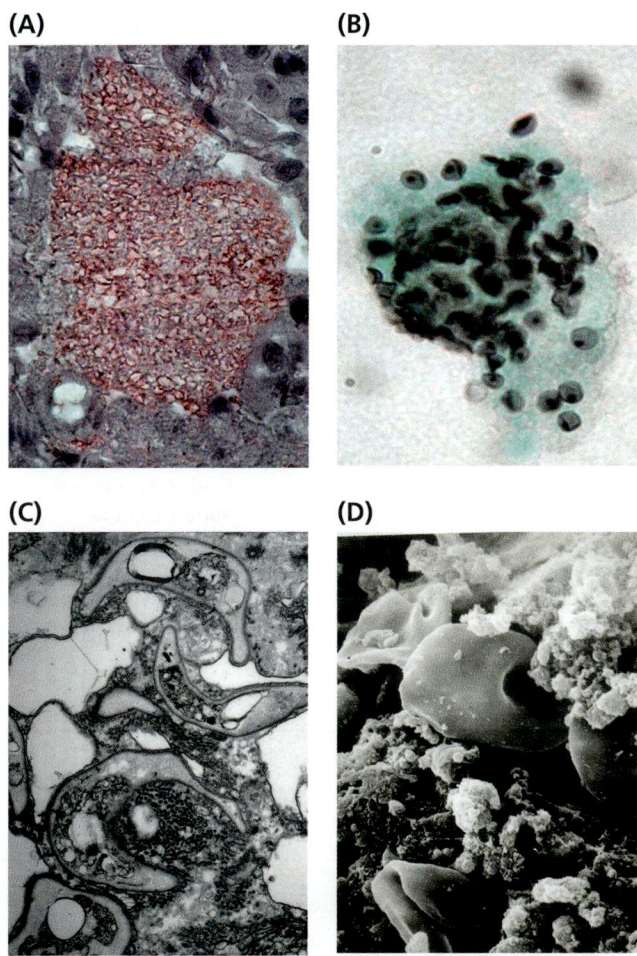

Figure 7.3 *Pneumocystis jiroveci* (PCP), in BAL. (A) Immunohistochemical stained foamy alveolar cast. (B) Organisms demonstrated with Gomori methanamine silver. (C) TEM with filopodia in their concave surface. (D) SEM showing hollow spaces responsible for foamy appearance by light microscopy.

category and are the preferred fixatives for slide-based IF study of samples.

As pathology may diagnose benign conditions, such as infections, the IF method is ideal for the rapid, reliable identification of microorganisms. A number of fungi, protozoa, bacteria, and viruses can be identified by IF, a procedure most often performed in the bacteriology laboratory. Certain fungi are autofluorescent, a property that can be used in their rapid diagnosis. The agent responsible for *Pneumocystis jiroveci* pneumonia (PCP) can be demonstrated in Pap-stained preparations examined under fluorescent light, with good correlation of methods that complement one another (Figure 7.3). A disadvantage of IF techniques, when compared to IHC, is the requirement of a special IF microscope not generally available in some pathology laboratories.

IF is ideally suitable for the analysis of cell suspensions either by flow cytometry or image analysis, particularly in the diagnosis and classification of lymphomas. Monoclonal antibodies bound to fluorescent dyes have affinity for cell surface markers that recognize clusters of differentiation (CD) at the exclusion of other antigens. The combination of expressed CD antigens can distinguish cell lineages, developmental stages, and functional subsets of the abnormal lymphoid cell population, and serves as the basis of classifying lymphomas and other hematopoietic malignancies. The CD-based immunoprofile of the lymphoma guides the clinicians in their choice of chemotherapy. To overcome IF's inherent inability to provide morphological information, one can take advantage of laser scanning cytometry (LSC). This technique combines the best features of flow cytometry and image analysis to produce both morphological appreciation and quantitative measurements of antigens expressed by the cell under scrutiny.

IMMUNOHISTOCHEMISTRY

IHC is a powerful tool; immunoperoxidase and the avidin–biotin techniques permit the simultaneous appreciation of cell morphology and the presence and distribution of various antigens. As such, this method can be helpful in a number of practical ways as listed in Tables 7.3 and 7.4. IHC can be applied to direct smears, cytospins, liquid-based cytology (LBC), tissue imprints, cell blocks, and small tissue biopsies from a number of anatomic sites. For cytology, the results are better in Papanicolaou-stained rather than Diff-Quik®-stained preparations. A crucial step for good results is the choice of fixative applied to air-dried smears and cytospins. These include alcohol, acetone, formalin, B5 and para-formaldehyde, and their choice depends heavily upon which marker is being investigated. In LBC preparations, cytoplasmic markers react as expected, but nuclear antigens are not as well detected as they are in cell blocks. Thus, most labs prefer to use formalin-fixed, paraffin-embedded cell blocks, and tissue. The methodology is adjusted for the marker being sought, as pretreatment influences the detection of various antibodies. Pre-treatment measures include: (1) proteolytic digestion via trypsin, pepsin, and other proteinases. This is a delicate step, as excessive digestion may result in the floating of the section or uneven distribution of the immunostaining; and (2) heat-induced epitope retrieval, via microwave irradiation or high temperature, using autoclaving or pressure-cooking the slide, which should be carefully de-paraffinized.

Table 7.3 Differential diagnosis of large cell neoplasms

	Poorly differentiated carcinoma	Germ cell tumor	Histicytic neoplasm	B-cell lymphoma	Melanoma	Sarcoma
CEA	+	+/−	−	−	−	−
EMA	+	−	−	−	−	−
Keratin	+	−	−	−	−	+/−
Vimentin	+/−	−	+/−	+/−	+	+
LCA	−	−	+/−	+	−	−
AFP	+/−	+	−	−	−	−
S-100	+/−	−	−	−	+	+/−
A₁AT/A₁ACT	+/−	+	+	−	−	+/−

AFP, alpha-fetoprotein; CEA, carcinoembryonic antigen; EMA, epithelial membrane antigen; LCA, leucocyte common antigen

Table 7.4 Antibodies useful in the study of non-epithelial neoplasms

Antibody	Applicable neoplasm
Vimentin	Mesenchymal tumors (general)
Keratin	Synovial sarcoma, epithelioid sarcoma
Desmin	Myogenous tumors (smooth muscle, striated muscle)
Myoglobin	Rhabdomyoma, rhabdomyosarcoma
Factor VIII-related antigen, Ulec europaeus agglutinin	Vasoformative tumors (excluding Kaposi's sarcoma)
a₁-Antitrypsin, lysozyme, a₁-Antichymotrypsin	Malignant fibrous histiocytoma
S-100 protein	Granular cell tumor, neurofibroma, schwannoma, clear cell sarcoma, malignant schwannoma, chondrosarcoma

Table 7.5 Common causes of false-positive and false-negative immunohistochemical reactions

False-positive	False-negative
Immuno-marker not as specific as originally believed	Non-representative sample (no tumor cells)
Neurotic debris, degenerated cells	Antigen expression below threshold detection level
Antigen phagocytozed by nearby macrophages	Antigen degeneration from delayed or improper fixation
Cross-reactive antibodies	Ineffective antigen retrieval
Ineffective blocking of peroxidose or biotin reaction	Unnecessary decolorization of Pap stain
Inappropriate specimen fixation	Antigen masking by over-fixation
Diffusion of antigen from normal cells	Thick preparations blocking antigen–antibody contact
Staining artifacts	Cell drying and other causes of desaturation
Too highly concentrated antibody	Too lowly concentrated antibody
Air-drying artifact	Lack of antigenic preservation due in defixation
Non-specific binding to background	

A growing number of antibodies assure the role of IHC in the study of small tissue samples. Cell blocks offer certain advantages, including (1) architectural detail; (2) tissue of the same cell population for multiple stains; (3) permitting comparison with results in surgical excision; (4) using standard protocols so that antibody reactivity is reliable and reproducible; and (5) standardized controls. It is important that cytological samples fixed in alcohol have proper quality controls slides. Table 7.5 lists the most common causes of false-positive and false-negative results in the application of IHC to cytological specimens.

CELL LINEAGE ELUCIDATION

In all mammalian cells the genotype residing in the nucleus pre-determines the protein biosynthesis in the cytoplasm, which is then reflected in the cellular phenotype. Although the nuclei of vastly diverse cell types may closely resemble one another, their active genetic make-up varies considerably and is biologically responsible for all cellular characteristics. Stem cells retain limitless biological pathways reflected in their potential for future differentiation into specialized cell types. As these cells are pluripotential, they may differentiate in a variety of directions, depending on the derepression of their regulatory mechanisms. During their neoplastic transformation, tumor cells may have multiple phenotypes, as carcinosarcomas and sarcomatoid carcinomas occur in various body sites and sarcomas may exhibit heterologous elements. The process of differentiation implies the gradual loss or restriction of these pathways, resulting in limited functional and morphological characteristics. Poorly differentiated cells are more primitive in their appearance so that their lineage is more difficult to discern by routine stains. Even a single cell population of undifferentiated cells can be further characterized by a combination of pattern recognition and appreciation of individual cell morphology, particularly when combined with appropriate immunophenotypic and genotypic studies, correlated with clinical findings. The first step in achieving this goal is to classify the cell population according to broad categories that facilitate their further subdivision into narrower subtypes. This classification of neoplasms includes at least seven different cell lineages with clinical significance: (1) hematopoietic; (2) melanocytic; (3) germ cell; (4) mesenchymal; (5) mesothelial; (6) epithelial; and (7) neuroglial. Once the cell lineage is defined, the tumor cell population can be further subclassified with the use of antibodies with more restricted specificity. Although this approach is potentially useful in any anatomic sample, it is most frequently applied to samples from serous cavities and fine needle and core biopsies with an abnormal cell population that defies initial classification.

HEMATOPOIETIC NEOPLASMS

Indications for lymph node fine needle aspiration (FNA) include the diagnosis of benign lymphoid proliferations, malignant lymphoma, metastatic non-lymphoreticular cancers, and infections. Benign proliferations and infections yield a heterogeneous cell population, which can be confirmed immunohistochemically as polyclonal. Special stains, including IF, aid in the identification of the offending microorganism. With metastates, a foreign cell population stands out from a background of lymphocytes. Such nodes can be assessed with an IHC profile obtained from a cell block preparation. In lymphomas, the diagnosis by FNA may be followed by an excisional biopsy if the FNA sample is insufficient for sub-classification. As such, when a lymphoma is suspected, additional tissue should be submitted for flow cytometry, molecular analyses, and cytogenetics, first to establish their hematopoietic lineage and clonality, and second to classify further the putative neoplastic proliferation. Direct smears for FISH analysis may be helpful. Antigenic substances that recognize hematopoietic differentiation are known as CD (clusters of differentiation) markers. CD-45 or Leucocyte-Common Antigen (LCA) can be considered a pan-hematopoietic marker that identifies the hematopoietic lineage. By cytomorphology, alone it is often possible to determine whether the lymphoma is a high-, intermediate- or low-grade neoplasm, simply by assessing the presence of predominantly small or large lymphocytes. When a malignant B-cell process is composed largely of cells with cleaved nuclei, a follicular lymphoma is likely and is usually CD-10 positive. Further characterization of a lymphoma can be obtained with an initial panel that classifies the neoplasm into main subtypes according to their cell-lineage differentiation. Non-committed hematopoietic stem cells express CD-34, terminal deoxynucleotidyl transferase (TdT) and HLA-DR. B-cell lineage markers include CD-10, CD-20, CD-19 and CD-22, whereas CD-2, CD-3 and CD-7 recognize lymphomas of the peripheral T-cell types. Thymocytes express CD-4, CD-8 and TdT, while CD-13 and CD-33 recognize the myeloid lineage of a lymphoid proliferation. B-lymphocytes mature into plasma cells, which can proliferate and give origin to plasma cell myeloma. These lesions, composed of monoclonal cell populations, are programmed to secrete a single type of immunoglobulin, with either kappa (K) or lambda (L) light chains. There are two important sub-types of end-stage T-lymphocytes, both of which can give rise to lymphomas, classified by their predominant CD expression. The helper-inducer T-lymphocyte expresses mainly CD-4; and the suppressor-cytotoxic T-lymphocyte expresses mainly CD-8. A third significant group of T-lymphocytes consists of "natural killer cells" (NK cells) and may be recognized by CD-7 and CD-56. The rapid, accurate, and precise diagnosis of lymphomas and their subtypes can be achieved by flow cytometry (Figure 7.4).

MELANOTIC TUMORS

Melanomas can be one of the greatest challenges in diagnostic pathology and are a major target of immunohistochemistry. Besides S-100 protein, other useful positive markers in the identification of melanoma include HMB-45, MART-1 and Melan-A. Melanomas are commonly positive for vimentin, but negative for keratin, desmin, Nuclear Factor (NF) protein, and GFAP (glial fibrillary acidic proteins). Cell membrane-associated glycoproteins

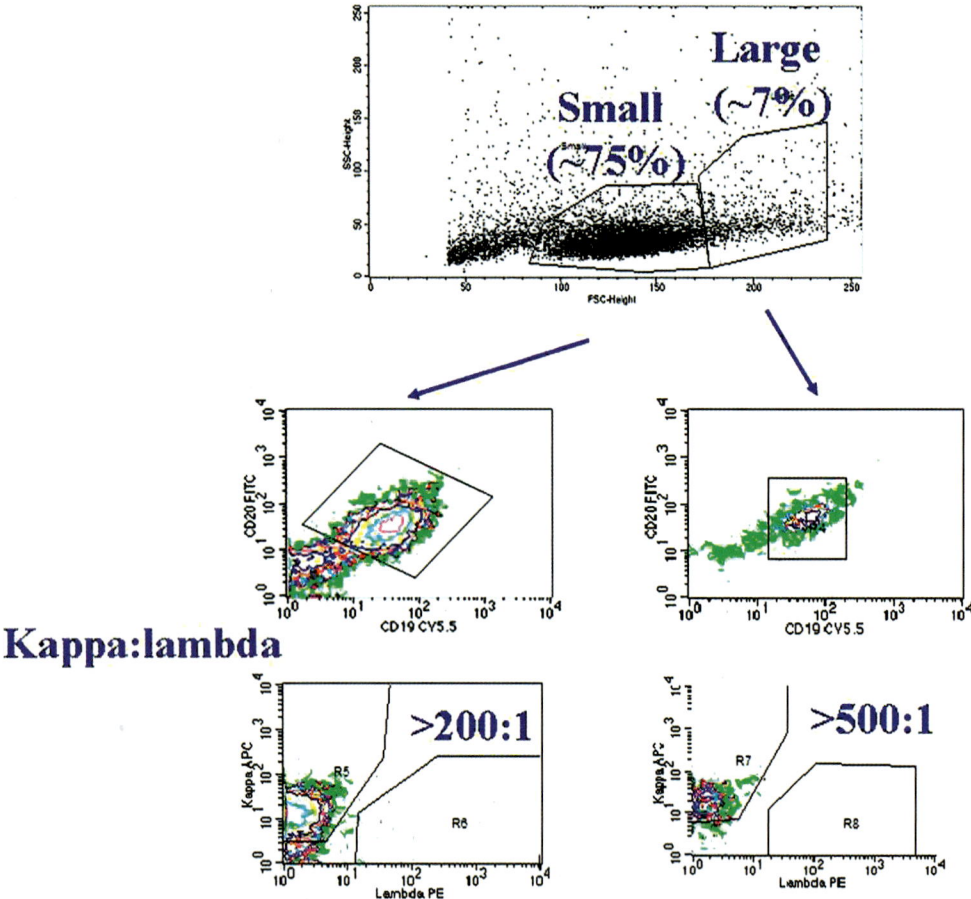

Figure 7.4 Flow cytometry analysis, small cell lymphoma. Lymph node FNA specimen collected in Normosol. Notice monoclonality for Kappa light chain. (Picture courtesy of Mariusz Wasik MD PhD, University of Pennsylvania, Philadelphia.)

CEA, EMA, TAG-72(B72.3), Ber-Ep4, and MOC-31 are absent in melanoma. Placental alkaline phosphatase (PLAP) positivity excludes melanoma and places the tumor in the germ cell category. Among the calcium-binding proteins, melanoma stains positively for the S-100 protein, but not for calmodulin or calretinin, which are useful in the study of mesothelioma.

GERM CELL TUMORS

Germ cell tumors (GCT) share antigenic characteristics with gonadal tumors and certain poorly differentiated carcinomas. A tumor of suspected germ cell lineage can be further classified based on its expression of certain serum tumor markers, with the caveat that poorly differentiated carcinomas must be excluded prior to accepting the tumor as either a gonadal or an extra-gonadal GCT. FNA of these tumors must include a number of FNA passes for adequate,

representative sampling, as mixed cell types often occur in the same neoplasm. All germ cell tumors are positive for PLAP, whereas alphafetoprotein (AFP) expression is almost exclusively confined to endodermal sinus tumor (yolk-sac tumor). Cytokeratins are usually negative in seminomas but positive in non-seminomatous germ cell tumors (NSGCT). In addition, (1) dysgerminoma and seminoma are positive for lactate dehydrogenase (LDH), OCT-3/4 (nuclear), D2-40 and CD-117 (c-Kit), but negative for EMA; (2) endodermal sinus tumor is positive for AFP and A1AT; (3) embryonal carcinoma is positive for OCT3/4 and CD-30; and (4) choriocarcinoma is positive for human chorionic gonadotrophin (HCG) and EMA. It should always be remembered that poorly differentiated carcinoma may ectopically secrete PLAP, AFP, HCG, and other GCT markers. Consequently, immunohistochemistry should be cautiously interpreted in concert with morphology and in light of clinical information, including the serum level of tumor associated markers.

MESENCHYMAL TUMORS

Sarcomas constitute a heterogeneous group of neoplasms that resemble mesoderm-derived tissues, although they do not necessarily originate from these tissues. These tumors can be classified according to their tissue differentiation pattern, which may be difficult to discern in FNA specimens or small tissue biopsies without the help of ancillary techniques. The clinical presentation and the radiographic pattern of the lesion play an important role in the diagnosis and classification of soft tissue lesions. Close cooperation between the pathologist and the individual performing the biopsy ensures that representative specimens are obtained for a variety of ancillary techniques, including cytogenetics, which is more important in the classification of soft tissue tumors than in the categorization of epithelial neoplasms.

No infallible marker exists to recognize mesenchymal differentiation. Although vimentin is positive in most soft tissue tumors, this antigen can be expressed by a number of carcinomas, melanoma, mesothelioma, and lymphomas. It is necessary to exclude other cell lineages in vimentin-positive neoplasms in order to classify soft tissue tumors into more specific categories. The sub-classification of sarcomas along differentiation pathways is not as crucial as the determination of their grade. Histologically, the degree of pleomorphism, the frequency of mitotic figures and the presence and extent of necrosis serve as the basis for grading soft tissue sarcomas. A greater number of translocations and other genetic alterations have been identified for various subtypes of sarcoma, especially in the pediatric age group. Once a benign, reactive process has been excluded, it is possible to classify a lesion according to its predominant cell population by the products that they elaborate. Soft tissue sarcomas that lack an obvious phenotype may be classified by their predominant cell population, including: (1) small round cells; (2) spindle cells; (3) epithelioid cells; and (4) pleomorphic large cells. Some of these tumors may be recognizable by their typical morphology. Most soft tissue neoplasms, however, require immunohistochemistry for their exact classification. This approach includes the study of soft tissue tumors with markers of restricted specificity, some of which may have diagnostic, prognostic, and therapeutic applications. Gastrointestinal stromal tumors (GIST) for instance express CD-117 (c-Kit) and respond well to chemotherapy with Gleevec (Figure 7.5).

A useful approach with non-epithelial neoplasms is to establish their reactivity to vimentin and keratin. In

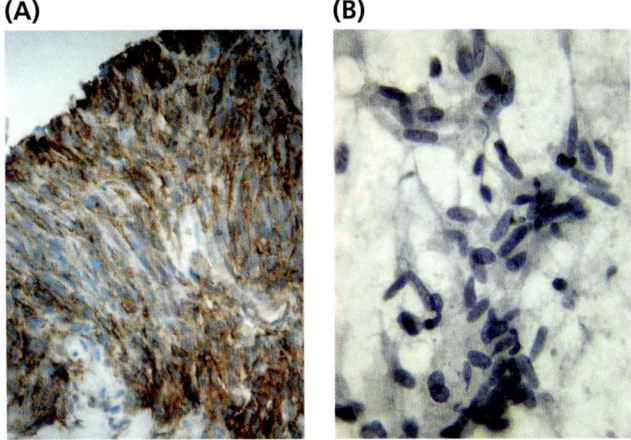

Figure 7.5 Gastrointestinal stromal tumor (GIST). (A) CD117 (cKit) immunostaining of a cell block. (B) Papanicolaou stain of FNA direct smear.

addition, a number of antibodies can then be applied to arrive at a more specific diagnosis. When dealing with soft tissue sarcomas, not only individual cell morphology but also the identification of substances in the extracellular matrix plays a significant role in their classification. These include: myxoid stroma in myxomas; chondroid matrix in cartilaginous tumors; osteoid in bone tumors; neurofibrils in neurofibromatosis; and free lipid in lipomas. None of these substances, however, are specific for any given tumor type, as soft tissue sarcomas may have heterologous elements in their composition.

Tumors defined by their cellular features. The classification of soft tissue tumors into cells that share the same size and shape is based upon the predominant morphology. However, this approach is very practical when considering the differential diagnosis of aspirates and small tissue samples with a predominant cell population. These include the following categories.

Small round cell tumors – this group of soft tissue neoplasms shares small, "blue" round tumor cells as their characteristic cell population. They occur typically in children and adolescents and include the following. (1) Embryonal rhabdomyosarcoma, a neoplasm that expresses desmin, HHF-35 (smooth muscle actin), myogenin, MYO-D1, and myoglobin (Table 7.6). (2) Extraskeletal Ewing's sarcoma, a neoplasm closely related to peripheral neuro-ectodermal tumor (PNET), with which it shares the t (11:22); (q24; q12) translocation. (3) PNET, a designation which includes a number of primitive small blue round cell tumors (SBRCT) that require clinical–pathological correlation for their identification, including neuroblastoma, retinoblastoma, medulloblastoma, ependymoblastoma, and

Table 7.6 Differential diagnosis of small blue cell tumors

Tumor category		NE	Ker	NF	Hormone	LCA	CD74/CD75	ACT	VIM
Neuroendocrine				−					
Epithelial	Carcinoid	+	+	+	+	−	−	−	−
	Intermediate	+	+	+	+	−	−	−	−
Neural	NE carcinoma	+	+	+	−	−	−	−	−
	Neuroblastoma	+	+	+	−	−	−	−	−
	Pheochromocytoma	+	+	+	−	−	−	−	−
	Paraganglioma	+	+	+	−	−	−	−	−
Non-neuroendocrine									
Lymphohistiocytic	Lymphoma	−	−	−	−	+	+	+/−	+/−
	Plasmacytoma	−	−	−	−	−	+	−	+/−
	Histiocytic	−	−	−	−	+	+/−	+	+
Mesenchymal	Wilms' tumor	−	−	−	−	+	+/−	+	+
	Ewing's sarcoma	+/−	+/−	−	−	−	−	−	+
	Rhabdomyosarcoma	−	−	−	−	−	−	−	+

NE, neuroendocrine marker; Ker, keratin; NF, neurofilament; LCA, leucocyte common antigen; ACT, antichymotrypsin; VIM, vimentin

pineoblastoma. (4) Desmoplastic small round cell tumor, a neoplasm characterized by well-demarcated nests of tumor cells surrounded by connective tissue. This tumor typically shows a reciprocal translocation t (11; 22), (p13; q12) associated with the chimerical EWS-WT1 gene fusion transcript. (5) Wilms' tumor, also known as nephroblastoma, comprises a mixture of blastemal, epithelial and spindle mesenchymal cells, sometimes with cross-striations. Yet, the tumor may also be monomorphous, with only undifferentiated blastemal cells. By flow cytometry this neoplasm may be near-diploid. (6) Polyphenotypic small round cell tumor is a rare neoplasm that can be positive for a variety of mesenchymal, epithelial, and myogenic markers and may also express neuro-ectodermal markers. Table 7.6 lists other neoplasms that share the SBRCT morphology.

Spindle cell tumors. As mentioned before, sarcomas with a predominance of spindle cells can appear remarkably similar morphologically, but run the gamut of the various mesenchymal cell lineages and include: (1) fibrosarcoma, a neoplasm that produces collagen but lacks a specific tumor marker. The close association of tumor cells with collagen is typical but not specific for this neoplasm. Most often, fibrosarcoma is a diagnosis of exclusion relying on clinicopathological correlation, such as a history of prior radiation; (2) leiomyosarcoma, when well-differentiated exhibits the smooth muscle phenotype, recognized by eosinophilic areas that correspond to the dense bodies at the ultrastructural level; (3) rhabdomyosarcoma may exhibit typical cross-striations or may be difficult to distinguish from leiomyosarcoma, as they are both positive for markers of muscle differentiation. However, myoglobin is positive only in rhabdomyosarcoma. A new marker, nestin, has been observed in poorly differentiated rhabdomyosarcoma. (4) High-grade liposarcoma may be recognized by the presence of rare lipoblasts that are positive with Sudan Black and Oil Red O lipid stains. (5) Peripheral nerve sheath tumors include schwannoma and neurofibroma. (6) Malignant peripheral nerve sheath tumors develop from pre-existing neurofibromas and carry the loss of chromosome 9p, along with the CDKN2 gene inactivation; tumors with both skeletal muscle and peripheral nerve components are known as Triton tumors. (7) Spindle cell angiosarcoma ranges from well-differentiated lesions which are positive for a number endothelium-related antigens, to markedly anaplastic tumors that may be positive for only EGFR-3. (8) Kaposi's sarcoma occurs in a number of clinical settings, such as chronic and Mediterranean, post-transplant, and long-standing lymphadenopathy, including HIV infection. This entire spectrum shares a similar phenotype including the positivity for vascular markers, including thrombomodulin. (9) Monophasic synovial sarcoma expresses CK-7 and occasionally, CK-19. These tumors may also express BCL-2 and demonstrate the t (X:18) translocation by FISH analysis. (10) Dermatofibroma (DF) is positive for factor XIIIa, but negative for CD-34.

This tumor requires careful interpretation of the immunostaining to ascertain that the factor XIIIa positivity occurs only in the lesional tumor cells and not in benign dermal fibroblasts. (11) Dermatofibrosarcoma protuberans gives results opposite to those in DF: negative for factor XIIIa and positive for CD34. Hemangiopericytoma (HPC) originally considered of pericytic origin, is now grouped with solitary fibrous tumor (SFT) with which it shares a striking immunohistochemical overlap. Markers frequently expressed in both entities include CD34 and CD99. (13) Solitary fibrous tumor (SFT) is a neoplasm of fibroblastic origin which may occur in any location, but is most frequently present in the subcutaneous tissue. While positive for CD34 and CD99, SFT negative for cytokeratin, S-100 protein and desmin. Immunohistochemistry is of limited value in recognizing benign, reactive fibroblastic/myofibroblastic lesions such as myositis ossificans, nodular fasciitis and proliferative myositis. They uniformly express vimentin, sometimes SMA and HHF35, but desmin is usually negative.

Epithelioid cell tumors – a number of soft tissue sarcomas contain polygonal-shaped tumor cells which may resemble epithelial cells. Since these tumors may co-express vimentin and keratin, they may be confused with metastatic carcinoma. Although cytomorphologically different, these tumors share a nearly identical immunoprofile with their spindle cell counterpart. This category includes: (1) epithelioid sarcoma (ES). ES tumor cells are positive for vimentin (peri-nuclear), cytokeratin (AE1/AE3), and EMA, CD-34, CD-31 and occasionally VE-Cadherin and CEA. Distinction of ES from a metastasis may not be achieved by immunohistochemistry, and requires careful clinico-pathological to avoid a misdiagnosis. (2) Epithelioid monophasic synovial sarcoma (EMSS) has an immunoprofile which recapitulates that of the polygonal cell element in biphasic synovial sarcoma. EMSS is positive for CD-99, EMA, Ber-EP4 and a variety of cytokeratins (AE1/AE3, CK-7, CK-8, CK-18 and CK-19); EMSS tumor cells are also positive for E-Cadherin and calretinin, which make their immunohistochemical distinction from malignant mesothelioma (MM) a most difficult task. This diagnostic dilemma can be resolved by the cytogenetic demonstration of the t(x; 18) (p11; q11) translocation and the molecular detection of the typical SYT–SSX fusion that occurs in EMSS but not in MM. (3) Epithelioid angiosarcoma expresses EMA and keratin (AE1/AE3), and vascular markers (CD-31, CD-34, UEA-I and Factor VIII-RA). This tumor may be confused with metastatic carcinoma since they also express the tumor-associated glycoprotein TAG-72, recognized by the B72.3 antibody. (4) Perivascular epithelioid cell tumor (PEComa) is positive for SMA and HMB-45. (5) Clear cell sarcoma (melanoma of the soft tissues). This tumor is invariably positive for melanocytic markers S100, HMB-45; and less consistently for Melan-A (Mart-1). Other positive markers include vimentin, CD57, and NSE. Variable results occur with c-Kit (CD117). (6) Epithelioid leiomyosarcoma (E-LMS), is positive for muscle markers, including desmin and SMA, but uniformly negative for markers of non-myogenic phenotype. (7) Alveolar soft part sarcoma (ASPS) is composed of epithelioid tumor cells with zonation, i.e. a granular perinuclear rim and a clear vacuolated periphery. Positivity for desmin, SMA, myosin, and z-band protein suggests myogenic differentiation. ASPS are often negative for myogenin and MyoD1. With the TPE-3 antibody it is possible to detect the (X; 17) translocation resulting in an ASPL 0150TPE3 fusion gene, diagnostic of ASPS.

Pleomorphic neoplasms – the most common pattern exhibited by soft tissue neoplasms consists of a mixed neoplastic cell population, including small round cells, spindle cells, large epithelioid cells, and multinucleated giant cells. Tumors in this category include: (1) malignant fibrous histiocytoma (MFH); some prefer the term pleomorphic undifferentiated sarcoma. MFH cells express antigens common to macrophages, e.g. CD68, alpha 1 anti-trypsin (A1AT), alpha-I-anti-chymotrypsin (A1ACT), and ferritin. If a putative MFH fails to express CD-68, an investigation may be in order as an MFH-like tumor may disclose evidence of a myogenic, neurogenic, or lipoblastic differentiation lineage. High-grade tumors that enter the differential diagnosis of MFH include pleomorphic rhabdomyosarcoma, high-grade leiomyosarcoma, high-grade malignant peripheral nerve sheath tumor, dedifferentiated liposarcoma, pleomorphic liposarcoma, angiosarcoma, metastatic carcinoma, extra-skeletal osteosarcoma, and malignant melanoma. IHC stains such as muscle-specific markers, S-100 protein, CD34, cytokeratin and HMB45, among others, are helpful in making MFH a diagnosis of exclusion. (2) Alveolar rhabdomyosarcoma combines immature small round cells with irregularly elongated "strap cells" (this could be considered a spindle cell tumor). (3) Pleomorphic rhabdomyosarcoma displays a more variegated cell population, which mimics that of MFH-like tumors. Both of these tumors express myogenic markers such as desmin, MSA, Myo-D1, myogenin, and myoglobin. However, only alveolar rhabdomyosarcoma displays cytogenetic abnormalities, such as a consistent t (2; 13) (q35; q14) translocation and a variant t (1; 13) (p36; q14) translocation. (4) Pleomorphic liposarcoma also resembles an MFH. Still, they may contain lipoblasts, are positive for S-100, and only rarely express CD-68; dedifferentiated liposarcoma resembles pleomorphic liposarcoma, except that it is clinically preceded by or includes simultaneously a well-differentiated liposarcoma lacking clear-cut pleomorphic features. These lesions may show cytogenetic abnormalities present in well-differentiated liposarcoma, including ring or giant marker chromosomes. Leiomyosarcoma, fibrosarcoma, and metastatic melanoma are additional tumors in the soft tissues that can rarely present with pleomorphic tumor cells, including multinucleated giant cells.

MESOTHELIAL PROLIFERATIONS

One of the most challenging diagnostic dilemmas can be the distinction between reactive mesothelial cells, malignant mesothelioma (MM), and metastatic adenocarcinoma. When properly collected and representative of the lesion with sufficient number of diagnostic cells, immunohistochemistry is very useful in elucidating the phenotypic identity of the cell populations at hand. If the phenotype is mesothelial, then the distinction between reactive mesothelial hyperplasia (MH) and MM is largely based on cytoarchitectural features in cytologic samples and on the pattern of invasion in tissues. Desmin and EMA are useful markers in distinguishing benign from malignant mesothelial proliferations. Desmin is preferentially expressed in MH, while EMA is preferentially expressed in MM. The combination of EMA negativity and desmin positivity favors MH over MM in cytological samples.

The distinction between MH and adenocarcinoma (AC) also can be difficult. Immunohistochemistry with a simple panel of calretinin, D2–40, desmin, and MOC-31 will distinguish between MH and AC. MOC-31 membranous reactivity occurs only in AC, it is negative in MH. Calretinin and D2–40 positivity in the nucleus and cytoplasm recognizes MH but can rarely be positive in the cytoplasm of AC. Desmin is also positive in MH but negative in AC, with the advantage that it is also negative in MM. A new antibody, GLUT-1, shows promise as a positive marker in MM but not MH. GLUT-1 cannot be used to distinguish MM from AC. Strong positive reactions for both p53 and Ki-67 favor MM (Figures 7.6 and 7.7).

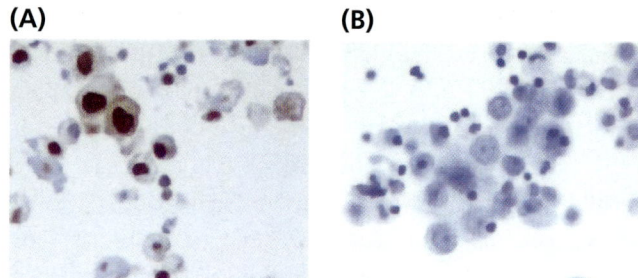

Figure 7.6 Proliferative markers of adenocarcinoma in pleural fluid. (A) Ki67 immunostaining of nuclei in cell block. (B) Lack of nuclear stain in liquid-based preparation.

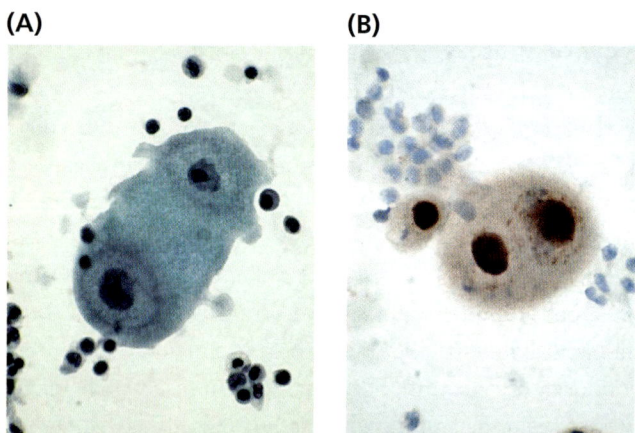

Figure 7.7 Expression of p53 in malignant mesothelioma. (A) Enlarged mesothelial cell with peripheral blebs, abundant two-tone cytoplasm and prominent nucleoli. (B) Despite bland cytological features, the nuclei of the tumor cells are positive for p53.

Tables 7.7 and 7.8 list a panel of biomarkers and ultrastructural features that are useful in making the distinction between MM and AC in histological sections and cell blocks. IHC should not be used at the expense of special stains, including PAS, PAS-D, mucicarmine, Alcian Blue, and Alcian Blue-H, which can differentiate between AC and MM in select cases, at a fraction of the cost of IHC. EM can also recognize MM and is considered by many the gold standard. MM is classified as epithelioid, mixed (biphasic) and sarcomatoid, according to the predominant cytomorphology present. Epithelioid MM is by far the most common type found in effusion specimens, but mixed and sarcomatoid MM may be sampled by FNA and core biopsies. A myriad of markers may assist in distinguishing AC and epithelioid MM. Our current preference for an initial immunoprofile includes the following antibodies, which are typically positive in AC but negative in epithelioid MM: CEA (monoclonal),

Table 7.7 Staining characteristics of mesothelioma and adenocarcinoma

Type of stain	Mesothelioma	Adenocarcinoma
Routine stains	Two-tone appearance with Papanicolaou stain	Homogeneously distributed stain
	Peripheral blebs with Romanowsky's stain	No peripheral blebs noted
Special stains	Cytoplasm contains PAS (+) digestible material	Glycogen content small
	Extracellular space contains Alcian Blue (+) material removable by hyaluronidase	No hyaluronic acid present in extracellular space

Table 7.8 Ultrastructural distinction between mesothelioma and adenocarcinoma

Location	Mesothelioma	Adenocarcinoma
Cell surface	Microvilli evenly distributed around entire cell	Microvilli concentrated at poles
	Slender bushy	Short stubby microvilli
	Microvilli	Glycocalyceal bodies noted
	No glycocalyceal bodies	
Cell junctions	Apical tight junctions	Terminal bars near lumen
	Well-developed desmosomes	Poorly developed junctions
Cytoplasm	Tonofilaments surrounding the nucleus	Irregularly distributed intermediate filaments
	Abundant glycogen	Variable amount of glycogen
	No secretory granules	Numerous secretory granules

Ber-Ep4, CD-15 (Leu-M1), MOC-31, and B72.3. In contrast, the following markers are usually positive in epithelioid MM but negative in AC: D2–40, beta-catenin (podoplanin), calretinin, CK-5/6, HBME-1 and WT-1. Depending on the differential diagnosis, antibodies specific for different types of carcinoma have to be added to the basic panel. Evidence-based criteria (EBC) have calculated the sensitivity, specificity, and post-test odds (PTO) for various putative antibodies that distinguish malignant mesothelial cells and exclude carcinoma cells according to their primary site of origin. The antibody panels that provide the best PTO for this purpose were different for male (calretinin, TTF-1, PSA, and CDX-2) and female (calretinin, TTF-1, ER, and CA125) patients.

Other antibodies can be used for other specific purposes, e.g. AE1/AE3 is valuable for determining the geographic distribution of epithelioid MM in a core biopsy, including invasion of the adipose tissue and the skeletal muscle of the chest wall. EMA with strong accentuation of the cell membrane favors epithelioid MM over MH, which may demonstrate a weakly positive membrane pattern. This is in contrast with AC, which exhibits cytoplasmic staining with EMA. Together, vimentin and AE1/AE3 positivity distinguish between sarcomatoid MM and a reactive fibrotic process.

EPITHELIAL NEOPLASMS

Carcinomas are one of the most common malignancies diagnosed in cytological specimens. Of the six main categories of neoplasms (carcinoma, sarcoma, mesothelioma, melanoma, lymphoma, and germ cell tumors), carcinomas comprise the single largest group of metastatic malignancies of unknown origin. It is no surprise, therefore, that a large number of immuno-markers have been developed for the diagnosis and classification of tumors with an epithelial cell lineage.

Main categories of epithelial neoplasms

Virtually all ectoderm- and endoderm-derived organ systems can produce epithelial neoplasms, which may remain undifferentiated or undergo further differentiation into four main types of epithelial tumors, classified according to the structures they form and the substances they elaborate: (1) adenocarcinoma, a gland-forming tumor that secretes muco-substances of various biochemical compositions; (2) squamous cell carcinoma, a solid tumor containing intracellular and extracellular keratins of different molecular weights; (3) neuroendocrine carcinoma, a tumor that secretes simple or complex polypeptides with neuroendocrine properties; and (4) undifferentiated carcinoma, which is often composed of large cells, without evidence of glandular, squamous, or neuroendocrine differentiation. An exact classification can sometimes be accomplished on purely cytohistological grounds utilizing routine stains. An initial cytohistological approach should provide a valuable preliminary impression of tumors without obvious differentiation. A differential diagnosis can be further refined by inexpensive special stains which should not be immediately ignored in favor of more costly and time-consuming ancillary techniques. Only after cytomorphology and special stains have exhausted their usefulness should IHC be utilized. In practice, however, intermediate filaments from the cellular cytoskeleton and glycoproteins secreted in the cytoplasm are the most common targets of immunostains.

Determinants of glandular differentiation

Glandular neoplasms can be identified by their contents of epithelial membrane antigens, cell adhesion molecules, and secretions including glycoproteins, polypeptides, and hormones. Adenocarcinoma, the most common of all cancers, is defined by its secretory capacity, a function that resides in the endoplasmic reticulum, the Golgi apparatus, and secretory vesicles which can coalesce and form vacuoles, visible by light microscopy. Muco-substances are the secretory products identified with mucus-producing adenocarcinoma. These tumors can be further categorized by their secreted muco-substances of variable viscosity, pH and chemical composition identifiable by special stains. Although essentially pathognomonic for adenocarcinoma, mucin production can also occur in non-epithelial neoplasms, e.g. myxo-papillary ependymoma.

Highly sensitive and specific markers for adenocarcinoma include: CEA (monoclonal or polyclonal), which identifies tumors of foregut derivation; in addition to BG-8, Ber-Ep4, B72.3, Leu M1 (CD-15), EMA, HMFG-2, E-Cadherin, and MOC-31 (Table 7.9). These are often used with varying molecular weight cytokeratin antibodies.

Markers of squamous differentiation

Squamous cells have a well-defined cytoskeleton, particularly rich in cytokeratins of various molecular weights. As accurate as these and other markers are, one should not interpret IHC results only as positive or negative. The distribution or pattern of the immunostaining reaction is very useful and reliable in conjunction with the morphological features. For instance, cytoskeletal proteins share the physical space with other organelles and are responsible for the foamy distribution of the rough endoplasmic reticular (RER) within the cytoplasm. Thus, the fluffy cytoplasmic texture of a secretory cell should be appreciated together with its positivity for any secretory marker. This is in contrast with the coarse and distribution of IF immune-positivity noted in all cell types. Likewise, the

Table 7.9 Metastatic workup applicable to FNA and other cytologic specimens

Primary neoplasm	Immunodiagnostic markers	Ultrastructural features
Lymphoma	CD45, CD3, CD10, CD30	No cell junctions, no surface specifications
Prostate	PSA, PAP	Short microvilli, abundant organelles
Thyroid	Thyroglobulin, calcitonin, CEA	Complex nuclear contours, electron-dense granules
Breast	Lactoalbumin, estrogen receptors	Intracytoplasmic lumina
Lung	CEA, surfactant apoprotein	Fluffy granules, lamellar bodies
Kidney	Secretory piece, URO series	Glycogen granules, lipid droplets
Liver	AFP, HbsAG, A1AT, CEA	Bile canaliculi, bizame mitochondria
Pancreas	Du-Pan 2	Small secretory granules, short microvilli
Ovary	OC-125	Peripheralized secretory granules, abundant microvilli

perinuclear distribution of the immunostaining and the dense texture of the cytoplasm of a keratinized cell are as much an indicator of its squamous differentiation as is its mere positivity for a pan-cytokeratin antibody. IHC is reflective of the underlying fine structure of the cell.

Intermediate filament proteins

These are classified on a biochemical and functional basis into five distinct types, all of which have diagnostic applications: keratins, vimentin, desmin, neurofilament proteins (NFP), and glial fibrillary acidic proteins (GFAP) (Table 7.10). Lamins, on the other hand, are nuclear envelope proteins, responsible for the shape of the nuclear membrane. Keratin and vimentin are widely used to recognize epithelial and mesenchymal differentiation, respectively. In addition, tumors can co-express keratin and vimentin, so that keratin-positive sarcomas and vimentin-positive carcinomas are recognizable phenotypes, useful in the identification of certain tumors. A keratin cocktail with antibodies against low and high molecular weight keratin recognizes most carcinomas, not only the squamous cell variety. A large number of keratin subtypes exist, which can be grouped according to their molecular weight and have wide application in the study of specimens. Although single keratin subtypes seldom if ever

Table 7.10 Intermediate filaments of diagnostic interest in cytopathology

IF class	Protein component and molecular weight	Occurrence in cells	Expression in tumors
1. Epithelial	Keratins (40 kDa (NF), 68 kDa)	Keratinizing and non-keratinizing epithelium	Carcinomas, some sarcomas
2. Neuronal	Neurofilament (68 kDa, 106 kDa, 200 kDa)	Neurons (CNS), peripheral nerve	Neuroblastoma, neuroendocrine carcinomas
3. Glial	GFAP (55 kDa)	Astroglial elements extra-CNS cells (i.e. salivary gland)	Astrocytotomas, pleomorphic adenomas
4. Muscular	Desmin (53 kDa)	Sarcomeric muscle (smooth, striated, cardiac)	Leiomyosarcoma, rhabdomyosarcoma
5. Mesenchymal	Vimentin (57 kDa)	Fibroblasts, chondrocytes, macrophages, endothelial cells	Sarcomas, some carcinomas

GFAP, glial fibrillary acidic protein

can be considered a specific tumor marker, combinations of two or more types can aid in the recognition of certain neoplasms. In particular, the combined use of CK-7 and CK-20 has emerged as a useful tool in the recognition and classification of epithelial tumors that share morphological features.

Desmin is very useful in the recognition of neoplasms that differentiate as smooth muscle. It can also occur in other tumors, such as malignant mesothelioma, desmoid tumor of the pleura, GIST, and pediatric SBRCT. NFP antibodies recognize tumors of both central and peripheral nervous system origin. They are very useful in neuropathology as well as in the classification of spindle cell sarcomas of unknown origin and the classification of neoplasms in the pediatric age group. Besides their helpful application in tumors of the central nervous systems, GFAP is also positive in pleomorphic adenoma, GIST, certain skin tumors, and lesions of the Creutzfeldt–Jacob disease. Interpretation of GFAP reactions, however, may be challenging, given its cross-reactivity with certain keratin antibodies.

Tumors with neuroendocrine differentiation

Neuroendocrine antibodies can be directed at all phases of the metabolic process involved in the elaboration of neuroendocrine substances. Thus, there are antibodies against enzymes (NSE), synaptic vesicle proteins (synaptophysin), contents of the neuroendocrine granule (chromogranin, secretogranin), genes associated with the neuroendocrine pathway (NP-Y, MOPC), neuroendocrine gene products (bombesin, other polypetides, and hormones), and neural cell adhesion molecules (CD-56). Of these, NSE has limited application due to its non-specific expression in non-neuroendocrine neoplasms. Synaptophysin is very reliable

in poorly differentiated neuroendocrine carcinomas, such as small cell lung cancer (SCLC), whereas chromogranin works best in well-differentiated neuroendocrine tumors such as carcinoid and pancreatic endocrine neoplasms. End-product hormones are useful in the sub-classification of tumors from the pituitary gland and the recognition of ectopic hormonal secretion in neuroendocrine carcinomas of the lung.

SITE-SPECIFIC MARKERS: IN SEARCH OF THE PRIMARY SITE

There are only a handful of immunomarkers which are specific for the site of origin of an epithelial neoplasm (Table 7.11). The combined use of CK 7 and CK 20 is helpful in narrowing the possible primary sites of metastatic tumors of unknown origin. Still, more precise recognition can be achieved with additional site-specific markers (Table 7.12).

FLOW CYTOMETRY AND IMAGE ANALYSIS

The IF technique is the backbone of quantitative morphology. Using cell suspensions as the target specimen and flow cytometry as the detection system, IF tags allow the quantification of antigen concentration within tumor cells, which can also be accomplished via image analysis. Flow cytometry and image analysis favorably combine the advantages of quantitation and automation. Table 7.13 compares flow cytometry (FC) to image analysis (IA) for the characterization of tumor cell populations. Although these methods are used primarily in tumors of the

Table 7.11 Combined expressions of cytokeratins 7 and 20 in carcinomas and mesotheliomas

	CK7 positive	CK7 negative
CK20 positive	Pancreas and biliary tract (2/3)	Colon and rectum
	Stomach (1/3)	Stomach (1/3)
	Ovary (mucinous)	Merkel
	Transitional cell carcinoma (2/3)	
CK20 negative	Epithelioid malignant mesothelioma (2/3)	Epithelioid malignant mesothelioma (1/3)
	Breast	Prostate
	Lung (adenocarcinoma)	Stomach (rare)
	Ovary (serous and endometrioid)	Hepatocellular carcinoma
	Pancreas and biliary tract (1/3)	Renal cell carcinoma
	Stomach (rare)	Adrenal carcinoma
	Endometrium	Squamous carcinoma
	Salivary gland	Lung (small-cell carcinoma)
	Thyroid gland	
	Transitional cell carcinoma (1/3)	

Table 7.12 Keratin antibodies according to molecular weights recognized

	Molecular weight recognized		
Antibody	Low	High	Antigenic source
AE1	40–48–50	51–56.5	Keratin from callus
AE3		58–65–67	Keratin from callus
CAM 5.2	39–43– 0	–52	Colorectal carcinoma
PKK 1	41	54–56	Kidney cell line
35 BH11	45	52	Hepatocellular cancer
34 BE12		57–66	Epidermis

hematopoietic system, considerable progress has been made in the study of solid tumors in the past few years.

Flow cytometry

FC has evolved into the benchmark for the diagnosis and the classification of lymphoid cell proliferations, including lymphomas and leukemia. It is an indispensable tool in their study. The diagnosis of lymphoma requires the correlation of morphology and cell surface antigen analysis by flow cytometry. FC is more sensitive than cytomorphology

Table 7.13 Comparison between flow cytometry and image analysis

Feature	Flow cytometry	Image analysis
Basis of analysis	Fluorescence and/or light scanner	Morphology and/or cell markers through transmitted light (absorbance)
Special preparation	Single cell suspension	Cytocentrifuge preparation, imprints, fine needle aspirates, tissue sections (frozen paraffin-embedded)
Morphologic correlation	Absent	Present and will facilitate the identification of specific cells of interest
Morphometry	Limited to light scatter measurement (size, granularity)	Large numbers of direct and derived morphometric parameters

and image analysis, permitting the detection of abnormal cells in the low range (1:1000 to 1:10 000) of concentration. As the results are expressed in quantitative terms, the method provides prognostic data as well as information for therapeutic monitoring. FC permits the determination of clonality, cell lineage, and the specific phenotype of lymphoid proliferations. In solid tumors, FC is used for the measurement of DNA in a large number of abnormal cells, which presumably represent a single tumor cell population. Aneuploidy is considered a reliable sign of malignancy in urinary bladder washings; tetraploid tumors behave worse than diploid tumors, whereas aneuploid tumors are biologically the most aggressive, with frequent high grade and a greater incidence of metastases. Multicolor FC can also be used for cell lineage determination and tumor phenotype identification in cytological samples. The combination of CD45 and Ber-Ep4 discriminates between large-cell lymphoma and carcinoma. Other combinations of markers can be used for the exact classification of solid tumors (Figure 7.8).

Image analysis

With automation, digital IA has been used to quantify characteristics of cells and their components, including: (1) cellular area, volume, and mass; (2) cellular components: nucleus, cytoplasm, and N:C ratio; (3) DNA content, including distribution (chromosome configuration) and quantification (DNA ploidy); (4) antigenic content, including cell surface receptors, tumor markers, and

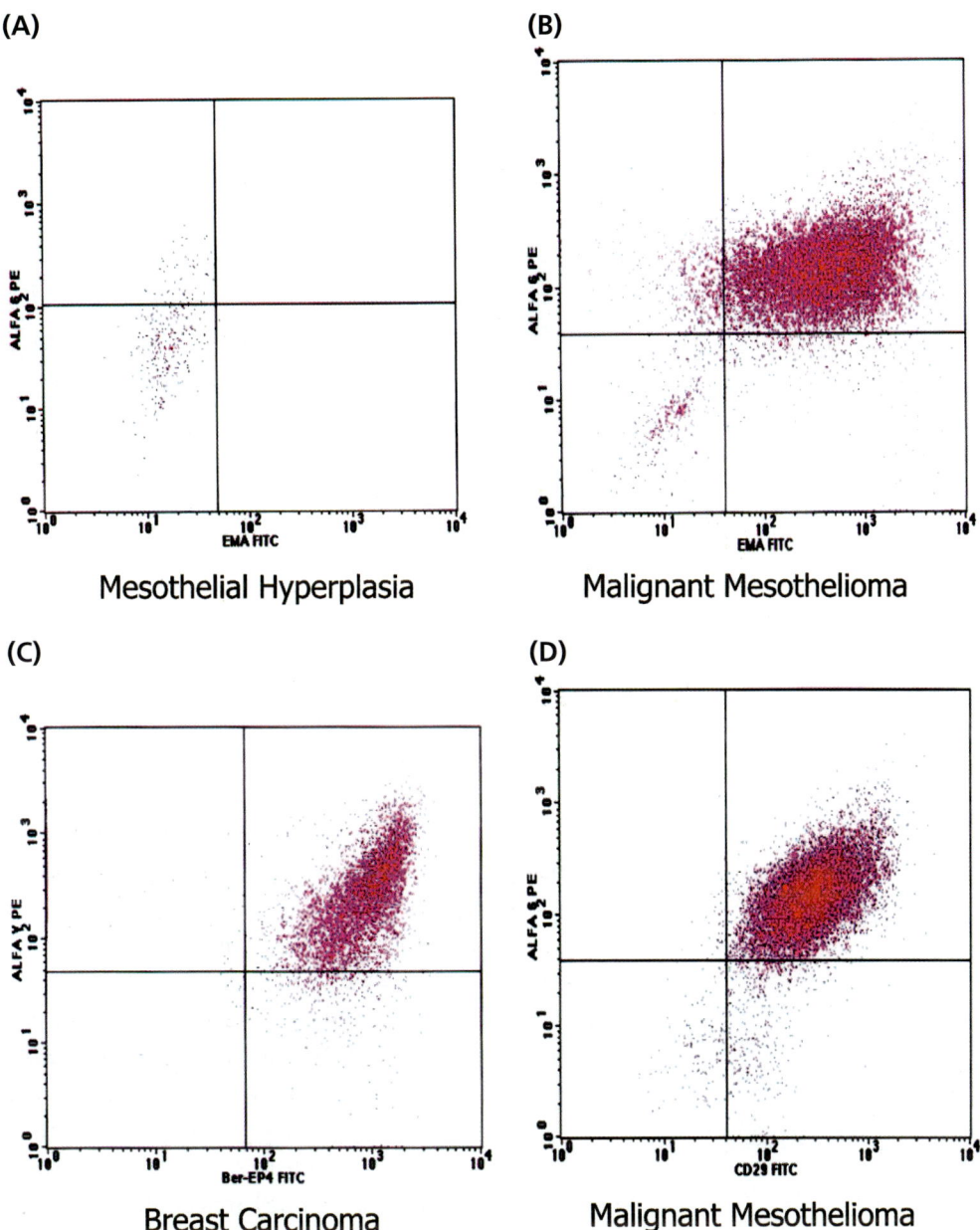

Figure 7.8 Flow cytometric analysis solid tumors. (A) Few EMA-stained cells in mesothelial hyperplasia. (B) Large numbers of EMA-positive cells in malignant mesothelioma. (C) BerEp4-positive cells in breast carcinoma. (D) FITC-labeled CD29 (Integrin B-1 chain) antibody in malignant mesothelioma.

phenotypic determinants. Cellular epitopes can be labeled with fluorescent molecules of chromatic dyes and their amount can be quantified in computerized systems. Thus, not only the detection of the presence, but also the amount of a given target substance, for instance, ER and PR, can be quantified in a computerized image analysis system. Although slower than FC, IA requires fewer cells and can be applied to slide-based tissue or cell block preparations. The method provides qualitative as well as quantitative data simultaneously, a great advantage with diagnostic,

prognostic, and therapeutic implications. Clinically relevant markers that can be measured by image analysis include: hormone receptors, such as ER/PR; prognostic markers, such as HER 2; proliferative factors, such as Ki-67; C-Kit (CD-117) MYC gene and EGFR in lung cancer; and the CDKN2 gene. The nuclear affinity for the Feulgen reagent can also be quantified by IA for the determination of DNA ploidy. The digital IA of comparative genomic hybridization (CGH) or chromosomal microanalysis (CMA) data, comparing a specific patient's genomic map to that of a bank of various tumors, is a powerful tool, as it allows the prediction of tumor behavior, natural history, and possible response to treatment modalities, including targeted molecular therapies. The technique includes the separate steps of image acquisition, processing, analysis, and interpretation, each with its own challenges in clinical practice. Laser scanning cytometry (LSC) combines flow cytometry and image analysis for the simultaneous cytomorphological characterization and the quantitative assessment of a given cell population. It can be used for the evaluation of hypocellular samples, unsuitable for conventional FC. LSC closely parallels IHC as it is slide-based and demonstrates cytological abnormalities. The method has the advantage of providing objective quantitation of antigen concentration, rather than the subjective grading of positive reactions (+ to ++++) or the semi-quantitative estimates of positive cell percentages. Applications of the digital IA include the analysis of IHC tissue arrays and the analysis of DNA and RNA micro-arrays at the cellular level. The use of digital imaging also renders itself to virtual pathology that allows the interactive sharing of expertise, including offsite consultations and extension of diagnostic services to geographically remote locations. Training of cytotechnologists and residents can also benefit from a remote broadcast of digitally acquired images of tissues and cells.

MOLECULAR ANALYSIS

This is the study of cell biology at the genetic and molecular level. This section is an overview of the methods and comment on their current and potential applications in diagnostic pathology.

Cancer cells evolve clonally from a single cell as the result of specific mutations (changes in DNA sequence) that affect basic cell processes leading to the detection of abnormal substances not expressed in benign cells. Normal cell differentiation is altered in cancer, so that poorly differentiated or undifferentiated tumor cells allow for their recognition as a malignant population. Cancer cells lose the ability to control cell proliferation, so that proliferative markers can be used in the separation between a reactive and a neoplastic process, with the caveat that a certain overlap occurs between these two processes. In general, an accumulation of mutational events leads to cancer, and malignant cells thus have high levels of genomic instability (rearrangements in chromosomes) which can be detected by cytogenetics.

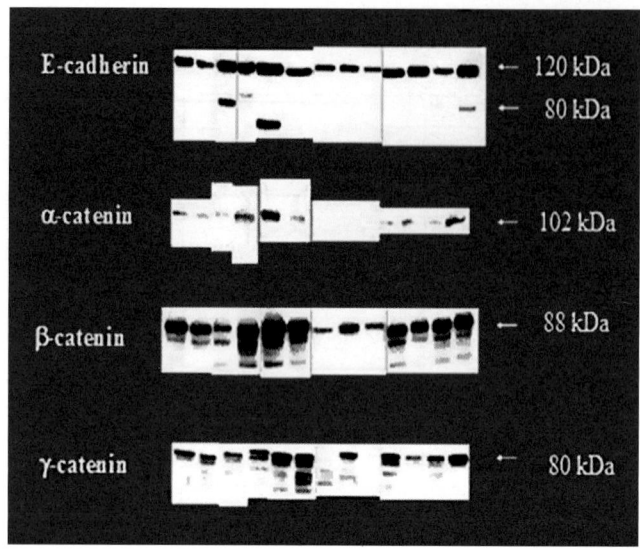

Figure 7.9 Immunoblotting analysis of cell adhesion molecules. Note different members of the E-cadherin family with a distinct pattern by electrophoresis.

Molecular analysis is concerned with the cloning of DNA coding for a specific protein, via restriction enzymes or PCR into plasmids, which then serve as the expression vectors for targeted protein molecules. Successful applications include attempts at detecting specific molecular pathways, genes, and larger DNA sequences as the aim of targeted cancer therapies. Among these, the c-Kit proto-oncogen and its susceptibility to Inatinib (Gleevec) is the first success story. Several other tyrosine kinase inhibitors are under investigation, leading clinicians and even patients to request c-Kit testing in clinical samples. PCR has found its niche in clinical microbiology for the identification of microorganisms by their molecular fingerprint. Numerous useful applications in surgical pathology and diagnostic cytopathology cannot be taken as evidence of failure of this methodology. PCR can detect somatic mutations, gene rearrangements, chromosomal translocations, and other cancer-related genetic abnormalities. The method plays an important role in the recognition and sub-classification of lymphomas. Alternative techniques of macromolecular blotting have been met with limited clinical usefulness. Immunoblotting is uncommonly used in the lab. The procedure requires DNA extraction, which destroys the cell, thus precluding correlation between molecular findings and morphology (Figure 7.9). In Western blotting, cancer-related proteins extracted from tumor cells can be separated by electrophoresis, and transferred to nitrocellulose sheets where they can be identified by their reaction with labeled antibodies. This type of

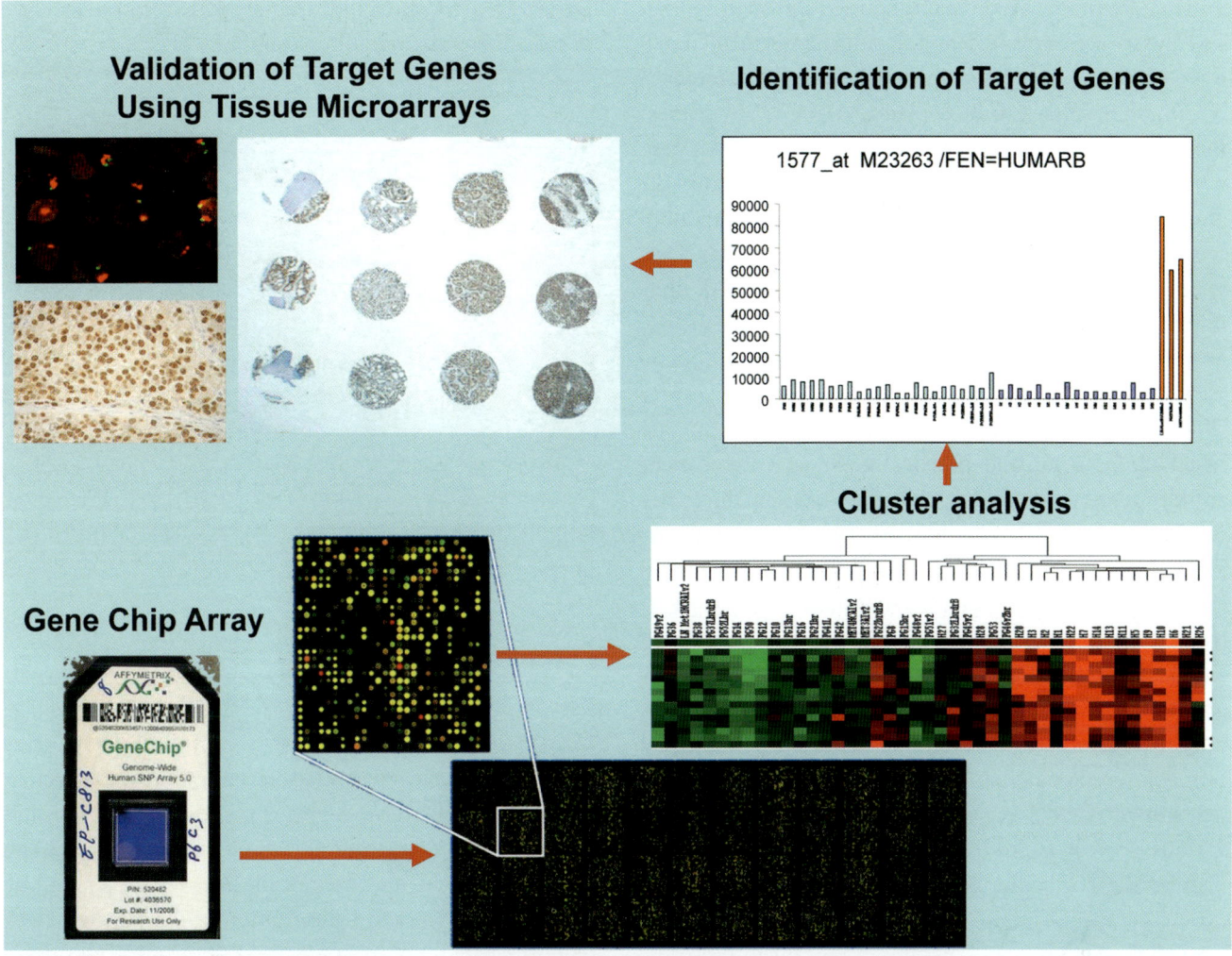

Figure 7.10 Microarray utilization. This composite picture summarizes the use of DNA microarray using single nucleotide polymorphism (SNP) is used to analyze thousands of genes. Sophisticated statistical methods identify target genes for validation by tissue microarrays. (Picture courtesy of Priti Lal MD, University of Pennsylvania, Philadelphia.)

analysis holds promise for future research applications, such as the elucidation of how epithelial tumor cells interact with the stroma and what factors contribute to their migration in the form of metastases.

DNA and tissue arrays are another tool with potential application in diagnostic pathology. The use of high-throughput technology allows for a multimodal approach to understanding the disease process in query. DNA microarrays use minute amounts of clinical samples to elucidate the differences in expression profiles of thousands of genes. Statistical analyses subsequently identify relevant genes. These findings can be simultaneously validated in many archival tissue samples represented on a single tissue microarray slide (TMA) by using various methods.

A DNA array is a collection of spots attached to a microscopic slide where each spot contains one or more oligonucleotide fragment of single-stranded DNA. It is also possible to test micro-arrays from histological and cytological samples, with potential diagnostic and prognostic applications using immunohistochemistry and FISH. Cross-testing of various putative phenotypic-restricted antigens may accelerate the characterization of the specificity of a new tumor marker. The pharmaceutical industry is utilizing molecular biology techniques with great gusto for the development of diagnostic "magic markers" and therapeutic "silver bullets." Cautious optimism pervades the medical community that waits its turn to test these innovations in the clinical arena (Figure 7.10).

Cytokines and growth factors

A central dogma of molecular biology is the notion that normal cells follow a pathway of information exchange initiated by the DNA and culminating in protein synthesis. This is accomplished by the so-called general transfers which control the normal flow of biological information: DNA can be copied to DNA (*DNA replication*); DNA information can be copied into mRNA (*transcription*), and proteins can be synthesized using the information in mRNA as a template (*translation*). Both the DNA and the mRNA of a cell can be tested for, have their structure elucidated, and can be measured, thus providing important biological information. In practice, however, the detection of the proteins (gene products) associated with a given DNA abnormality has greater clinical application, and therefore is more frequently relied upon in clinical practice. Cytological specimens are ideal targets for this type of investigation, since they can be obtained in a non-invasive fashion and can originate from rather small, incipient tumors and at an early stage, when the lesion is more amenable to treatment. A particular group of proteins act as growth factors, playing a crucial role in stimulating cellular growth, proliferation, and *differentiation*. Data are beginning to accumulate regarding the detection of amplified estrogen receptor alpha (ESB1) in breast cancer; epidermal growth factor receptor (EGFR) in lung cancer and various growth factor receptors in other categories of neoplasms, which play the role of molecular targets in novel therapeutic strategies currently being developed. Growth factors and cytokines are important in the regulation of a variety of cellular processes, by acting as signaling molecules between cells by binding to specific receptors on the surface of their target cells. Growth factor implies a positive effect on cell division; a cytokine is a neutral term with respect to whether a molecule affects proliferation. While some cytokines can be growth factors, others have an inhibitory effect on cell proliferation. Some cytokines have the role of "death" signals; they cause target cells to undergo programmed *cell death* or apoptosis. An abbreviated list of apoptosis regulators includes Bcl-2 protein, p53, RAS, caspase-8, heat shock proteins (HSP) and inhibitor of apoptosis proteins (IAP). Several growth factors, on the other hand, often promote cell differentiation and maturation, which varies between specific growth factors, making them and their receptors ideal markers for specific cell abnormalities. Many of these may be unique to a certain type of cancer cell. Table 7.14 depicts various growth factors whose receptors are potential candidates for targeted molecular therapies.

Table 7.14 Growth factors and targeted receptors involved in cell differentiation and maturation

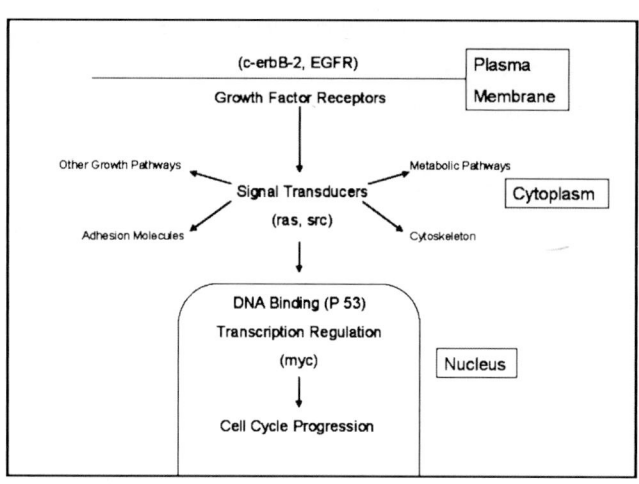

Cytogenetics

Karyotyping is an integral part of the diagnostic practice, particularly after the advent of banding techniques. This method has been supplanted partially by two molecular techniques: fluorescent in situ hybridization (FISH) and comparative genomic hybridization (CGH) (Figure 7.11). FISH involves the uncoiling of the double DNA strand by heat denaturation and hybridization of the targeted DNA sequence with a complementary DNA probe. The precise location of this unique sequence is then revealed by fluorescent-labeled antibody, which can be observed with a fluorescent microscope, but with little data about cytomorphology. A chromogen-labeled antibody can also be utilized in the related technique chromogenic in-situ hybridization (CISH), with the advantage of allowing the appreciation of cell morphology but with reduced sensitivity. FISH is currently more commonly utilized than CISH because of its higher detection rate and its greater repertoire in color-labeling, which allows for the simultaneous detection of multiple points in the chromosome. The ends of human chromosomes, called telomeres, consist of specialized nucleoprotein structures essential for their stability. Telomeres play a fundamental role in the regulation of cellular lifespan, which is measured by the number of generations, not by the chronological time of their viable existence. Without new synthesis of telomeres, the chromosome ends progressively shorter with each cell division and are associated with the cell aging process. Therefore, telomeres are crucial for the intrinsic molecular

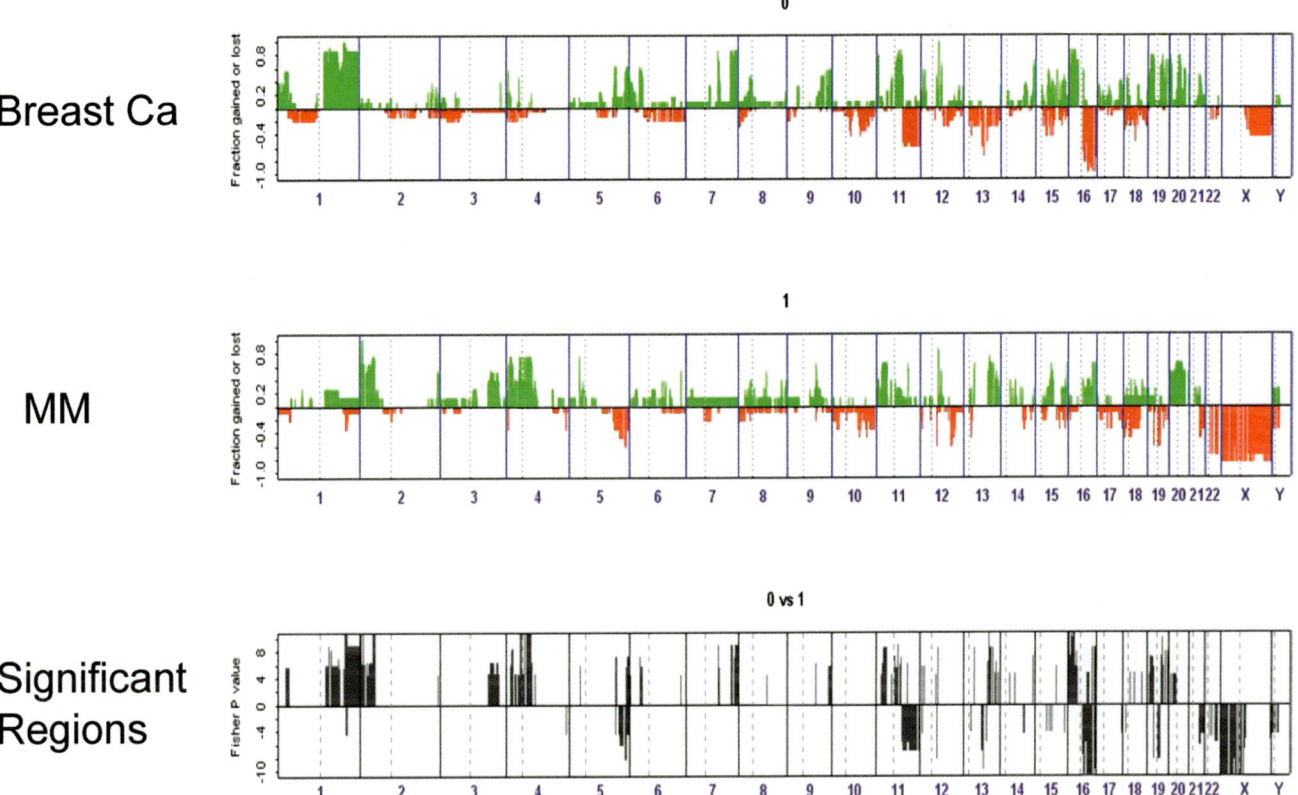

Figure 7.11 Comparative genomic hybridization (CGH) analysis of malignant mesothelioma and adenocarcinoma, breast. Notice multiple gains and losses in both types of tumor.

counting mechanism which controls cell growth and culminates in the cessation of cell division. Normal cells divide for a limited number of times before they undergo replicative arrest (senescence) or cell death (apoptosis) when the length of telomeres becomes too short. By contrast, tumor cells do not experience shortening of telomeres and proliferate indefinitely (immortalization). Telomerase, an enzyme that protects the integrity of telomeres, is tightly repressed in normal cells, but becomes activated during cell immortalization. FISH-based detection of increased telomerase activity can be used both as a diagnostic marker and a prognostic factor in breast cancer and a number of other neoplasms. Effective forms of treatment that inhibit telomerase show promise as novel types of anti-neoplastic targeted therapy.

Urine cytology suffers from low accuracy in the detection of early stage urothelial carcinoma. The UroVysion™ Bladder Cancer Kit (Abbott Molecular Inc.) detects aneuploidy for chromosomes 3, 7, 17, and loss of the 9p21 locus by FISH in urine specimens from patients with persistent hematuria and a suspicion of bladder cancer. As such, the method may detect urothelial carcinoma despite negative cytological changes. Other detection systems exist, such as the Urocyte method, applied to Hologic's liquid-based Preparations (ThinPrep). These methods have been successful in monitoring patients previously diagnosed with bladder cancer for the presence of tumor recurrence. However, these techniques should be used in conjunction with rather than in lieu of current standard diagnostic procedures, including conventional urine cytology.

Microsatellites are segments of non-coding DNA which are fixed for life in all tissues of an individual. The microsatellites on both alleles may be different from one another, a phenomenon referred to as heterozygosity. Deletion of one of the two alleles, leads to loss of heterozygosity (LOH), which can be detected by PCR amplification. LOH analysis of microsatellites linked to tumor suppressor genes can detect malignant transformation, prior to the morphological changes of malignancy being recognized by conventional microscopy.

Since both FISH and CISH are applicable only to cells in metaphase, they offer limited information when compared to CGH, which demonstrates the totality of the

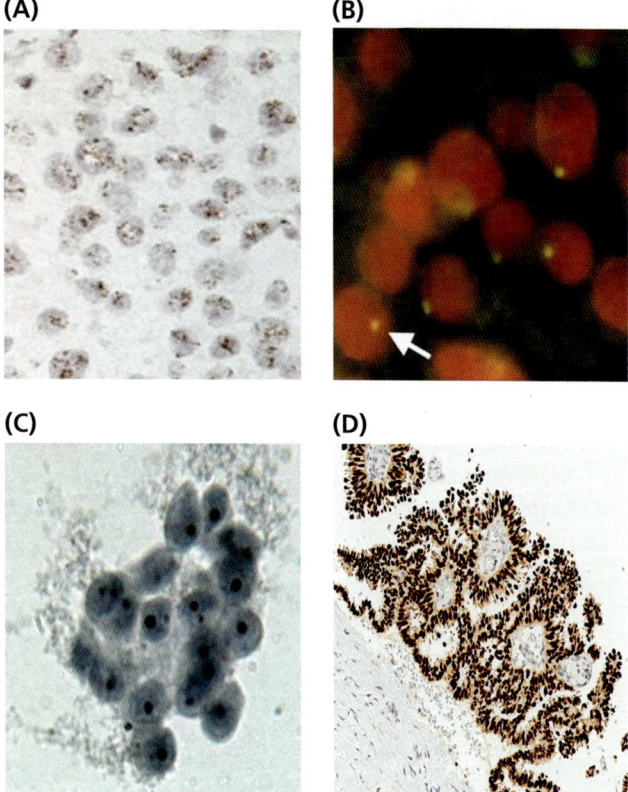

(A) **(B)**

(C) **(D)**

Figure 7.12 Prognostic factors in breast cancer. (A) CISH demonstrating amplification of Her2-Neu. (B) FISH showing amplification of chromosome 17. (C) Positive ER in core biopsy (IHC). (D) Expression of telomerase in smear from breast FNA (IHC).

genomic tumoral DNA. In this method, the tumoral DNA and a normal reference DNA are hybridized together to normal human metaphases and compete with one another for immunolabeling by green and red fluorescent probes. The ratios of these two colors are measured along the entirety of every chromosome allowing for the detection of copy number alterations, so that gains and losses of DNA sequences in neoplastic cells can be mapped on normal chromosomes. The method, therefore, is capable of detecting both amplified genomic regions harboring oncogenes and deleted genomic regions, which harbor suppressor genes. Although the method is capable of detecting DNA imbalances, it has a disadvantage: its inability to detect balanced chromosomal translocations, where no losses or gains of chromosomal material occur. Our knowledge of chromosomal alterations in neoplasms has grown exponentially since the advent of FISH/CISH and CGH. Certain tumors, particularly sarcomas and pediatric tumors, have been fertile territory for the elucidation of cytogenetic abnormalities. It is beyond the scope of this discussion to list these genetic alterations in greater detail.

Clinical value of the use of these molecular makers is best demonstrated in the evaluation of breast adenocarcinoma and is illustrated in Figure 7.12. This field is rapidly evolving as newer makers and technologies are being added continuously.

FURTHER READING

Akhtar, M., C. W. Bedrossian, et al. (1992). "Fine-needle aspiration biopsy of pediatric neoplasms: correlation between electron microscopy and immunocytochemistry in diagnosis and classification". *Diagn Cytopathol* **8**(3): 258–65.

Anagnostou, V. K., A. W. Welsh, et al. (2010). "Analytic variability in immunohistochemistry biomarker studies". *Cancer Epidemiol Biomarkers Prev* **19**(4): 982–91.

Baker, M. S., J. L. Knuth, et al. (2008). "Pancreatic cystic neuroendocrine tumors: preoperative diagnosis with endoscopic ultrasound and fine-needle immunocytology". *J Gastrointest Surg* **12**(3): 450–6.

Beaty, M. W., P. Fetsch, et al. (1997). "Effusion cytology of malignant melanoma. A morphologic and immunocytochemical analysis including application of the MART-1 antibody". *Cancer* **81**(1): 57–63.

Bedrossian, C. W. (1989). "Ultrastructure of *Pneumocystis carinii*: a review of internal and surface characteristics". *Semin Diagn Pathol* **6**(3): 212–37.

Bedrossian, C. W. (1992). "Asbestos-related diseases: a historical and mineralogic perspective". *Semin Diagn Pathol* **9**(2): 91–6.

Bedrossian, C. W. (1992). "Electron microscopy: the neglected tool of cytopathology". *Diagn Cytopathol* **8**(3): iv–vi.

Bedrossian, C. W. (1998). "Diagnostic problems in serous effusions". *Diagn Cytopathol* **19**(2): 131–7.

Bedrossian, C. W. (1998). "Special stains, the old and the new: the impact of immunocytochemistry in effusion cytology". *Diagn Cytopathol* **18**(2): 141–9.

Bedrossian, C. W., S. Bonsib, et al. (1992). "Differential diagnosis between mesothelioma and adenocarcinoma: a multimodal approach based on ultrastructure and immunocytochemistry". *Semin Diagn Pathol* **9**(2): 124–40.

Bedrossian, C. W., R. M. Davila, et al. (1989). "Immunocytochemical evaluation of liver fine-needle aspirations". *Arch Pathol Lab Med* **113**(11): 1225–30.

Bedrossian, C. W., E. A. De Arce, et al. (1985). "Herpetic tracheobronchitis detected at bronchoscopy: cytologic diagnosis by the immunoperoxidase method". *Diagn Cytopathol* **1**(4): 292–9.

Bedrossian, C. W., M. A. Luna, et al. (1973). "Ultrastructure of pulmonary bleomycin toxicity". *Cancer* **32**(1): 44–51.

Bedrossian, C. W., M. R. Mason, et al. (1989). "Rapid cytologic diagnosis of *Pneumocystis*: a comparison of effective techniques". *Semin Diagn Pathol* **6**(3): 245–61.

Bedrossian, C. W., R. Verani, et al. (1979). "Pulmonary malignant fibrous histiocytoma. Light and electron microscopic studies of one case". *Chest* **75**(2): 186–9.

Bhan, R., L. R. Pisharodi, et al. (1998). "Cytological, histological, and clinical correlations in intravesical Bacillus Calmette-Guerin immunotherapy". *Ann Diagn Pathol* **2**(1): 55–60.

Bocking, A., N. Pomjansky, et al. (2009). "[Immunocytochemical identification of carcinomas of unknown primaries on fine-needle-aspiration-biopsies]". *Pathologe* **30**(Suppl 2): 158–60.

Bourtsos, E. P., C. W. Bedrossian, *et al.* (2000). "Thyroid plasmacytoma mimicking medullary carcinoma: a potential pitfall in aspiration cytology". *Diagn Cytopathol* **23**(5): 354–8.

Carbone, M. and C. W. Bedrossian (2006). "The pathogenesis of mesothelioma". *Semin Diagn Pathol* **23**(1): 56–60.

Cavaco, B. M., F. Torrinha, *et al.* (2003). "Preoperative diagnosis of suspicious parathyroid adenomas by RT-PCR using mRNA extracted from leftover cells in a needle used for ultrasonically guided fine needle aspiration cytology". *Acta Cytol* **47**(1): 5–12.

Chell, S. E., R. Nayar, *et al.* (1998). "Metaplastic breast carcinoma metastatic to the lung mimicking a primary chondroid lesion: report of a case with cytohistologic correlation". *Ann Diagn Pathol* **2**(3): 173–80.

Chen, J. C., D. R. Gnepp, *et al.* (1988). "Adenoid cystic carcinoma of the salivary glands: an immunohistochemical analysis". *Oral Surg Oral Med Oral Pathol* **65**(3): 316–26.

Chen, W., R. Bardhan, *et al.* (2010). "A molecularly targeted theranostic probe for ovarian cancer". *Mol Cancer Ther* **9**(4): 1028–38.

Chhieng, D. C., J. F. Cangiarella, *et al.* (2001). "Use of thyroid transcription factor 1, PE-10, and cytokeratins 7 and 20 in discriminating between primary lung carcinomas and metastatic lesions in fine-needle aspiration biopsy specimens". *Cancer* **93**(5): 330–6.

Constantinou, M., A. Binka-Kowalska, *et al.* (2006). "Application of multiplex FISH, CGH and MSSCP techniques for cytogenetic and molecular analysis of transitional cell carcinoma (TCC) cells in voided urine specimens". *J Appl Genet* **47**(3): 273–5.

Dai, Y., C. W. Bedrossian, *et al.* (2005). "The expression pattern of beta-catenin in mesothelial proliferative lesions and its diagnostic utilities". *Diagn Cytopathol* **33**(5): 320–4.

Davidson, B. (2007). "Expression of cancer-associated molecules in malignant mesothelioma". *Biomark Insights* **2**: 173–84.

Davidson, B., H. P. Dong, *et al.* (2007). "Flow cytometric immunophenotyping of cancer cells in effusion specimens: diagnostic and research applications". *Diagn Cytopathol* **35**(9): 568–78.

Davidson, B., B. Risberg, *et al.* (2006). "The biological differences between ovarian serous carcinoma and diffuse peritoneal malignant mesothelioma". *Semin Diagn Pathol* **23**(1): 35–43.

Davidson, B., B. Risberg, *et al.* (2003). "Effusion cytology in ovarian cancer: new molecular methods as aids to diagnosis and prognosis". *Clin Lab Med* **23**(3): 729–54, viii.

Davila, R. M., C. W. Bedrossian, *et al.* (1988). "Immunocytochemistry of the thyroid in surgical and cytologic specimens". *Arch Pathol Lab Med* **112**(1): 51–6.

De Las Casas, L. E., M. Gokden, *et al.* (2004). "A morphologic and statistical comparative study of small-cell carcinoma and non-Hodgkin's lymphoma in fine-needle aspiration biopsy material from lymph nodes". *Diagn Cytopathol* **31**(4): 229–34.

de Matos Granja, N., R. Soares, *et al.* (2002). "Evaluation of breast cancer metastases in pleural effusions by molecular biology techniques". *Diagn Cytopathol* **27**(4): 210–3.

Diaz, L. K., A. Okonkwo, *et al.* (2002). "Extensive myxoid change in well-differentiated papillary mesothelioma of the pelvic peritoneum". *Ann Diagn Pathol* **6**(3): 164–7.

Ellison, D. A., J. F. Silverman, *et al.* (1996). "Role of immunocytochemistry, electron microscopy, and DNA analysis in fine-needle aspiration biopsy diagnosis of Wilms' tumor". *Diagn Cytopathol* **14**(2): 101–7.

Facundo, D. J., G. Quinonez, *et al.* (2003). "Transmission electron microscopy of fine needle aspiration biopsies of metastases. Accuracy of both techniques as established by biopsy diagnoses". *Acta Cytol* **47**(3): 457–62.

Ferra, S., R. Denley, *et al.* (2009). "Reflex UroVysion testing in suspicious urine cytology cases". *Cancer Cytopathol* **117**(1): 7–14.

Fetsch, P. A. and A. Abati. (2001). "Immunocytochemistry in effusion cytology: a contemporary review". *Cancer* **93**(5): 293–308.

Filho, A. L., F. Baltazar, *et al.* (2007). "Immunohistochemical expression and distribution of VEGFR-3 in malignant mesothelioma". *Diagn Cytopathol* **35**(12): 786–91.

Gong, Y., X. Sun, *et al.* (2003). "Immunocytochemistry of serous effusion specimens: a comparison of ThinPrep vs cell block". *Diagn Cytopathol* **28**(1): 1–5.

Granja Nde, M., S. A. Ricardo, *et al.* (2005). "Potential use of loss of heterozygosity in pleural effusions of breast cancer metastases using the microsatellite marker of the 16q22.1 region of the CDH1 gene". *Anal Quant Cytol Histol* **27**(2): 61–6.

Grote, H. J., V. Schmiemann, *et al.* (2003). "DNA extraction from bronchial aspirates for molecular cytology: which method to take?" *Anal Cell Pathol* **25**(2): 83–8.

Halling, K. C., W. King, *et al.* (2002). "A comparison of BTA stat, hemoglobin dipstick, telomerase and Vysis UroVysion assays for the detection of urothelial carcinoma in urine". *J Urol* **167**(5): 2001–06.

Halperin, D., M. R. Fairfax, *et al.* (1995). "*Wuchereria bancrofti* in BAL fluid of a woman with a concomitant breast lesion". *Diagn Cytopathol* **12**(3): 285–7.

Hanna, A., Y. Pang, *et al.* (2010). "Podoplanin is a useful marker for identifying mesothelioma in malignant effusions". *Diagn Cytopathol* **38**(4): 264–9.

Jhala, N. C., D. Jhala, *et al.* (2004). "Endoscopic ultrasound-guided fine-needle aspiration biopsy: a powerful tool to obtain samples from small lesions". *Cancer* **102**(4): 239–46.

Jin, L., T. J. Sebo, *et al.* (2006). "BRAF mutation analysis in fine needle aspiration (FNA) cytology of the thyroid". *Diagn Mol Pathol* **15**(3): 136–43.

Johnson, T. L., C. L. Joseph, *et al.* (1994). "Prevalence of HPV 16 and 18 DNA sequences in CIN III lesions of adults and adolescents". *Diagn Cytopathol* **10**(3): 276–83.

Kaleem, Z., G. White, *et al.* (2001). "Critical analysis and diagnostic usefulness of limited immunophenotyping of B-cell non-Hodgkin lymphomas by flow cytometry". *Am J Clin Pathol* **115**(1): 136–42.

Khan, W. A., H. Attal, *et al.* (2001). "Cytodiagnosis of a meningeal fibrosarcoma metastatic to the thyroid gland". *Semin Diagn Pathol* **18**(2): 104–09.

Khayyata, S., S. Yun, *et al.* (2009). "Value of P63 and CK5/6 in distinguishing squamous cell carcinoma from adenocarcinoma in lung fine-needle aspiration specimens". *Diagn Cytopathol* **37**(3): 178–83.

Krishnamurti, U., E. Sasatomi, *et al.* (2007). "Analysis of loss of heterozygosity in atypical and negative bile duct brushing cytology specimens with malignant outcome: are 'false-negative' cytologic findings a representation of morphologically subtle molecular alterations?" *Arch Pathol Lab Med* **131**(1): 74–80.

Kulshrestha, R. and V. K. Vijayan. (2009). "Immunohistochemical staining on fine needle aspiration biopsy-cell block specimens in the differential diagnosis of lung cancers". *Indian J Chest Dis Allied Sci* **51**(1): 21–5.

Levine, P. H., A. Joutovsky, *et al.* (2006). "CDX-2 expression in pulmonary fine-needle aspiration specimens: a useful adjunct for the diagnosis of metastatic colorectal adenocarcinoma". *Diagn Cytopathol* **34**(3): 191–5.

Lozano de Arce, E. A., C. W. Bedrossian, et al. (1985). "Detection of herpesvirus cervicovaginitis by a sequential Papanicolaou–immunoperoxidase technique". Diagn Cytopathol 1(1): 23–7.

Mai, K. T., D. G. Perkins, et al. (2006). "ES1, a new lung carcinoma antibody–an immunohistochemical study". Histopathology 49(5): 515–22.

Maksem, J. A., C. W. Bedrossian, et al. (2005). "Resolving ASCUS without recourse to HPV testing: manual reprocessing of residual automated liquid-based cytology (ALBC) material using manual liquid-based cytology (MLBC)". Diagn Cytopathol 33(6): 434–40.

Maksem, J. A., V. Dhanwada, et al. (2006). "Testing automated liquid-based cytology samples with a manual liquid-based cytology method using residual cell suspensions from 500 ThinPrep cases". Diagn Cytopathol 34(6): 391–6.

Maldonado, F. and J. R. Jett. (2010). "Advances in the diagnosis of lung cancer: contribution of molecular biology to bronchoscopic diagnosis". Curr Opin Pulm Med 16(4): 315–20.

Marchevsky, A. M., R. Gupta, et al. (2010). "Diagnosis of metastatic neoplasms: a clinicopathologic and morphologic approach". Arch Pathol Lab Med 134(2): 194–206.

Mason, M. R., C. W. Bedrossian, et al. (1987). "Value of immunocytochemistry in the study of malignant effusions". Diagn Cytopathol 3(3): 215–21.

Mennemeyer, R., M. Bartha, et al. (1979). "Diagnostic cytology and electron microscopy of fine needle aspirates of retroperitoneal lymph nodes in the diagnosis of metastatic pelvic neoplasms". Acta Cytol 23(5): 370–3.

Michael, C. W. and J. A. King (1997). Confocal laser scanning microscopy and tridimensional reconstruction of cell clusters in serous fluids. Diagn Cytopathol 17(4): 272–9.

Mullins, J. M. (1999). "Overview of fluorochromes". Methods Mol Biol 115: 97–105.

Naryshkin, S. and C. W. Bedrossian. (1995). "Selected mimics of malignancy in sputum and bronchoscopic cytology specimens". Diagn Cytopathol 13(5): 443–7.

Nayar, R., C. Breland, et al. (1999). "Immunoreactivity of ductal cells with putative myoepithelial markers: a potential pitfall in breast carcinoma". Ann Diagn Pathol 3(3): 165–73.

Ng, W. K., A. S. Li, et al. (2003). "Significance of atypical repair in liquid-based gynecologic cytology: a follow-up study with molecular analysis for human papillomavirus". Cancer 99(3): 141–8.

Nguyen, C. T., D. B. Litt, et al. (2009). "Prognostic significance of nondiagnostic molecular changes in urine detected by UroVysion fluorescence in situ hybridization during surveillance for bladder cancer". Urology 73(2): 347–50.

O'Hara, M. F., C. W. Bedrossian, et al. (1984). "Flow cytometry in cancer diagnosis". Prog Clin Pathol 9: 135–53.

Ohar, J. A., F. Jackson, et al. (1992). "Bronchoalveolar lavage cell count and differential are not reliable indicators of amiodarone-induced pneumonitis". Chest 102(4): 999–1004.

Ohori, N. P., A. Khalid, et al. (2002). "Multiple loss of heterozygosity without K-ras mutation identified by molecular analysis on fine-needle aspiration cytology specimen of acinar cell carcinoma of pancreas". Diagn Cytopathol 27(1): 42–6.

Onofre, A. S., N. Pomjanski, et al. (2007). "Immunocytochemical diagnosis of hepatocellular carcinoma and identification of carcinomas of unknown primary metastatic to the liver on fine-needle aspiration cytologies". Cancer 111(4): 259–68.

Ordonez, N. G. and B. Mackay. (1998). "Electron microscopy in tumor diagnosis: indications for its use in the immunohistochemical era". Hum Pathol 29(12): 1403–11.

Osamura, R. Y. (2009). "Molecular cytopathology: a new era of clinical cytology". Acta Cytol 53(3): 245–6.

Pajor, G., N. Sule, et al. (2008). "Increased efficiency of detecting genetically aberrant cells by UroVysion test on voided urine specimens using automated immunophenotypical preselection of uro-epithelial cells". Cytometry A 73(3): 259–65.

Pisharodi, L. R. and C. Bedrossian. (1998). "Diagnosis and differential diagnosis of small-cell lesions of the liver". Diagn Cytopathol 19(1): 29–32.

Pisharodi, L. R. and C. W. Bedrossian. (1996). "Cytologic diagnosis of pseudomyxoma peritonei: common and uncommon causes". Diagn Cytopathol 14(1): 10–3.

Pomjanski, N., H. J. Grote, et al. (2005). "Immunocytochemical identification of carcinomas of unknown primary in serous effusions". Diagn Cytopathol 33(5): 309–15.

Raber, M. N., B. Barlogie, et al. (1982). "Ploidy, proliferative activity and estrogen receptor content in human breast cancer". Cytometry 3(1): 36–41.

Rada, T., R. L. Reis, et al. (2010). "Distinct stem cells subpopulations isolated from human adipose tissue exhibit different chondrogenic and osteogenic differentiation potential". Stem Cell Rev. Epub.

Reich, R., L. Vintman, et al. (2005). "Differential expression of the 67 kilodalton laminin receptor in epithelioid malignant mesothelioma and carcinomas that spread to serosal cavities". Diagn Cytopathol 33(5): 332–7.

Saad, R. S., D. L. Essig, et al. (2004). "Diagnostic utility of CDX-2 expression in separating metastatic gastrointestinal adenocarcinoma from other metastatic adenocarcinoma in fine-needle aspiration cytology using cell blocks". Cancer 102(3): 168–73.

Safley, A. M., P. J. Buckley, et al. (2004). "The value of fluorescence in situ hybridization and polymerase chain reaction in the diagnosis of B-cell non-Hodgkin lymphoma by fine-needle aspiration". Arch Pathol Lab Med 128(12): 1395–403.

Salla, C., P. Chatzipantelis, et al. (2007). "Endoscopic ultrasound-guided fine-needle aspiration cytology diagnosis of solid pseudo-papillary tumor of the pancreas: a case report and literature review". World J Gastroenterol 13(38): 5158–63.

Savic, S., N. Franco, et al. (2010). "Fluorescence in situ hybridization in the definitive diagnosis of malignant mesothelioma in effusion cytology". Chest 138(1): 137–44.

Schindler, S., R. Nayar, et al. (2001). "Diagnostic challenges in aspiration cytology of the salivary glands". Semin Diagn Pathol 18(2): 124–46.

Shultz, T., W. C. Miller, et al. (1979). "Clinical application of measurement of angiotensin-converting enzyme level". JAMA 242(5): 439–41.

Sigstad, E., H. P. Dong, et al. (2004). "The role of flow cytometric immunophenotyping in improving the diagnostic accuracy in referred fine-needle aspiration specimens". Diagn Cytopathol 31(3): 159–63.

Sigstad, E., H. P. Dong, et al. (2005). "Quantitative analysis of integrin expression in effusions using flow cytometric immunophenotyping". Diagn Cytopathol 33(5): 325–31.

Simsir, A., P. Fetsch, et al. (2001). "Absence of SV-40 large T antigen (Tag) in malignant mesothelioma effusions: an immunocytochemical study". Diagn Cytopathol 25(4): 203–07.

Singh, G., S. L. Katyal, et al. (1983). "Pulmonary alveolar proteinosis. Staining for surfactant apoprotein in alveolar proteinosis and in conditions simulating it". Chest 83(1): 82–6.

Sivertsen, S., A. Berner, et al. (2006). "Cadherin expression in ovarian carcinoma and malignant mesothelioma cell effusions". Acta Cytol 50(6): 603–07.

Strojan Flezar, M. and I. Srebotnik Kirbis. (2009). "Identification of carcinoma origin by thyroid transcription factor-1 immunostaining of fine needle aspirates of metastases". *Cytopathology* **20**(3): 176–82.

Visscher, D. W. and C. W. Bedrossian. (1995). "c-erbB-2 in retrospect: is it time for molecular cytology?" *Diagn Cytopathol* **12**(2): 145–7.

Warth, A., T. Muley, *et al.* (2010). "A histochemical approach to the diagnosis of visceral pleural infiltration by non-small cell lung cancer". *Pathol Oncol Res* **16**(1): 119–23.

Westfall, D. E., X. Fan, *et al.* (2010). "Evidence-based guidelines to optimize the selection of antibody panels in cytopathology: pleural effusions with malignant epithelioid cells". *Diagn Cytopathol* **38**(1): 9–14.

Willmore-Payne, C., L. J. Layfield, *et al.* (2005). "c-KIT mutation analysis for diagnosis of gastrointestinal stromal tumors in fine needle aspiration specimens". *Cancer* **105**(3): 165–70.

Wolman, S. R., J. S. Sanford, *et al.* (1995). "Genetic probes in cytology: principles and applications". *Diagn Cytopathol* **13**(5): 429–35.

Wu, M., A. H. Szporn, *et al.* (2005). "Cytology applications of p63 and TTF-1 immunostaining in differential diagnosis of lung cancers". *Diagn Cytopathol* **33**(4): 223–7.

Wurlitzer, F., C. Bedrossian, *et al.* (1973). "Problems of diagnosing and treating infiltrating lipomas". *Am Surg* **39**(4): 240–3.

Yang, B., S. Z. Ali, *et al.* (2002). "CD10 facilitates the diagnosis of metastatic renal cell carcinoma from primary adrenal cortical neoplasm in adrenal fine-needle aspiration". *Diagn Cytopathol* **27**(3): 149–52.

Yoder, B. J., M. Skacel, *et al.* (2007). "Reflex UroVysion testing of bladder cancer surveillance patients with equivocal or negative urine cytology: a prospective study with focus on the natural history of anticipatory positive findings". *Am J Clin Pathol* **127**(2): 295–301.

Zeppa, P., I. Cozzolino, *et al.* (2009). "Cytologic, flow cytometry, and molecular assessment of lymphoid infiltrate in fine-needle cytology samples of Hashimoto thyroiditis". *Cancer Cytopathol* **117**(3): 174–84.

Zhu, L. C., G. S. Sidhu, *et al.* (2005). "Fine-needle aspiration cytology of pancreatoblastoma in a young woman: report of a case and review of the literature". *Diagn Cytopathol* **33**(4): 258–62.

Zografos, G. N., A. Stathopoulou, *et al.* (2005). "Preoperative imaging and localization of small sized insulinoma with EUS-guided fine needle tattoing: a case report". *Hormones (Athens)* **4**(2): 111–6.

INDEX